Praise For *Thugs, Drugs and the War On Bugs*

"Dr. Case's book does an outstanding job of explaining, not only why vaccines aren't safe, but why they aren't necessary."

JOHN GRAY, PH.D., Bestselling author of *Men Are from Mars, Women Are from Venus* and *The Mars & Venus Diet & Exercise Solution*

"Dr. Case's book is so important in this toxic world! Everything, from food additives to vaccines, medical drugs, and even water is poisoned with the excuse that it serves the public. Dr. Case also helps us to understand the terrible truth behind medical drugs, their "side effects," which even include death, and the unending string of poisons in our lives. This book should be in every mother's hands to protect, not only her children, but the whole family!"

CHARLOTTE GERSON, Daughter of Dr. Max Gerson, Founder and Director of the Gerson Institute, Author of *The Gerson Therapy* and *Healing the Gerson Way*

"Dr. Brad's book is an extensively researched indictment of Western medicine's practices and the parasitic industry that, under the guise of promoting health, has plundered the wealth of those it has been imposed upon. Leaving no stone unturned he has highlighted the sinister effects of pharmaceuticals and the sinister nature of the organizations that profit from their distribution. And for the reader, most importantly, Dr. Brad provides readily available alternatives for all those seeking true whole-health."

GERALD CELENTE, Publisher of the *Trends Journal*, Founder and Director of the Trends Research Institute, Bestselling Author of *Trend Tracking* and *Trends 2000*

"This book serves as a powerful wake-up call with documented evidence that the medical-pharmaceutical industry has violated healthcare's first commandment: Do No Harm. We have the knowledge and ability to bring true wellness to our country and the world, but first we must reject the fear-based medical paradigm. This book will go a long way to making sure that happens."

TERRY A. RONDBERG, D.C., CEO, World Chiropractic Alliance, Publisher of *The Chiropractic Journal*, Author of *Chiropractic First*

"Medicine has become big business, with 'drugs for everything, and nothing but drugs for anything' being the medical/pharmaceutical mantra. Dr. Case's book clearly outlines all the sordid details, and gives alternatives that you, the patient, desperately need."

DR. BRUCE WEST, Founder, "Health Alert" Newsletter

"Brad Case's book is entertaining, thought-provoking and well researched—a fine read. I could not put it down until I had finished it. It will suit those who wish to make informed health decisions for themselves, rather than simply accept medical products that one can only guarantee to be highly profitable—and often risky. He covers vaccines, antibiotics, cancers, AIDS, Big Pharma and more. As he says: 'Toxic chemicals cannot make you well; only nature can.' The shame is that these toxins are often in the very products that are supposed to make us healthy. The final chapter, on the nature of viruses, will definitely be an eye-opener for many!"

JANINE ROBERTS, Author of *Fear of the Invisible, How Scared Should We Be of Viruses and Vaccines, HIV and AIDS?*

"Our society, which has grown up thinking health will be found in drugs, is in for a rude awakening as health continues to decline and the U.S. healthcare system fails to meet society's expectations. Let me make it personal—if you care about your health, you must read this book!"

JAMES WINTERSTEIN, D.C., D.A.C.B.R.
President, National University of Health Sciences

"Dr. Case is an important, energetic voice in the American healthcare reform debate. Not only is he unique among the chiropractic profession in his understanding of the historical, political and economic factors, which have accumulated into the present difficulties, he is a superb, seasoned clinician whose unrelenting personal mission and professional practice begin and end with his patients. This book elucidates, explains, clarifies, shocks, and helps. It points us in a very positive direction and will be understood as a beacon of insight in the healing of America's fragmented, commoditized healthcare landscape."

DR. DAVID J. SCHLEICH, PH.D.,
President, National College of Natural Medicine

"*Thugs, Drugs and the War On Bugs* reads like a crime novel. It's so scary and so real that you can't put it down. Dr. Case uses Western medicine's own journals to prove that what they're doing doesn't work most of the time. He shows us that the way Western medicine is currently being practiced by mainstream doctors, it's not really healthcare at all. It is instead 'disease management.' This book is sure to make some mad and others much enlightened, but it is a must for those who want to reclaim their health and then maintain it. I have been thoroughly un-brainwashed. Thank you Dr. Case."

JOHN W. BRIMHALL, D.C., Author of
Solving the Health Puzzle with the 6 Steps to Wellness

BOOK 1 in the WHY WE'RE SICK™ Series

THUGS, DRUGS AND THE WAR ON BUGS

How the Natural Healthcare Revolution Will
Lead Us Past Greed, Ego, and Scary Germs

DR. BRAD CASE

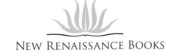

NEW RENAISSANCE BOOKS

NEW RENAISSANCE BOOKS
17811 Countryside Ct.
Prunedale, CA 93907

ISBN-13: 978-0-9819895-0-1
ISBN-10: 0-9819895-0-0

Library of Congress Control Number: 2009904651

Book jacket text by Graham Van Dixhorn,
Write to Your Market, Inc.

Book interior design and typesetting by
Shannon Bodie, Lightbourne, Inc.

Index by Phyllis Linn, INDEXPRESS

This book is dedicated to Dr. D. D. Palmer,
Dr. B. J. Palmer, Dr. Andrew Taylor Still, Dr. Samuel Hahnemann,
Dr. Benedict Lust, Dr. Chester Wilk, Dr. Harvey Wiley,
Dr. Royal Lee, Dr. Antoine Béchamp, Royal Rife, Gaston Naessens,
Barbara Loe Fisher, and all the other unsung heroes throughout
history who've stood up in the face of tyranny and said,

"No more!"

CONTENTS

Foreword

Skating to Where the Puck is Going to Be

David J. Schleich, Ph.D.

President, National College of Natural Medicine, Portland, Oregon
Former President, the Canadian College of Naturopathic Medicine, Toronto, Canada

B rad Case is on the frontline of healthcare in America and he has something important to tell us from there. Every day at his Holistic Healing Center in Prunedale, California, his experience with patients reinforces what he wants to teach us about the shifts occurring in primary healthcare. Those shifts are making patient-centered therapies more important than ever. These include, in summary, altered patterns of illness (e.g., more chronic disease and reduced infectious risks), the demographic changes resulting from increased life expectancy, and the inherent challenges of living in a chemical-laden environment, further compounded by industrial farming methods and desperately poor nutritional habits. But there's more. Dr. Case fearlessly challenges the status quo of orthodox biomedicine and its paradigm of symptom-suppression and disease management rather than focusing on prevention and cure.

Dr. Case bravely declares once again, as if for the first time, what has been rebounding in the current American health debate. Healthcare in America has been co-opted by the richest industry on the planet, "Big Pharma." He documents with passion and precision that the powerful biomedical locomotive long ago crashed into its limits, and despite its "I think I can" attitude, is now floundering in its efforts to carry an exponentially heavier load of chronic diseases such as cancer, diabetes, asthma, and Alzheimer's up the mountain. Dr. Case tells us, in his dramatically titled book, that the dominant healthcare profession, often called "Western medicine," "allopathic medicine," or "scientific medicine," is undergoing a grass-roots level shake up as patients by the millions are discovering that there is a better way.

Ironically, Dr. Case predicates his concerns and the values underlying them on principles that an earlier generation of medical doctors knew, even as they systematically took control of healthcare in North America during the early decades of the last century. As recently and as far back as seventy-five years ago, medical academics and teaching hospital clinicians saw what was evolving. As Dr. K. Ludmerer pointed out in his 1999 book *Time to Heal,* the social contract which gave medical doctors the lead role in healthcare, has long been broken. Over seventy years ago, in something called the "Western Reserve" curriculum, there was already alarm at the distance developing between doctor and patient. Overall, the goal of this curriculum was to repair the dehumanizing effects of the rapidly emerging dominance of scientific specialization, while still retaining the best science had to offer. The modern medical student, heavily invested in the well-beaten pathway of the dominant medical paradigm, will find Dr. Case's alarm bells jolting as he challenges the failure of a Western Reserve curriculum to take root in America's medical schools.

The detail, the documentation, and the delivery in Dr. Case's book about what the healthcare marketplace really looks like and who is really pulling the strings is gripping for any student of medicine, patient, health administrator, or politician numb and paralyzed with the complexity of the American healthcare landscape. The reader needs to fasten his or her seatbelt and be ready to take on topics such as what happened to homeopathy; how the chiropractic profession took on the American Medical Association; and how big business took over medicine.

Get ready to move along with him as his argument regarding the brainwashing of the American people accumulates into an exposé about the utility and safety of drugs, and the collusion between Big Pharma and the FDA. Dr. Case lingers on the topic long enough to put a spotlight on how so much money is being made by so few for so long for reasons and goals completely unrelated to wellness, longevity, and human survival. He's not afraid to declare that these relationships and privileges have created "bad medicine" and the arrogance of a guild-like control over the health of individuals. Sprinkled among the evidence are shocking details about the dramatic presence of iatrogenic (doctor-caused) death in America and unnecessary, high-cost surgery and treatment. Dr. Case does not pull punches and you can count on him to choreograph more than enough credible data to substantiate his conclusions and insights.

Dr. Case is relentless in scouring the biomedical landscape to take on topics and territory which the mainstream medical profession can no longer defend, ethically or historically. Ranging from controversial conversations about pleomorphism to the sinister dangers of antibiotic overuse and the massive invasiveness of vaccinations in the lives of men, women, and children, his allegations of healthcare mismanagement by the medical establishment not only gain momentum, but volume, credibility, and purpose.

Dr. Case took seven years to generate this first offering in the *Why We're Sick™* series because there is a story that needs to be told. The ennui medical students are experiencing these days, which lead these apprentice healers away from an earlier certitude about how their chosen discipline is secure in its received concepts, is part of what is evolving. The American Medical Association knows that the entire biomedical profession is an applied science. More specifically, as Wyngaarden put it in 1982, "medical science is a branch of applied biology."* The modern physician is painfully aware that his

or her profession is stumbling ahead in the twenty-first century
on foundations that belong to an earlier time when Galilean-
Cartesian-Baconian-Newtonian science was the best that we had.
But with our new, deeper understanding of how the universe
functions, especially at the quantum level, these foundations are
now crumbling. And while biology has evolved to include the
concepts of quantum physics, medical science has not. Meanwhile,
the so-called "alternative" branches of medicine have *embraced* this
new model, as have many patients who are eager for a more holistic
approach to their wellness. Now, "alternative" practitioners find
themselves on firmer scientific ground than the average, orthodox
medical doctor.

What place in the modern physician's repertoire of skills is held
by the classic intuition of the doctor who respects the healing power
of nature? Apart from defining more precisely what comprises the
form and content of that intuition, what opportunities are there for
modern medical educators to make available the "clinical pearls"
of the nature-cure doctor within the dense, intense curriculum
of North America's medical schools? Scary though it may be for
proponents of the biomedical paradigm, a curriculum which
propels students right into the conflicted claims of biomedicine
and more natural approaches to wellness, longevity, and balance is
precisely where we need to be headed.

Dr. Case's book is definitely helpful in that continuum of
debate. Our modern medical students will not settle for a one-sided
academic and clinical journey focused on morbidity and mortality;
they want to know more about the causes of *health*, too. Why is
it not surprising that nutrition is not studied routinely in medical
programs? The modern medical student wants a balance between
pathogenesis (the cause of disease) and salutogenesis (the cause
of health and well-being). They are fed up with the perspective of
physicalism, which dominates and bullies human medical science.
They want to know more about psychosocial variables in human

ailment. They want to know how the mind, the body, and the spirit work together to generate lifelong wellness. At a more specific level, they want to know whether vaccines are at the root of the current autism epidemic in America.

Modern medical students know from other disciplines such as cybernetics, biosemiotics, systems theory, and chaos theory that the age of reductionism is giving way to the upward and downward mutual causation of a self-organizing universe. The biomedical doctor's time of dominance is on borrowed time, owing at least in part to their breaking of the social contract which puts patient focused care ahead of profit. Dr. Case knows that and this is his message to us in the first instalment of *Why We're Sick*™.

David Schleich
Montreal, Quebec
February 23, 2010

*Citation: Wyngaarden J.B., Smith, L.H. (eds). *Cecil Textbook of Medicine,* vol. 1, 16th ed. Philadelphia: W.B. Saunders, 1982.

Acknowledgments

I'd like to tip my hat and raise a glass to a few people who have helped make this book possible. First of all, to Dr. John Donofrio for introducing me to the world of medical conspiracy and setting me on this quest to educate the world about the truth. To Dr. Fred Hult for showing me what a chiropractor *can* be. To Dr. Devi Nambudripad, Dr. Ellen Cutler, Dr. Victor Frank, Dr. Timothy Francis, Dr. Freddie Ulan, Dr. John Brimhall, Dr. Michael Dobbins, and my late friend Dr. David Nilmeier for teaching me so much about natural health. To Dr. Jim Winterstein, for his kind words, help, and encouragement regarding this book, and for continually raising the bar within our profession. To Dr. David Schleich, whose enthusiasm for this book and its message touched me so that I asked him to write the foreword for it—and he did a bang-up job. To my parents Mel and Judy Case for recognizing my talents, for encouraging me to go into natural healthcare, and for all their help along the way. To my editing team Beth Kirkman, Renée Jourdenais, Nichole Rodriguez, James Smith, Howard Straus, and Drs. Eric Haag and Stephen Gunter for all their comments and suggestions and for helping me to make this book better than it was. To Graham Van Dixhorn, George Foster, Phyllis Linn, and Shannon Bodie for helping to make this book a real work of art. I'd also like to thank the editors and contributors of the *Journal of the American Medical Association, British Medical Journal, New England Journal of Medicine, the Lancet, Science,* and many other journals cited in this book without which this story would not be nearly so credible. And of course, thanks to my lovely wife Maria, for her endless encouragement and patience, for her wisdom (both grammatical and otherwise), for being my toughest critic, and my best friend.

Introduction

"We are apt to shut our eyes against a painful truth, and listen to the song of that siren till she transforms us into beasts. Is this the part of wise men, engaged in a great and arduous struggle for liberty? Are we disposed to be the number of those who, having eyes, see not, and having ears, hear not, the things which so nearly concern their temporal salvation? For my part, whatever anguish of spirit it may cost, I am willing to know the whole truth; to know the worst, and to provide for it."

—Patrick Henry, March 23, 1775

A recent survey of 12,000 primary care physicians found that 66 percent of them were either less-than-satisfied or unsatisfied with the practice of medicine. Sixty percent said they would not recommend medicine as a career. Approximately one-third of those who participated said they planned to stop seeing patients in the next one to three years and another 14 percent planned to cut back on patient care to part-time. Tying in with this lack of job satisfaction, M.D.s also suffer from the highest rate of suicide among professionals. Many others are saddled by drug and alcohol addiction.

For many, it may seem odd that people who've dedicated their lives to helping others, who cared so much about humanity that they were willing to spend $100,000 and 11 or more years of grueling education to learn a job that most would assume to be highly rewarding and high-paying, would be so dissatisfied. But the realities of practicing medicine are far from what's depicted on TV medical dramas. Besides never-ending piles of paperwork, loads of stress, and utterly ridiculous insurance games, there's the shocking reality that for the most part, medicine does little for its patients other than mask symptoms. If you've ever gone to the doctor and been disappointed with the service you received, imagine how your doctor must feel, knowing s/he's dedicated his/her life to that dog and pony show.

You may also think, "Well, that's just the way it is. Healthcare sucks the world over. There are too many sick people and not enough doctors." But that's not really the case either. Shockingly, the World Health Organization reports that in the United States, we spend more on healthcare per capita than any other country *by far*, and yet they rate our healthcare system 37th in the world—out of 37 industrialized countries. So we spend the most, but fare the worst. In fact, it appears that the more we spend on medical care the worse our health gets.

Despite all this spending, chronic diseases of all sorts are on the rise and they're occurring in younger people all the time. Children are obese. They're being diagnosed with adult onset diabetes and high cholesterol and put on meds for life. Children are also being diagnosed with neurological disorders at an alarming rate. They're being declared autistic, learning disabled, or ADHD and put on psychiatric drugs. Genetic and autoimmune diseases are also on the rise. Though the American Cancer Society claims we're "winning the war on cancer," more people are diagnosed and die from cancer every year. In fact, cancer recently replaced heart disease as the nation's number one killer disease. As the rates of all these diseases continue to rise, sperm counts and fertility are on the decline. Clearly, what we're doing is not sustainable. A few more generations of heading in this direction and the human race could be done for.

Sadly, not only are Western medicine's attempts to treat these diseases ineffectual, their efforts often prove deadly. Using very conservative estimates, the *Journal of the American Medical Association (JAMA)* actually admits that M.D.s kill well over 280,000 people per year—more than all other accidental deaths combined! But when more realistic numbers are used, we find that M.D.s are actually killing around 784,000 people every year. That's the equivalent of more than seven jumbo jets crashing into the ground every day. This puts Western medicine at the top of the list—killing more people every year than *any* disease, including every type of cancer put together. Amazingly, most of this isn't even due to medical *mistakes*. In fact, according to another study in *JAMA*, "properly prescribed drugs" by themselves are the fourth leading cause of death in America, killing an estimated 106,000 people per year. (And that study only included the drugs given in the hospital.) In other words, these are the *expected* "side effects" of using this type of healthcare system, if one can call such a system "healthcare."

Findings like these have led the Institute of Medicine to say, "The American healthcare system is in need of a fundamental change." The National Roundtable on Healthcare Quality stated in *JAMA*, "Our present efforts [to improve the system] resemble a team of engineers trying to break the sound barrier by tinkering with a Model-T Ford. We need a new vehicle, or perhaps many new vehicles." In other words, we need a whole new healthcare paradigm.

Western medicine is *one* healthcare paradigm. It's not the *only* healthcare paradigm, but it *is* the most dominant one in this country right now. Unfortunately, it also happens to be a paradigm that doesn't work for the kind of diseases we're currently plagued with. While it works fairly well for certain problems, such as bacterial infections, and extremely well for emergency situations, surgeries, and the like, it's all but useless for handling the chronic diseases we now find ourselves plagued with. Most shocking of all, Western medicine, with its all-for-drugs-and-drugs-for-all approach to healthcare, is actually *causing* many of the diseases it's charged with curing. Using more drugs to treat these new diseases is like throwing gasoline on an already raging fire.

Playing around with who pays for such a system is not healthcare reform; this is merely re-arranging deck chairs on a rapidly sinking ship. While the insurance system *certainly* needs an overhaul, it's not the insurance companies causing all of this death and disease—it's medicine. It's time to get off of this sinking ship and find a new vessel—one that can actually take us to the destination of our choosing—health.

This book and the rest of the *Why We're Sick*™ series will outline the basic tenets of that new healthcare paradigm. If we want to be healthy as individuals and healthy as a species, we must first understand and then change our backwards system of healthcare. This will necessarily require stepping on some toes and bruising some egos, but this is a small price to pay for a healthcare system that actually makes people healthy instead of simply masking symptoms and making the drug companies wealthy.

This book is not a cookbook approach to treating illness because I find cookbook approaches rarely work. Using vitamins and herbs to treat individual diseases in the place of drugs is just a safer way to fail at getting people well. Diseases are merely groups of signs and symptoms. There are thousands of different diseases and many more groupings of symptoms that haven't been named yet. Treating a disease is really the same thing as treating symptoms, and *symptoms* are your body's way of dealing with the actual problem. That means treating diseases, whether with drugs, vitamins, or herbs, is actually fighting against what your body is trying to do. Take this fight to the most extreme level and you can easily see why medicine is killing so many people.

The truth of the matter is, health is a relatively easy thing to achieve *if* you know what you're doing. There are a finite number of things that cause ill health and when you remove these causes, the effects cease. In other words, find the problem, remove the problem, then stand back and watch nature perform miracles. It really doesn't matter what symptoms you have or what your diagnosis is. When you fix the problem, the body will begin to heal itself. This is the only way healthcare actually *works*. Putting foreign chemicals into the body or cutting out bad parts will *not* create health. Doing these things may save your life in certain circumstances, but that's not the same thing as making someone healthy. Therefore, Western medicine should not be wholly discarded, but it *should* be scrutinized and used only for what it can truly benefit.

This book and the books that follow will delineate the problems that occur (i.e., the real causes of disease) and the things that will fix them. It will also propose solutions to fixing the healthcare system because only when the system is set up to *work*, can we have true health as a species.

I was told long ago that if people knew what I knew, they would do what I do. That is why I wrote this book and the ones that follow. I want you to enjoy the type of health that I have. Listen to what I say with an open mind. Do what I recommend and your body will respond by giving you your health back. Depending on where you are right now, your road to health may be a long one or a short one. The point is to get on the right road and start heading in the right direction. You cannot get healthy if you're heading down the road of disease. And *that's* where Western medicine will take you. Toxic chemicals *cannot* make you well; only nature can.

Good luck in your journey back.

In health,

Brad Case, D.C.

DISCLAIMER:

The statements made in this book are based entirely on the study of anatomy, physiology, pathology, histology, biochemistry, biomechanics, quantum physics, hundreds of thousands of hours of clinical practice, common sense, logic, and other modes of scientific study. The book is heavily referenced and uses quotes from the most respected medical and scientific journals in the world, as well as leading experts in each field of study. However, the statements contained herein have not been evaluated by the FDA, and therefore they insist that I tell you that they should not be considered or substituted for medical advice. But more importantly, I would encourage you to educate yourself and use your personal judgment in *all* matters of health, including advice coming from me, your doctor, and statements that *have* been evaluated by the FDA.

PART I

The Anatomy of the Medical Mafia

"Great spirits have always encountered
violent opposition from mediocre minds."

—Albert Einstein

1

Genesis of the Medical Monopoly

Monopoly, n. Exclusive control by one group of the means of
producing or selling a commodity or service.

Cartel, n. A combination of independent business organizations
formed to regulate production, pricing, and marketing
of goods by the members.

—*American Heritage Dictionary*, Second College Edition

There have always been multiple schools of thought in healthcare
and these opposing factions have always been at war with one
another. For over 150 years, however, healthcare in America
has been almost completely dominated by one group of healthcare
practitioners. Currently, this faction of healthcare providers
holds a virtual monopoly over the competing schools of thought.
They carry immense political clout through their own lobbying
organizations and they are supported by the largest, richest
corporations in the world. Further, those huge corporations have
massive political power themselves, holding in their deep, fur-
lined pockets, not only politicians, but the very organization that is
supposed to be regulating them as well. They spend $11 million a
day to convince the public to buy their products; and through their
massive advertising budgets, which accounts for about one third of
all advertising, they have major influence on the mass media and
their regulating agency as well. The type of healthcare I'm speaking
of is, of course, Western medicine, and their corporate sponsors are
the pharmaceutical companies.

For all intents and purposes, healthcare in America is now under the control of a vast and corrupt medical monopoly. Because medicine is not run by a single company, you may not think of it as being a monopoly in the traditional sense, but the effect is just the same. When multiple companies, very often *competing* companies, work together to create a monopoly over some product or service, we call it a cartel. These competing companies work in concert to eliminate the outside competition and thereby strengthen the cartel as a whole. A good analogy of what I'm talking about might be competing oil companies banding together to suppress alternative energy sources. In the case I'm talking about here, we have competing pharmaceutical companies (and their affiliates) working together to suppress alternative medicine.

The idea behind creating a monopoly, as I'm sure you know, is so that money can be continuously and effortlessly funneled into the pockets of those in control. That sounds great, right? Who wouldn't want that? But there's a downside, as I'm sure you also know. The downside of a monopoly is, by definition, there is no competition; therefore, no choice for the consumer. When there's no competition and no choice, there is often corruption. When one group has *that* much power, greed inevitably rears its ugly head; and when that happens, prices escalate and quality suffers.

Those things are all bad enough, but with the *medical* monopoly, things are actually much worse. *This* monopoly isn't just dangerous economically, it's just plain *dangerous*. That's because, the two main products/services this healthcare monopoly offers, drugs and surgery, are actually dangerous and detrimental to your health. A choice between the cholesterol drugs Lipitor and Zocor isn't much of a choice if both of them are toxic to your liver, destroy your muscle tissue (including your heart), and do nothing but harm your body. The medical monopoly would rather you not know that there are safe, natural ways to lower your cholesterol (let alone the fact that cholesterol was never the problem to begin with). They would

much rather you not see a chiropractor, acupuncturist, or massage therapist for back pain, but just go right in for the surgery. Natural alternatives such as these have an amazing safety record, but they *are* dangerous in one way. They're dangerous because they threaten the unanimity of the medical monopoly—that singular voice that says drugs and surgery are the only ways to health. So, this healthcare cartel works very hard at preventing information about the benefits of alternative therapies from making it to the masses, or discrediting any positive information that ever does get out.

As scary as it sounds, the cartel that runs healthcare in America has actively suppressed, and attempted to destroy or eliminate, several valid forms of healthcare. Negative propaganda, often completely made-up information, is circulated to the media regarding competing healthcare fields. The same can be said of many safe and effective therapies, including *several* cancer cures, many of which have been confiscated and/or destroyed in Gestapo-like raids. Because these competing forms of healthcare and alternative therapies threaten the medical monopoly, each has been branded "quackery" and quickly pounced upon by organized medicine. Many of these alternative therapies have been hypocritically labeled as dangerous; others have simply been declared an ineffective waste of money. Still others, some of the best and safest, have actually been made illegal!

If one looks with an objective eye, it becomes glaringly obvious that what the traditional healthcare advocates are doing is purely about eliminating the competition and has nothing at all to do with "protecting the public from quackery." This cartel has worked hard over the course of many years to lead the public into a tunnel-visioned way of thinking about healthcare. They've tried very hard to convince people that there are only two valid forms of healthcare—drugs and surgery—and that all other forms of healthcare are "quackery" at worst, and "alternative" at best. And to a large extent, their plan has worked. They truly have become the

dominant form of healthcare, despite the fact that their products/
methods are inherently dangerous and largely ineffective.

We've seen some amazing advancements in medical
technology in the last 60 years or so. Through the use of that
technology, medical doctors can truly do amazing things in the
fields of emergency medicine and surgery. Also through the use of
technology, M.D.s are very adept at diagnosing certain problems
and keeping sick people alive. Antibiotics, no doubt, save lives as
well. M.D.s are also reasonably good at alleviating symptoms like
pain or depression. All of these things I grant them. In other words,
if you're severely injured, gravely ill, or dying, medical doctors are
worth their weight in gold. But none of these things actually make
you *healthy*. Shocking your heart back to life or keeping you alive
on a respirator is not health care—it's sick care. Medical doctors
can keep you on this side of the line between life and death, but in
terms of actually promoting *health*, they have very little to offer.
Prescribing a toxic medication to alleviate a symptom cannot be
considered healthcare any more than removing the oil light from
your car's dashboard when it goes on, can be considered auto
mechanics.

All these technical advances are great. I'm glad we have them
for the people who really need them. But as you'll read throughout
this book and the ones that follow, many of the problems requiring
all this technology were actually created by the system that is now
being forced to handle them. In other words, the medical monopoly
has begun to feed on its own carnage.

An example might go something like this: Certain chemical
companies produce artificial fertilizers and pesticides for
agriculture. Other chemical/pharmaceutical companies produce
growth hormones and antibiotics for cows and other livestock.
Still other companies produce the chemical "vitamins" they spray
on processed, "enriched" foods like breads and cereals. People eat
all this non-nutritious, toxic food for years and eventually develop

diseases because of it. These people then go to their doctors and receive a drug (another chemical) to help with their illness. That drug is toxic as well. It also suppresses the body's symptoms so the people no longer realize they're sick; therefore, they see no reason to change their ways. So, they continue to eat the same toxic foods and take their new toxic drugs. After a few years, new diseases crop up and more drugs are needed. Because the people have been thoroughly brainwashed, they never realize that their illnesses are being caused by the drugs and chemicals they are consuming every day. This cycle continues until a major illness hits (stroke, heart attack, cancer, etc.). Now, surgery and long hospital stays come into the picture. Eventually, organ transplant, dialysis, or other life support mechanisms may be needed just to keep the patients alive. These people are now medical invalids, reliant on a constant stream of medical care and medications made by the very same companies (or subsidiaries of the companies) that made the fertilizers and pesticides, hormones and antibiotics that started the ball rolling in the first place. This is how the medical cartel operates.

So, yes, this century has seen some amazing things in the world of healthcare. I won't deny this, but there's something wrong. Everyone who understands the system says that it's broken almost beyond repair. One of the main reasons they're saying this is because more people are chronically ill than ever before. Just look at all the different types of illness that are on the rise: diabetes, obesity, cancer, heart disease, hypothyroidism, multiple sclerosis, Parkinson's, Alzheimer's, autism, depression, acid reflux, AIDS, attention deficit disorder, learning disabilities, lupus, chronic fatigue syndrome, fibromyalgia, allergies, asthma, environmental illness... Why, with all this expensive medical care, are so many chronic diseases on the rise?

Is it because there are no solutions to these problems? Is it because humankind is just doomed to disease? Well, if you've never read anything on this subject before, I can understand how you might think that, but I'm here to tell you that there *are* solutions to these problems and they are being *kept* from you by the medical monopoly. Why would they do that? Because if you knew how to deal with these problems yourself, they would no longer have any power over you. They can only control you and make money off of you if you're sick.

Who are *they*? Who *is* this cartel? The organizations include the American Medical Association (AMA), the Food and Drug Administration (FDA), the Centers for Disease Control and Prevention (CDC), the National Institutes of Health (NIH), the National Cancer Institute (NCI), the American Cancer Society (ACS), and others. The corporations include all of the major chemical/pharmaceutical companies in the world, collectively known as Big Pharma. Also involved in this cartel are medical schools, research facilities, universities, hospitals, insurance companies, other doctors' organizations, and individual M.D.s. These are the main players in this game of Monopoly®.

If you and everyone you know were to follow the advice given in this book and the books that follow, in a short time you would no longer need medical care (or only need it infrequently) and the monopoly on healthcare would start to erode. The need for heart-lung machines, dialysis machines, and many of their other forms of biotechnology would gradually decline. Very few would ever need angioplasty, bypass surgery, or to have their hearts shocked back to life again, and all this amazing medical technology would start to collect dust in the corners of our hospitals' ERs and ICUs.

Like I said, it's *wonderful* that we have such amazing technology; and there are some amazing drugs out there as well, but I don't ever want to use them if I don't *have to*. These machines, procedures, and drugs are designed to save your life in an emergency—but wouldn't you rather not *need* them?

Listen, I don't want to get *rid* of medicine. I just want to get rid of the *monopoly*. I want a more logical system of healthcare. But, wait, I'm already getting ahead of myself. Before we go into all of that, let's first take a look back at how this monopoly developed in the first place.

As I mentioned, Western medicine, also known as allopathic medicine, is made up of two distinct branches, which use two different types of treatment. There's the medical side, which uses drugs as its main form of treatment, and then there's surgery, which involves using scalpels and other sharp instruments to cut into the body. These two forms of treatment have not always been under the umbrella of "medicine" nor have they always been practiced by doctors. They each evolved from very humble beginnings and along very different routes, finally coming together under the banner of the M.D. fairly recently. In fact, they are still sometimes referred to separately, such as in the phrase "physicians and surgeons."

Throughout this book, many pieces of this long, sordid story will fall into place more securely, but for now, let's just take a brief look back at how these two diverse forms of medical treatments came to monopolize healthcare today.

A BRIEF HISTORY OF MEDICINE

The Condensed Version

2000 B.C.	"Here, eat this root."
1000 A.D.	"That root is heathen! Here, say this prayer."
1850 A.D.	"That prayer is superstition. Here, drink this potion."
1940 A.D.	"That potion is snake oil. Here, swallow this pill."
1985 A.D.	"That pill is ineffective. Here, take this antibiotic."
2000 A.D.	"That antibiotic doesn't work. Here, eat this root."

—Unknown source, found on Internet

The Slightly Longer Version

For millennia, all the world over, herbal medicine was the one universally accepted form of medicine. In those early days of medicine, women were the healers more often than not. This ancient knowledge of herbs and their healing properties was reverently passed down from one healer to the next.

In the early part of the Middle Ages, religion began its reign over the world. In those days, also known as the "Dark Ages," the Roman Catholic Church had its hand in everything. The leaders of the Church knew that knowledge was power, so they guarded and hoarded information of all kinds with a jealous fervor. Strange as it sounds today, back then, even medicine and surgery were practiced by the clergy.

In the days of Hippocrates and the ancient Greeks, people believed illness came from an imbalance of the humors (blood, phlegm, choler, and black bile). But in the Dark Ages, illness was blamed on sinfulness. In other words, it was a punishment from God.

The men who ran the Catholic Church would not allow women to read, vote, be members of the clergy, or be involved in healthcare. In Christianity, only men were allowed to hold such important places of power because women have always been blamed for the fall of mankind. Because Eve ate fruit from the tree of *knowledge* (see box below), the Bible says that God cursed her with the pain of childbirth. It also says that because of this evil act, man should rule over her.

Notice how it is the quest for *knowledge* that is being punished here. This is a very important point. Recall that since the beginning of recorded history, back to the very first civilizations on Earth, the serpent has always represented wisdom, not evil, and certainly not Satan. In fact, the Bible never says the serpent is either of those things.

The symbol of the medical profession is usually described as "the serpent on the staff" (see below). Surely this serpent isn't representing the devil—it represents wisdom. And doesn't it make sense that the creature that represents wisdom be the one to offer knowledge to God's newest creatures? God tells Adam and Eve they will die if they eat the fruit of the tree of knowledge, but the serpent tells Eve she won't die if she eats it. He says that her eyes will be opened and she will become "like God, knowing good and evil." And indeed, this is what happens, as God later states, "The man has now become like one of us, knowing good and evil." [1]

So in the *Old Testament*, wisdom (the serpent) and knowledge (eating from the tree) are presented as being "evil." They are punishable offenses. But the Bible also says that through gaining this knowledge Adam and Eve became like God, and here is the truth of the matter. Just as God did in the story of Adam and Eve, the Church wants to hoard knowledge and the power that comes with it, retaining Godlike status only for itself. In other words, knowledge will set you free—free from the bondage of the Church, free from the bondage of Western medicine, and free from the bondage of all the other corporate and political oppression that rules your life as well.

Perhaps ignorance is bliss, but only if you prefer slavery to sovereignty. Being sovereign requires taking responsibility for your own life. Slavery requires giving up that responsibility. If you want to be sovereign, if you want to be more "Godlike," you must seek out and acquire knowledge. I have eaten of the tree of knowledge. My eyes have been opened. I now see with eyes that see, and in this book I am passing some of this knowledge on to you. Knowledge is not evil; knowledge is power. There are many people and many organizations who would rather you remain ignorant to the things revealed in this book. It is your lack of knowledge that allows them to control and manipulate you. If you prefer to remain ignorant and blissful, I suggest you put this book down right now. But if you want to understand and have some control over your own life and your health, then by all means, keep reading.

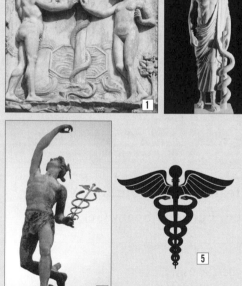

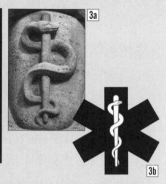

1. Adam and Eve being tempted by the serpent
2. Asclepius, the Greek god of medicine holding the traditional serpent on the staff
3. The original medical symbol, the staff of Asclepius: a) Ancient carving in stone, b) modern graphic illustration
4. Hermes or Mercury, conductor of the dead, god of commerce, protector of merchants and thieves
5. The commonly used medical caduceus, the magic wand of Hermes or Mercury

It's interesting to note that the original symbol of medicine, and the one still used by most of the world, is the staff of Asclepius, an ancient Greek physician who was deified as the god of medicine. The medical caduceus used by most American medical organizations today is actually the staff of Hermes (Mercury), who was the messenger of the gods, conductor of the dead, the god of commerce, and protector of merchants and thieves.

Midwives and healers of the day knew of herbs that would lessen the pain of childbirth. Perhaps this was seen as heretical back then. Not only did these women have more knowledge than the priests were comfortable with, but they were also interfering with God's punishment of women for seeking out such knowledge in the first place. Since the Bible says that men were supposed to rule over women, these priests apparently saw it as their duty to put a stop to all this depravity. Whether this was the reason for their actions or not, the fact of the matter is, priests began accusing women healers and midwives of being witches.

In reality, this was the beginning of the healthcare monopoly. These healers were the Church's competition. Those who can heal the sick have always been held in high regard, and the jealous Church could not abide in women or, for that matter, anyone outside of the clergy holding this powerful position. As a result, millions of these "witches" were hanged or burned at the stake by these religious men.

During the Renaissance, certain people, men mostly, began experimenting by using poisons or toxins in small quantities in an attempt to cure different ailments. These people were viewed by most as "charlatans," or "snake oil salesman." One of the poisons these charlatans would use quite frequently was mercury, which was sold as a salve. It was a popular remedy for syphilis, but was sold as a cure-all. You may know that mercury also goes by the name of quicksilver. You may also know that mercury is a neurotoxin and is one of the most toxic elements on earth. Because many of these charlatans sold quicksilver salve, people began referring to them as "quacksalvers" or simply "quacks." [2] Thus, "snake oil salesman," "charlatan," and "quack" became synonymous terms.

The murdering of healers and midwives by the Church worked gloriously to the advantage of the quacks. Thanks to the Church's efforts, over time, traditional herbal medicine began to be seen as "folklore," "witchcraft," or "voodoo." Those healers who weren't killed, either abandoned the practice of herbal medicine or practiced it very quietly "underground." And with all these healers out of the way, the profitable practice of medicating people with poisons could kick into high gear. As a result, despite the fact that these quacks' poisons were dangerous and many people died as a result of them, this vastly inferior alternative to herbal medicine managed to gain a foothold in healthcare.

Besides fast-talking sales pitches and pie-in-the-sky promises, this group of charlatans had some major support. As luck would have it, the makers of these poisons were very shrewd businessmen. With the investments of some well-known international businessmen (J. D. Rockefeller among them) and lots of deception, suppression, cover-ups, and lies, the pharmaceutical industry grew into what is today the biggest industry on earth. (For more detail on how this happened, see Appendix A: "How Big Business Took Over Medicine.")

In order to continue growing, these pharmaceutical companies needed a more credible sales force than "snake oil salesmen," so medical schools were taken over. The physicians who attended these "allopathic" medical schools were taught how to use pharmaceuticals (i.e., chemicals), or mild poisons to treat the sick. These schools were, of course, run by men. Women were not allowed in. Just as in the Dark Ages, women were to be subservient to men and were only allowed to be nurses. With some education, a clean white coat, and a stethoscope draped casually about the neck, suddenly the image of these poison peddlers went from dastardly to dashing. These "quacks" were now "Doctors of Medicine."

As you'll read in the next chapter, medical doctors went on to organize and form the American Medical Association (AMA), a lobbying group for doctors. Ironically, one of this group's stated goals was to fight against "quackery." Unfortunately, their definition of quackery was anything that competed with their brand of healthcare. Through the sales of advertising in their journal and other ties, the AMA is, and has always been, intimately connected to the Big Pharma. Chapter 4 describes the incestuous ties between the pharmaceutical companies and the FDA. Together, these groups and others now form the gigantic cartel that holds a monopoly on healthcare in America. And just as the Church did long ago, this cartel is always trying to find new ways of eliminating the competition, while still coming off looking like everyone's protector.

The history of surgery follows an interesting path as well. As mentioned previously, during the Dark Ages, God was given credit for much of the illness of the day; however, bad humors, or an imbalance of the humors, were still known to get much of the credit as well. Blood was the humor blamed most often, so many of the early medical treatments involved ridding the body of excess blood. Thus, bloodletting and leeches were popular medical treatments back then. Bloodletting involved opening up the veins and draining a certain amount of blood from the victim. This was an early form of surgery and like all medical treatments of the day it was performed by the clergy. In 1215, however, the pope ruled that priests could no longer perform surgery.

Early physicians disdained surgery, perhaps because they felt it was too barbaric and somehow beneath them, or perhaps they just didn't believe it worked. But regardless of the reason, they refused to do it, so the job of surgeon often fell to the barbers because it was assumed that they were good with a razor. (Barbers were the original dentists as well.) There *were* surgeons who were not barbers, but they were the minority in those days. The surgeons and the barbers maintained a constant feud with one another for many years, but the two groups were officially united under Henry VIII in 1540 under the name "The United Barber Surgeons Company." They remained thus united for two centuries.

Speed, strength, and a strong stomach were the skills most needed to be a surgeon back then. Before the advent of anesthesia in 1842, patients would often use whiskey as an anesthetic. Assistants would then hold the screaming, writhing, oftentimes vomiting patients down. If the patients managed to survive the operation, many of them died from infection.

During bloodletting, the barber would use a bandage as a tourniquet and patients would squeeze a pole to encourage blood flow. When not in use, the barber would wind the bandage around the pole and hang it outside as a "sign" that he was available. This was the origin of the striped barber pole we know today. Though it is now a patriotic red, white, and *blue*, it was originally just red and white, which signified blood and bandages.

Eventually, as knowledge progressed, surgeries became more complicated. The barbers were forced to rob graves in order to study anatomy and couldn't keep up with the surgeons. By then, surgeons were receiving some medical training and were attempting to establish themselves into a distinct, separate profession from the barbers. Some surgeons began referring to themselves as "surgeons of the long robe" to distinguish themselves from the barbers, who were called "surgeons of the short robe." In 1745, the surgeons officially separated from the barbers and became a distinct profession.

Bloodletting continued to be practiced for many years, with the surgeon often draining up to 80 percent of the patient's blood. When this was combined with the use of toxic metals like mercury, the results were often devastating, as was the case with former President George

Washington. Washington woke in the middle of the night on Friday, December 13th, 1799, with a sore throat and a fever. He asked his staff to call for a bleeder, who promptly came and relieved the president of about 14 ounces of blood. In the morning, Washington was attended by three physicians who drained him of another 80 or 90 ounces of blood, bringing the total to about half of the blood in his body—a medical emergency by today's standards. He was then given large doses of calomel (about 650 milligrams of mercurous chloride—a fatal dose of mercury) both orally and injected. He was also given emetic tartar (antimony—another toxic heavy metal). Additionally, blisters were applied to his extremities and his throat. His doctors had him inhaling vapors of water and vinegar, and applied a poultice of bran and vinegar to his throat as well. The *Reformed Medical Journal* reported that, "the afflicted general, after various ineffectual struggles for utterance, at length articulated a desire that he might be allowed to die without interruption!" Twenty-four hours after waking up with a sore throat, George Washington died at the hands of his doctors.[3] Unfortunately, this sort of thing was all too common in the early days of Western medicine.

Surgeons eventually became full-fledged physicians, attending medical school alongside their medical colleagues. Both now use the designation Doctor of Medicine, or M.D., but there is still some competition and rivalry between the two factions of "medicine." In other words, many physicians still disdain surgery.

Medical doctors like to think of themselves as practicing scientific medicine, but this is not really the case. In fact, much of what medical doctors do is actually in direct contradiction to what science is telling them. Another large portion of what they do is simply not backed up by any science whatsoever, such as the prescribing of drugs for "off label" uses. In reality, medicine is a profession based largely on faulty logic, bad science, and dogma. In fact, as you'll read in the chapters on vaccines, M.D.s are still using quicksilver, one of the most toxic elements on earth! Using "scientific medicine," they kill, by their own admission, over 280,000 people every year. That's more than all other accidental deaths combined.[4] Yet this medical cartel has the gall to call anyone who opposes their deadly "all for drugs and drugs for all" approach to healthcare "quacks!" It's hypocrisy in its purist form.

> *"Only 15 percent of all medical procedures*
> *are scientifically validated."*
>
> —*David Eddy, M.D., Ph.D.*[5]

So yes, the *face* of medicine has changed dramatically since the snake oil days and the days of the barber surgeons, but these quacks are still just peddling poisons, despite what the slick TV ads for pharmaceuticals try to convince you of.

Dogma & the Religion of Medicine

As you will see throughout this book, organized medicine bears a striking resemblance to both organized crime and organized religion. Allopathic medicine has such a monopoly on healthcare today, that to oppose them is practically professional suicide, and to challenge their authority or philosophy is tantamount to heresy. In essence, they have become just like the religious leaders were back in the Dark Ages. They've traded the black robes of religion for the white coats of medicine, but the rest is virtually identical. No one must speak out against the dogma of the religion of medicine!

"Science" has become institutionalized and is largely regulated by an establishment community that governs and maintains itself… In recent times there has been a narrowing of perspectives resulting in a growing dogmatism, a dogmatic scientism. There is arrogance bordering on worship of contemporary scientific concepts and models…taught in our schools in a deadening way, which only serves to perpetuate the dogma…

Strangely, the contemporary scientific establishment has taken on the behavior of one of its early oppressors: the church. Priests in white lab coats work in glass-and-steel cathedral-like laboratories, under the rule of bishops and cardinals who maintain orthodoxy through mainstream "peer review."

—Beverly Rubik, Ph.D., director of the Center for Frontier Sciences at Temple University[6]

New ideas have always been a threat to the establishment; therefore, there are always groups bent on suppressing the free flow of such information. In the days of Copernicus, Bruno, and Galileo, it was the religious leaders who were in control and who stood to lose if new ideas were allowed to enter the people's minds. Ideas of a solar system that revolved around the sun rather than the earth threatened the status quo, and, therefore, the power and authority of the Church which had believed and taught otherwise for so long. These men, these thinkers, these *scientists* had their very lives threatened for their ideas. Many were imprisoned, such as Galileo, and some, such as Bruno, even died because of their ideas—ideas that threatened the Church's dogma—ideas, which we now know were correct.

Today we have the same thing going on, but instead of, or rather in *addition to* the Church's suppression of the free flow of new ideas, now we have medicine's as well.

Notice, I say medicine rather than science, because "science" implies impartiality. There can be no dogma in true scientific thinking; and dogma is exactly what we're talking about here. Dogma, not religion, is the real enemy of science. At the outer reaches of science in the field of quantum physics, science is now confirming what many of the world's oldest religions and great spiritual leaders have been saying for eons. So science and spirituality *can* peacefully coexist, but science and dogma cannot.

Whenever money or egos become invested in a certain way of thinking or doing, anything that opposes that action becomes dangerous. It's dangerous to the establishment because it threatens its monopoly, and because of that, it can often become dangerous to *do* as well. It matters not what profession we're talking about here. We tend to think of church people as having our best interests at heart, just as we do people of medicine. However, these two fields are not immune to the lure of power, money, and ego any more than other professions are. As a result, both of these powerful institutions, religion and medicine, have greatly hindered advances in science because of their participants being so entrenched in an old way of thinking.

For centuries after the heliocentric universe had been proposed, despite overwhelming evidence in support of it, the Church continued to deny this theory. Only recently, in 1992, did it admit to the mishandling of Galileo's case. Likewise, for hundreds of years after it was discovered that foods containing vitamin C would prevent and cure scurvy, the medical community denied that this horrible disease, which killed millions, could be caused by nutritional deficiency and continued to search in vain for a germ or some other cause to explain it. Other diseases, such as pellagra, have very similar histories.

"The heresy of one age becomes the orthodoxy of the next."

—Helen Keller

In the early 1800s, 16 percent of women who gave birth died from a disease known as puerperal sepsis, or childbed fever. Dr. Ignaz Semmelweis (1818–1865) discovered by watching midwives that simply by washing his hands and having his students do the same before handling the patient, he could reduce the death rate of these women to only one percent. This was the lowest mortality rate ever experienced in his hospital.

In 1847, he proclaimed his discovery to the world, no doubt expecting the world to embrace him. But instead of thanking him for his contribution to science and medicine, he was immediately labeled a "quack." Doctors, who claimed to revere the scientific method, would not even listen to one of their own, and rejected his teaching entirely. Dr. Semmelweis went on to write a book called *The Etiology, the Concept, and the Prophylaxis of Childbed Fever,* which provided overwhelming proof of his theory. This heretical book caused even greater hostility by his colleagues.

Semmelweis died in obscurity, driven insane by persecution and lack of recognition from his peers. It wasn't until several years after his death, which was around the same time that germs were being discovered, that others became convinced of his wisdom and finally began washing their hands between patients.[7] Because of this stubborn, dogmatic way of thinking, thousands of children were brought into this world without a mother to raise them, and just as many husbands lost their loving spouses at a time which should have been one of great joy.

Unfortunately, this steadfast resistance to change, even in the face of overwhelming evidence, is a very familiar pattern in medical "science." You will read of many others with similar stories in the pages that follow.

> *"All truth goes through three steps:*
> *First it is ridiculed;*
> *Second it is violently opposed;*
> *Finally, it is accepted as self-evident."*
>
> —Arthur Schopenhauer, German Philosopher

Dogma severely hinders the forward march of progress, and when that dogma pertains to our health, that hindering of progress can mean the loss of millions of innocent lives. Countless new ideas and cures to horrible diseases have been suppressed, quashed, or otherwise pushed aside because they challenged the dogma and the current, flawed, incomplete theories of traditional Western medicine. Millions have suffered and died because of doctrine, or more precisely, because of money and ego.

Today, very little has changed from the time of Galileo, for pioneer scientists are still being persecuted. Some are charged with crimes and imprisoned just as he was, for presenting a new idea that challenges the dogma of the day. Healers are still being hunted down like witches and summarily put out of business. Others have died very suspicious deaths. Many healers have fled this country for Mexico and other countries where the oppression from the medical monopoly is less severe and a modicum of freedom still exists.

Without the murder of countless healers and midwives over the years; the ruthless tactics of the AMA and the FDA to crush the competition; the medical community's monopoly on the use of antibiotics; and without some amazing marketing and brainwashing of the public, allopathic medicine would never have become the majority party it is today. In other words, if healthcare systems were judged purely by their merits instead of by the public's deluded perceptions, allopathic medicine would have been marginalized long ago in favor of safer, more effective, and more logical approaches to healing. Perhaps by the time you've finished reading this book, you'll join me in this sentiment.

2

The American Medical Association's War on the Competition

"Strive to preserve your health, and in this you will the better succeed in proportion as you keep clear of the physicians."

—Leonardo Da Vinci

The American Medical Association (AMA) was founded in 1847 under the guise of improving medical education and to fight against "quackery." Its driving purpose, however, was and still is to improve (or protect) the financial status of the practicing M.D. Hard as it is to imagine now, medical doctors have not always had the best reputation nor have they always produced a living wage. In fact, in 1900, 53 years *after* the creation of the AMA, the average allopath (Western medical doctor) was still only earning about $750 annually. They also suffered the shortest life expectancy of any profession and about 40 physicians committed suicide every year.[1] (See box below.) Of course, their money woes *weren't* because people weren't sick. People feared them and rejected their practices, which still consisted largely of bloodletting, using leeches, and prescribing poisons like mercury. As the saying goes, the cure was often worse than the disease. In fact, the "cure" often killed the patient.

Today between 300–400 physicians kill themselves every year—about one a day.[2] According to several studies, medical doctors commit suicide about twice as often as other professionals. Female doctors are much more susceptible to suicide than their male counterparts, putting them at about four times higher risk than the average professional. M.D.s also suffer higher rates of alcoholism and drug addiction than other professions.[3]

"Allopathy, marked by the use of medicine and surgery and by an allegiance to the scientific method, holds itself up in near religious terms as the one true faith, dismissing as cults groups that subscribe to other approaches."

—From *The Serpent on the Staff* by Howard Wolinsky & Tom Brune[4]

One of the primary ways the AMA went about trying to improve things for their members was to viciously (and hypocritically) attack the competition, labeling them "quacks," "irregulars," or "cultists." Of course, these attacks had nothing to do with the safety or effectiveness of what today would be considered "alternative" techniques. In fact, by comparison almost *all* techniques were safer and more effective than allopathy at that time. The attacks were purely about eliminating the allopaths' competition.

Let's Play "Who Are The Cultists?"

Forget everything you know about healthcare for a moment. I know you can't, but just play along for a minute, okay? Now, I'm going to tell you about two different types of healthcare providers, and you're going to tell me which you think are the "cultist quacks" and which ones you think are the "healers." Here we go.

Members of Group One use harsh chemicals or mild poisons, which are toxic and foreign to the body, to counteract what the body is trying to do to heal; thereby, suppressing the body's cries for help and creating a new layer of disease. When that doesn't work, they often cut the body open and remove organs or parts of organs, then sew it back together. When that doesn't work, they try more chemicals and more cutting. Group One members use cancer-causing radiation to test for cancer; and when they find it, they often use more cancer-causing radiation to *treat* cancer. Similarly, they use toxic chemicals to treat conditions that were caused by other toxic chemicals. This group's two main theories of disease causation are that 1.) Microscopic bugs attack certain people, and in doing so, make them sick, and 2.) The person was born with it (or with a predetermined predilection for it).

In either case, it's just a matter of bad luck. Of course, they claim to have the only treatments that will help with your condition, dismissing all others as worthless or even dangerous. Ironically, *their* treatments kill hundreds of thousands of people every year, placing their treatment methods firmly within the top three causes of death in the country. They also sacrifice hundreds of thousands, if not millions of animals every year, infecting them with viruses and cancers or testing new concoctions of chemicals on them.

Members of Group Two work with the body's own healing mechanisms. They try to restore balance to the organism using proper nutrition, and by helping the body to detoxify. Occasionally, healing herbs or the oils of certain plants are used to treat patients. They refuse to use anything that's not found in nature. Some practitioners work to restore and balance the subtle energies of the body; others work to restore the proper biomechanics of the body. The vast majority of their practices are rooted in the sciences including anatomy, physiology, biochemistry, and quantum physics. Their remaining practices are based on empirical evidence—often hundreds or thousands of years old. Their over-riding philosophy is that a body that is toxic, malnourished, or out of balance with nature, becomes sick, and that germs prey on the sick. Rarely, if ever, does one of their treatments kill or harm a patient in any way.

Okay, now which group consists of "cultist quacks" and which one has the "healers"? Do I oversimplify, or do I simply tell the truth?

Healthcare: The "Alternative" to Symptom Suppression & Disease Management

Let me say at this point that I object to the term "alternative medicine." I know this is the "en vogue" term to describe anything outside of mainstream allopathic medicine, but I object to what the word "alternative" implies. It implies that allopathic medicine is the "real medicine" and that everything else is this sort of kooky, non-scientific quackery; or that we are the "other guys" off on the sidelines. I prefer to call it "natural medicine" or "natural healthcare," as these terms are more descriptive of what we actually do and because there is no implicit comparison between the two groups.

I consider myself a holistic chiropractor. I say "holistic" because I take a whole-person approach to treating patients. In my assessment of patients, I look at their diet, medications, supplements, the function of all of their organs and glands including blood pressure, pH, heart rate variability, blood, hair, and urine tests. I look at their emotions, the arches of their feet, the length of their legs, and many other factors, in *addition* to the status of their muscles, spine, ligaments, and nervous system. This sets me apart from chiropractors who only focus on the spine or musculoskeletal system. So holistic healthcare is a branch of natural medicine that attempts to treat the whole person rather than simply treating that person's individual parts.

Perhaps I'm making a big deal over semantics, but it's more important than that. We have to be very careful about the labels we put on things. To view what natural healthcare practitioners do as "alternative," you have to have a pretty myopic view of the world of healthcare. As you've just seen, Western medicine, or the use of mild poisons and surgery as a form of healthcare, evolved from rather humble beginnings, and as a "scientific profession," it really hasn't been around for all that long. So to view things like acupuncture as "alternative healthcare" is completely absurd. The Chinese have been practicing acupuncture for over 5,000 years. To call *herbs* "alternative medicine" is even worse. Herbs were the *first* medicines and are still the *best* medicines if safety is a part of your criteria. In fact, many of today's drugs were borne out of herbal medicine. In many cases, scientists found an herb that had a certain effect on the body, isolated the so-called active ingredient, synthesized it, patented it, and gave it a fancy drug name.

The process of isolating and synthesizing the "active ingredient" of an herb allows for the application of a patent (you can't put a patent on a naturally occurring substance), but it also causes the majority of the drugs' side effects. By removing all the synergistic co-factors associated with the active ingredient, you make the drug less effective and more dangerous. It also makes it more expensive. By taking the whole herb, you have true synergy—the whole being much greater than the sum of its parts.

Spinal manipulation has been around for eons as well. In fact, in Point le Merd in southwestern France, there are prehistoric cave paintings of "adjustments" being given dating back as far as 17,500 B.C. The ancient Chinese were using spinal manipulation at least as far back as 2700 B.C. Many ancient villages had "bonesetters" who could cure by straightening the spine. Ancient Japanese, Tibetans, Babylonians, Hindus, Egyptians, and Syrians all practiced some form of spinal manipulation. The North, South, and Central American Indians all used some form of spinal manipulation. In fact, virtually every society on earth has developed some brand of spinal manipulation.[5]

> ### *"Get knowledge of the spine, for this is the requisite for many diseases."*
>
> —Hippocrates

Hippocrates, (460–377 B.C.), the famed Greek physician, believed not only in spinal manipulation, he also espoused a similar philosophy to that of chiropractors today. He felt that only nature could heal, and that it was the physician's duty merely to remove any obstruction that would prevent the body from healing. He spoke of a vital spirit or "vitalism" that was the essence of life and the natural healing ability of the body. He said, "The natural force within each one of us is the greatest healer of disease."[6]

This concept of vitalism has occurred throughout countless ancient writings and cultures. The Chinese use the term Qi (pronounced "Chee") for this same concept. Chiropractors use the term "Innate Intelligence." In India, they speak of "Prana." Indeed, all *true* healing modalities teach this concept.

> ### *"Intelligence is present everywhere in our bodies… our own inner intelligence is far superior to any we can try to substitute from the outside."*
>
> —Deepak Chopra, M.D.

Western medicine has a word for a similar concept. They speak of "homeostasis," which is basically defined as the body's ability to self-regulate. The difference between homeostasis and vitalism, et al., is that homeostasis lacks any spiritual context, assuming Newtonian physics and chemistry hold the ultimate answer to the source of life. Also, and perhaps more importantly, rather than *embracing* the concept of self-regulation as we "alternative practitioners" do, Western M.D.s tend to ignore it, or worse, regard it as something that must be overcome. Rather than working with the body's wisdom, they often go directly against it, attempting to force it into submission through the action of harsh drugs which actually suppress the body's attempts to heal.

This is not healthcare. Drugs and surgery do not make a person healthy. They may alleviate symptoms. They may even save a person's life in an emergency, but they do *not* make a person healthy. Therefore, to call Western medicine "healthcare" is a misnomer. I would call what they do "sick care," "symptom suppression," or "disease management." But more on that later.

These alternatives to Western medicine also have amazing safety records, especially when you compare them to "real" medicine. Most of them have been practiced for thousands of years by skilled practitioners. Oriental medical doctors still use acupuncture and herbs as the mainstays of their treatment protocols. Doctors in Europe prescribe herbs as well as pharmaceuticals. Medical doctors in the U.S. are even starting to learn about these alternative practices in school. Some are recommending vitamins or even trying to learn how to adjust their patients' spines in weekend seminars. Clearly, their problem with alternative treatments is not that they are unsafe or ineffective. Clearly, their problem is, and always has been, that we are the competition.

With that in mind, let's take a closer look at a few of the larger "competing" forms of healthcare, and see what the AMA has done in an effort to suppress, eliminate, or destroy them.

Homeopathy

"The physician's high and only mission is to restore the sick to health, to cure as it is termed. The highest ideal of cure is rapid, gentle, and permanent restoration of health, or removal and annihilation of the disease in its whole extent, in the shortest,

*most reliable, and most harmless way, on easily comprehensible
principles."*

—Samuel Hahnemann, Founder of Homeopathy [7] (1755–1843)

In the early nineteenth century, Dr. Samuel Hahnemann
founded the once very popular form of medicine known as
homeopathy [*Homeo*=similar + *path*=disease]. Homeopaths work
using the law of similars; in other words, they believe that "like
cures like." This was a concept similar to another medical treatment
that was just getting underway (vaccination), whereby the infected
pus from cowpox lesions was being injected into humans in an
attempt to ward off smallpox.

Dr. Hahnemann and his followers found herbs that at higher
doses would elicit symptoms similar to those of disease and
theorized that by giving the body a *very* diluted remedy of that
substance, it would spur the body's own defenses to fight against
that disease.

Most of the remedies used in homeopathy are so diluted, in fact,
that one could accurately say that the remedy no longer contains
any of the substance at all—merely the *energy* of that substance.
Thus, homeopathy is essentially a branch of energy medicine. This
means homeopathy is incredibly safe. But how could this work, you
ask? Though this explanation is perhaps a little over simplified, you
could say that the more diluted the remedy is, the deeper it's able to
penetrate into the body. This may seem counterintuitive to the Western
mind where if a little is good, a lot must be better, but the more diluted
a homeopathic remedy is, the more potent it is.

Pharmaceuticals, on the other hand, are treated as toxins by the body. In an effort to protect itself, the body tries to block or eliminate these drugs from the bloodstream as quickly as possible. Drug companies know this. They *know* that the body will strip a significant portion of the effectiveness out of their drugs on each pass through the liver and kidneys, so they must be given in high enough quantity and frequency that they actually overload the body's ability to fully detoxify that drug. Over time, this damages the liver, kidneys, and other organs. Damage to these vital organs puts stress on all other organs and inevitably leads to more disease. Let me say that again: Drugs given long-term *inevitably* lead to more disease.

Comparing homeopathy to Western medicine is a little like comparing Don Juan's dating style to a caveman's. One method seduces you and wins you over with subtlety; the other hits you over the head with a club and has its way with you.

The allopaths [*Allo*=opposition + *path*=disease] by contrast, use harsh chemicals in an effort to directly *oppose* what the body is doing to fight off disease. This is a very important distinction to be made so let me say that again. Allopaths treat disease by opposing what the body is trying to do. But even this description overly glorifies what M.D.s do because for the most part, medical doctors do not treat disease at all; they merely treat the *symptoms* of disease, attempting to mask them or cover them up. This is like putting a rug over a stain instead of removing the stain.

What the homeopaths knew back in the early 1800s that the allopaths *still* do not know is that symptoms are actually beneficial to the healing process. They serve a purpose. Symptoms are not the problem. Symptoms are the body's way of *dealing* with a problem. Fever, for example, is an attempt by your body to handle an infection. Western medicine would have you take aspirin or Tylenol™ to bring your fever down; thereby, going directly against what your body is attempting to do to heal.

High blood pressure, likewise, is not a mistake by the body. It is a legitimate attempt by your body to adapt to a situation. Here, your body has detected that your brain and other organs are not getting enough blood and oxygen because of narrowed arteries, and it's doing its level best to keep those organs working properly and to keep you alive. Again, Western medicine intercedes by treating the symptom instead of the problem, using drugs to fight directly against what the body naturally wants to do. As a result, the brain and other organs end up starved for blood and oxygen. Thus, the side effects of most blood pressure drugs reflect blood and oxygen starvation.

These are just two examples of Western medicine's ongoing battle against the body's innate intelligence. The reality of the situation is that outside of the emergency room or surgical suite, medical doctors do very little other than treat symptoms. This only prolongs the illness or sends it deeper into the body. Treating symptoms creates a whole new layer of disease, making it harder and harder to fix, until eventually the patient dies not from his/her ailment, but from the cure.

The only difference between now and the late 1800s is the speed with which their treatments kill you. The drugs and techniques may have changed, but the flawed philosophy of allopathic medicine has *never* changed and this is the problem. So creating new and better drugs will not solve the healthcare crisis we are currently facing. The only thing that *will* solve the problem is to use allopathic medicine only for what it's good for (see box below) and to otherwise avoid it like the plague.

Many procedures that medical doctors perform, such as jumpstarting someone's heart after cardiac arrest and emergency appendectomies, are undoubtedly life-saving; however, they do nothing to handle the actual *cause* of the problem. This doesn't make them unnecessary. In fact, they are an integral part of our healthcare system. But they do fall well short of what I would call *healing*. These procedures fall into the category of "crisis management," which is the arena where Western medicine truly shines. Logic would dictate then that medicine should be used only as a crutch; something you use in a crisis in order to buy yourself some time until you're able to get into an actual *healer* who can set you back on the right track again—the track to self-healing.

Homeopathy does the exact opposite of allopathy. Homeopaths literally *embrace* symptoms and sort of nudge them along in an effort to *speed* healing rather than counteract it. The result is that symptoms go away, albeit slightly slower, because the body actually heals. Practically every non-medical approach to healthcare, including that used by Hippocrates, embraces the fact that the body knows how to heal itself if all obstacles are removed. Only Western medicine distrusts the body's natural healing potential, believing they are somehow smarter than nature.

British and European royalty, William James, Henry Wadsworth Longfellow, Louisa May Alcott, Charles Darwin, Presidents James Garfield and William McKinley, and many others used homeopathic doctors. Most surprisingly, John D. Rockefeller, who lived to be 99 years old, used homeopathy to the complete exclusion of allopathic medicine. He apparently believed that homeopathy was best for healing people and allopathy was best for making money.

War on the Homeopaths

When the AMA was founded in 1847, the men in charge quickly established ethical prohibitions against consulting with homeopaths and other "irregular" physicians. In 1882, after some medical establishments refused to abide by these rules, the AMA forced its members to sign a pledge agreeing to adhere to their ethical code, which barred these inter-professional exchanges.

In the 1870s bacteria were discovered and the germ theory quickly became the new paradigm of Western medicine. This ushered in a new scientific legitimacy to allopathy, whose members soon began abandoning many of their common practices such as bloodletting and purging—part of the old "bad humors" paradigm.

As antibiotics become more and more ineffective, we are seeing the arrival of the newest allopathic paradigm—genetics—or the "you were born with it" excuse for bad health. As such, M.D.s are now blessedly abandoning the use of antibiotics for everything.

But they still had their problems. There were too many medical schools cranking out far too many M.D.s and because of this oversupply, doctors were starving. Also, prior to 1910, medical schools were unregulated and the education doctors received often left much to be desired. In fact, up until that time some schools were still offering mail order medical degrees. And then of course, there was the competition from the quacks.

The AMA recognized these problems and actually stated in its journal *JAMA* in 1902, "What the medical profession needs is a leader, to take it out of the valley of poverty and humiliation..." [8]

They found this leader in Dr. George Henry Simmons, a former homeopath, who made his way up to become the president of the AMA. Dr. Simmons acknowledged that the two key sources of the profession's woes were the oversupply of doctors and competition from quackery. Thankfully, he had plans to address both issues.

To solve the latter problem, Dr. Simmons created a Trojan horse. He opened the doors of the AMA to these "quack sectarians," as he called them, offering membership in their elite club. Not sensing the trap, large numbers of homeopaths, osteopaths, and other natural health practitioners joined the AMA in the hopes of gaining professional acknowledgment. The result, however, was that the lines between the two schools of thought began to blur. The public began to see homeopathy more as a specialty of allopathy and rather than gaining influence, the homeopaths and osteopaths ended up losing political leverage along with their identity as natural drugless healers.

Simmons next began designing medical standards that strongly favored the allopaths. In 1907, he created the Council on Medical Education, which was commissioned to evaluate the education at medical schools throughout the United States and Canada and then make specific recommendations for its improvement. Because the AMA now encompassed natural healers, the homeopathic schools were evaluated right alongside medical schools. You can probably guess what happened.

The "Flexner Report" was released in 1910. This report, which was backed by pharmaceutical interests (see box below), strongly favored the use of pharmaceuticals in healthcare. It also recommended the closing of most of the homeopathic schools along with the less desirable medical schools. Despite the fact that there were vested interests involved in the obviously biased outcome, the report was taken as law. The overall result was improved medical education, fewer medical schools (and therefore fewer M.D.s), and the virtual death of homeopathy. It also forever tied medical education to the nearly exclusive use of pharmaceuticals. This meant medicine would be forever backed by the powerful and growing pharmaceutical industry. It was the perfect solution to all of medicine's troubles, with one exception. It was now completely locked into a flawed paradigm that simply does not and cannot work.

The "Flexner Report" was funded largely by Andrew Carnegie and supported by his ally J. D. Rockefeller along with the AMA. Using this report as a springboard, which was followed by millions in "philanthropic donations," these two men eventually took control over medical education. Why would two international investors care about medical education, especially Rockefeller, who would only see a homeopath for his own health? They did it to support their other investments, namely pharmaceuticals. For more details, please read Appendix A: How Big Business Took Over Medicine.

Osteopathy

"You as osteopathic machinists can go no further than to adjust the abnormal condition in which you find the afflicted. Nature will do the rest... Order and health are inseparable...when order in all parts is found, disease cannot prevail."

—*Andrew Taylor Still (1828–1917)*

In 1874, osteopathy was born. Dr. Andrew Still, a disgruntled, frontier medical doctor set out to develop his own version of healthcare, which was based on a divine revelation and his own study of bones, which he dug up from Indian burial grounds. He believed that misalignments of the vertebrae impinged the nerves, which in turn caused a decrease in blood flow to the organs. Dr. Still developed a form of spinal manipulation and abandoned the harsh medicines of allopathy. He did, however, continue to use minor surgery and the practice of obstetrics so that osteopaths would still be seen as primary care physicians. Later, osteopaths began rejecting some of Dr. Still's ideas and became more and more like allopaths, eventually prescribing drugs and performing major surgeries.

In the 1920s the AMA began to describe osteopaths as cultists and forbade their members from associating with them, just as they had with the homeopaths. But over the years, osteopathic schools gradually shed Dr. Still's "bone lesion" philosophy and became more and more like medical doctors. This decrease in emphasis on spinal manipulation, along with a concomitant increase in emphasis on drugs and surgery, led to a gradual, although still reluctant acceptance by the medical community. Around the 1960s, many states came to consider the two degrees as being equal. California saw that the two degrees were so similar that they actually converted all of their osteopathic schools into medical schools.

Today, osteopaths still receive some training in spinal manipulation during their schooling, but otherwise their education is virtually indistinguishable from that of a medical doctor. The same can be said of the way most osteopaths practice. While some still embrace the value of the osteopathic manipulation, most practicing D.O.s (Doctors of Osteopathy) use it only infrequently, favoring instead the use of prescription drugs.

Naturopathy

"In a word, Naturopathy stands for the reconciling, harmonizing, and unifying of nature, humanity, and God. Fundamentally therapeutic because men need healing; elementally educational because men need teaching; ultimately inspirational because men need empowering, it encompasses the realm of human progress and destiny. Dietetics, Physical Culture, and Hydropathy are the measures upon which Naturopathy is to build; mental culture is the means, and soul-self-hood is the motive."

—*Benedict Lust (1872–1945)*

While many of its methods have been in existence for millennia, the profession we know as naturopathy was created in the early 1900s by Dr. Benedict Lust. While working as a waiter, Lust contracted tuberculosis. He sought help from Father Sebastian Kneipp in Germany, who cured him using water-cure therapies, known also as hydrotherapy—a form of treatment that involves water (mineral baths, water-massage, bathing in water laced with essential oils or flowers, etc.).

Lust returned to the United States determined to study natural methods of healing and spread the word about "nature cures." He attended and graduated from the New York Homeopathic Medical College and the Universal College of Osteopathy, thus earning both M.D. and D.O. degrees. He purchased the term "naturopathy" from John Scheel, M.D. and in 1901(at the age of 29) he opened the American School of Naturopathy in New York City. He also founded the Naturopathic Society of America (later re-organized as the American Naturopathic Association, ANA) and in 1918 published the Universal Naturopathic Encyclopedia for drugless therapy. He became known as "The Father of Naturopathy."

The philosophy and practice of naturopathy is governed by six core values:

1. *Primum non nocere*
    First, do no harm; provide the most effective healthcare available with the least risk to patients at all times.
2. *Vis medicatrix naturae*
    Recognize, respect, and promote the self-healing power of nature, or "vitalism" inherent in each individual human being.
3. *Tolle causam*
    Identify and remove the cause of illness, rather than eliminate or suppress symptoms.
4. *Docere*
    The physician's major role is to educate and encourage the patient to take responsibility for her/his own health.
5. *In perturbato animo sicut in corpore sanitas esse non potest*
    Treat each person by considering all individual health factors and influences. Treat the whole person.
6. *Principiis obsta: sero medicina curator*
    The emphasis is on building health for the individual, the community, and the world rather than on fighting disease. Health promotion is the best prevention.

Besides using hydrotherapy, herbal medicine, homeopathy, massage, and spinal manipulation, he introduced the West to the Indian concepts of Yoga and Ayurveda. He also promoted nude sunbathing, not overeating, and giving up coffee, tea, and alcohol. (Naturopaths are also trained in acupuncture, clinical nutrition, physiotherapy, lifestyle counseling, minor surgery, midwifery, and mind-body medicine.) As a result of his unorthodox approaches to health he was frequently harassed by medical associations and was arrested and imprisoned at least 19 times by New York and Federal authorities.

During the first three decades of the twentieth century, naturopathy grew steadily until at one point, naturopaths were licensed in 25 states as drugless healers. Many chiropractic colleges at that time began offering both Doctor of Chiropractic (D.C.) and Doctor of Naturopathy (N.D.) degrees, as the two complemented each other so well. However, several forces combined and led to a temporary shrinking of the profession.

First, the Flexner Report came out in 1910, which, in addition to challenging the standards of many allopathic medical schools, put serious pressure on all non-allopathic schools of health. Then, of course, there was the AMA's long-term war against all things natural, whose leadership considered naturopathy a "cult." In 1945, Benedict Lust died and with the loss if its founder, the ANA diffused into multiple splinter groups. And, of course, around the same time, the miracle drug penicillin was saving lives, which led to a dramatic increase in the public's confidence in allopathic medicine.

For decades, all the naturopathic schools in North America were housed within chiropractic colleges, but in the 1940s and 50s, in an effort to scrub their own image (as chiropractic was busy fighting for its own existence, as you'll read in the next section), one-by-one chiropractic colleges began dropping their naturopathic programs and distancing themselves from naturopaths. This, of course, led to a serious decline in naturopathic graduates. Western States Chiropractic College was the last to offer the N.D. degree, closing its doors to naturopaths in 1955. This very nearly spelled the end of naturopathy. By 1958, only five states licensed naturopaths.

But in 1956, the National College of Naturopathic Medicine opened in Portland, Oregon, providing an educational platform to sustain the profession. This school was the only source of naturopathic doctors in North America for the next two decades. During that entire time, it graduated only 70 students. The 1970s, however, brought with it the holistic/alternative medicine movement, which breathed new life into the naturopathic profession. Little by little, new schools sprung up and with additional naturopaths out looking for work, more states began to license them again.

Today, there are six accredited naturopathic colleges in North America. (My alma mater, National University of Health Sciences has also received candidacy for accreditation for their N.D. degree.) Fifteen U.S. states now grant licenses to naturopaths. These include: Alaska, Arizona, California, Connecticut, Hawaii, Idaho, Kansas, Maine, Minnesota, Montana, Vermont, New Hampshire, Oregon, Utah, and Washington. Florida and Virginia also license naturopathy under a grandfather clause. Additionally, naturopathy is licensed in the District of Columbia, Puerto Rico, and the U.S. Virgin Islands. Twelve states/jurisdictions allow naturopaths access to prescription medicine and 10 allow them to do minor surgeries. Naturopathy is specifically prohibited in Tennessee and South Carolina. Naturopathy is also licensed in British Colombia, Manitoba, Ontario, Saskatchewan, and Nova Scotia, Canada. The American Association of Naturopathic Physicians (AANP) and the Canadian Association of Naturopathic Doctors (CAND) are actively supporting licensing and credentialing efforts in numerous American states and several Canadian provinces as the profession continues to expand once more.

Chiropractic

"The science of chiropractic has modified our views concerning life, death, health, and disease. We no longer believe that disease is an entity, something foreign to the body, which may enter from without, and with which we have to grasp, struggle, fight, and conquer, or submit and succumb to its ravages. Disease is a disturbed condition, not a thing of enmity. Disease is abnormal performance of certain functions...a change in the amount of energy and function

performed. The body in disease does not develop any new form of energy; what it already possesses is diminished or increased, perverted or abolished."

—Daniel David Palmer (1845–1913)

The chiropractic profession was founded in 1895 by a man named D. D. Palmer. Unlike homeopathy and osteopathy, which were both founded by disgruntled medical doctors, Palmer had no formal medical training. He was working at the time as a magnetic healer, when he came upon the janitor in his building who had been completely deaf for 17 years. Palmer adjusted the man's spine and his hearing miraculously returned. Palmer described the incident this way:

> Harvey Lillard…could not hear the racket of a wagon on the street or the ticking of a watch. I made inquiry as to the cause of his deafness and was informed that when he was exerting himself in a cramped, stooping position, he felt something give way in his back and immediately became deaf. An examination showed a vertebra racked from its normal position. I reasoned that if that vertebra was replaced, the man's hearing should be restored. With this object in view, a half hour's talk persuaded Mr. Lillard to allow me to replace it. I racked it into position by using the spinous process as a lever; and soon the man could hear as before.[9]

Palmer became excited by his discovery and began doing research as to the cause of the man's deafness. He theorized that there had been a nerve impingement brought on by a misaligned vertebra, a theory very similar to that of Dr. Still. (See box below.) He called these misalignments "vertebral subluxations" [*sub*=less than + *luxation*= dislocation]. He named his new discovery "Chiropractic," from the Greek, meaning to practice by hand [*Chiro*=hand].

Palmer was soon treating people with all sorts of afflictions. Under his care, pain ended, infections healed, stomach disorders disappeared, vision improved, and fevers broke.

The nerve directly involved in hearing, the Cochlear nerve, never leaves the skull and therefore never comes anywhere near a vertebra. This has created somewhat of an enigma for chiropractors to explain. It *may* be that the Harvey Lillard story is nothing more than a legend, as I know of no other chiropractor curing deafness in the 100 plus years that have passed, nor do we have Mr. Lillard or his medical records to study. The truth is we don't even know what vertebra(e) Palmer adjusted. There *are* other theories for how an adjustment could restore hearing though. For example, there are many nerves of the autonomic nervous system, which *do* come in close contact with vertebrae, and these could definitely have some *indirect* control over hearing—perhaps even as Dr. Still (of osteopathy) suggested by increasing blood flow to the ear. Since we don't know what vertebra was adjusted, it's very possible that Palmer affected one or more of these nerves with his adjustment. But also, and perhaps more importantly, as we learn more and more about how the nervous system works, we're finding that it's much more complex than we originally thought and far beyond the scope of this book. I will tell you that the bone impinging on a nerve theory is vastly over-simplified to the point that it's really not even accurate, much as the models of atoms we all studied in science or high school chemistry class weren't. However, inaccurate as they are, these simplified theories *do* serve a purpose and that is to educate people on very complex ideas without the need for imparting them with a Ph.D. on the topic. And regardless of the accuracy of chiropractic theory, I've had innumerable patients get off of my table and tell me that they could see clearer, hear better, smell better, breathe fuller, that they get sick less often, etc. The point is, chiropractic *does* work, whether you, I, or the AMA understand why or not.

How Chiropractic Took on the AMA and Won

In 1905, after a decade of seeing Palmer and others cure people the allopaths had failed with, the medical profession had him arrested and put in jail for practicing medicine without a license. He became the first of many chiropractors to be jailed for this crime and was locked up on numerous other occasions as well. Each time his patients would protest his incarceration, and soon, he would be released.

He went on to form The Palmer School of Chiropractic and began teaching others to become chiropractors. It started out as a very brief schooling and at first required only a high school diploma to enter, but the program progressed quickly to include more and more training. Among those he trained was his son, B. J. Palmer. B. J. and his father disagreed on many things, but it was largely B. J.'s marketing skills that caused chiropractic to grow from its infancy into the profession it is today.

B. J. Palmer eventually became the president of the Palmer School of Chiropractic. In 1926, he also became president of the International Chiropractors Association (ICA). He remained president of both organizations until his death in 1961. During his term of presidency at the ICA, he maintained a constant feud with Dr. Morris Fishbein, who was a long-time editor of the *Journal of the American Medical Association*.

Morris Fishbein has probably been natural healthcare's greatest enemy. He was a true medical fascist. In addition to attacking chiropractic, he also attacked the naturopaths, homeopaths, and virtually anyone else who threatened pharmaceutical medicine. He was one of the main players in the suppression and destruction, or eventual exile of several proven cancer cures, including those of Royal Rife, Max Gerson, and Harry Hoxsey, stories which will be covered in a future *Why We're Sick*™ book. The suppression, destruction, and exile of these treatments, all of which were for financial reasons, has meant the death of millions of people, putting Morris Fishbein squarely in the ranks of one of history's greatest butchers.

In 1925, Fishbein (who never practiced medicine a day in his life) wrote a book entitled *The Medical Follies*, a book on quackery, wherein he described chiropractic as a "malignant tumor" and belittled its theories as a reversion to the original ideas of osteopathy, "so simple that even farm-hands can grasp it." [10] He also wrote, "It has been said that Osteopathy is essentially a method of entering the practice of medicine by the back door. Chiropractic, by contrast, is an attempt to arrive through the cellar. The man who applies at the back door at least makes himself presentable. The one who comes through the cellar is besmirched with dust and grime; he carries a crowbar and he may wear a mask." [11]

After World War II, many veterans entered chiropractic college and the profession began to take on a higher profile. As a result, chiropractors began to be seen as competition for the almighty dollar. In the 1950s, Doctors of Chiropractic and individual Doctors of Medicine were still known to cooperate peacefully with one another, but in the early 1960s, around the time of B. J. Palmer's death, all that changed.

In November 1962, Robert Throckmorton, general counsel to the Iowa Medical Society, gave a speech at the North Central Medical Conference in which he addressed "the chiropractic problem" and issued a call to arms against the "menace of chiropractic." He called for a "positive program of containment" and said, "Action taken by the medical profession should be firm, persistent, and in good taste [and] behind the scenes whenever possible." [12] In his speech, he listed several areas that he thought were important for this effort: 1. Oppose chiropractic efforts to be covered by health insurance and worker's compensation. 2. Oppose chiropractic efforts to get hospital privileges. 3. Contain chiropractic schools. 4. Encourage ethical complaints against chiropractors. 5. Resist chiropractic efforts to enhance its position through legislation. 6. Encourage disunity between the "straights" and "mixers." [13]

The terms "straight" and "mixer" refer to the two main philosophies within chiropractic and are somewhat analogous to the terms liberal and conservative. Straight chiropractors stick to using the spinal adjustment as their only form of treatment. Mixers use whatever their state's scope of practice allows, which can include physiotherapy, nutrition, massage, herbal medicine, detoxification, homeopathy, acupuncture, rehabilitation, etc.

Within a few months of his speech, the AMA hired Throckmorton as their general counsel. In September 1963, Robert Youngerman, a lawyer for the Department of Investigation (the AMA's quackbusting department) sent a memo to Throckmorton saying that chiropractors "present a clear and present danger to the health and welfare of the public, and it would seem that as guardians of our nation's health, doctors of medicine should be dedicated to the total elimination of any unscientific cult." [14]

By November 1963, the AMA had established a Committee on Quackery whose stated goal was to "contain and eliminate" the chiropractic profession.[15] In January 1965, Throckmorton hired H. Doyl Taylor, an attorney and city editor of the *Des Moines Register*, and set him loose on the chiropractic profession. Taylor helped write a position statement, adopted by the AMA's policy-setting House of Delegates in 1966, which stated, *"It is the position of the medical profession that chiropractic is an unscientific cult whose practitioners lack the necessary training and background to diagnose and treat human disease. Chiropractic constitutes a hazard to rational health care in the United States because of the substandard and unscientific education of its practitioners and their rigid adherence to an irrational, unscientific approach to disease causation."* [16] (Please see Appendix B: *A Comparison of Medical and Chiropractic Education.*)

The AMA represented, at most, half of all medical doctors in practice at that time, and yet they were making statements as if they *were* the medical profession.[17] But regardless of their numbers, this political lobbying organization, designed to protect the interests of medical doctors by eliminating the competition, declared war on the chiropractic profession under the *guise* of protecting the public from unscientific cultists.

AMA ETHICS

The AMA has the second biggest lobbying group in Washington. (The pharmaceutical companies have the biggest.) Where does the AMA get the money to fund such efforts? Well, *some* of it comes from membership dues, but about half of the AMA's total income comes from selling advertising space in its journal *JAMA*.

From the mid-1930s to the mid-1950s, under the leadership of Dr. Morris Fishbein, tobacco products were advertised in *JAMA* as health elixirs. In fact, in the 1940s Phillip Morris was the AMA's biggest advertiser. Through these advertisements, Big Tobacco convinced medical doctors to encourage their patients to smoke after meals to help with digestion. Because they were being funded in part by Big Tobacco, the AMA not only promoted cigarette smoking, but they continued to protect and defend tobacco companies long after it had been proven that smoking caused lung cancer.[18] These are the ethics and moral standards of the noble AMA.

Today, all of the ads in *JAMA* are for pharmaceuticals. But *these* drugs are poisons too, many of them addictive poisons, just like tobacco. Like smoking, these drugs slowly poison you to death, even while they help to mask your symptoms. Just like Big Tobacco, these companies will vehemently deny any wrongdoing or knowledge that they are harming us. To the contrary, they will pledge that they are fighting the common enemy, disease, with every resource they have. But these massive corporations are not the altruistic big brothers we'd like to think they are. These companies are only looking out for their own interests. As you'll see in the next chapter, you are nothing but a means to an end for them, and that end is increasing their stock prices.

Once again, we have poisons being promoted for their supposed health benefits by an organization (the AMA) that is being supported largely by the poison manufacturers. Because of this incestuous set up, and a hundred other reasons, the AMA cannot be considered a credible organization to rely upon for healthcare advice. The only real difference between Big Pharma and Big Tobacco is that Big Pharma has better PR. Because of that, the public hasn't yet come to the realization that pharmaceuticals are inherently bad for you. I predict that someday we'll look back on the days when doctors prescribed drugs for cancer, heart disease, depression, hyperactivity, etc., just like we now view doctors of the past suggesting having a smoke after dinner. Someday, we will realize that poisons, whether they come in sticks you light on fire and inhale, or in pills to swallow, or fluids to drink or inject—no matter how they are administered, poisons cannot make you well. They can only make you sick.

Taylor contacted hundreds of medical groups and encouraged them to adopt ethical prohibitions against M.D.s referring to or consulting with chiropractors. If you remember, we've seen this tactic already when it was used against the homeopaths: Cut off communication, and then paint the other side as a bunch of unscientific quacks.

Manufacturing the Evidence

In 1967, Congress asked the Department of Health, Education, and Welfare (HEW) to appoint a panel to advise the government on whether or not chiropractic should be reimbursed under Medicare. The panel consisted of two committees, which included medical doctors, osteopaths, hospital administrators, medical school officials, nursing officials, etc., but not a single chiropractor.[19] The AMA was prevented from being on the panel, but as they had an insider, this didn't really matter.

Dr. Samuel Sherman was the AMA's insider on the HEW panel. At Taylor's behest, Sherman orchestrated a study that was *supposed* to be an independent government study performed by the HEW. In actuality, the study was a complete sham. Sherman, a loyal puppet of the AMA, wrote a letter to Taylor, dated March 11, 1968, advising him of the outcome of the study. The problem was, the study wasn't scheduled to begin until *August* of 1968! How could he possibly have known the outcome of the study five months before it had even begun?[20]

The results of the study: Chiropractic was found to have no merit and had no place within the Medicare system. Well surprise, surprise! Apparently, in the late 1960s, the AMA was powerful enough (and corrupt enough) to have an "independent government study" fabricated in order to prove that chiropractic was worthless. (So much for that allegiance to the scientific method.) Thanks to this made-up study, the HEW panel voted against chiropractic being covered under Medicare.

For *years* after this study was exposed as a sham, the AMA continued to use it in their negative propaganda smear campaign against chiropractic, supposedly showing how an independent government study had proven chiropractic to be ineffective![21]

In further effort to sway public opinion against Doctors of Chiropractic, Dr. Joseph A. Sabatier, chairman of the AMA's Committee on Quackery, and others, would often make disparaging speeches against chiropractic. Sabatier was once quoted as saying that, "rabid dogs and chiropractors fit into about the same category... chiropractors were nice people but...they killed people." He also said "...it is very important to point out to members of the medical profession that it is considered nothing less than totally unethical to refer patients to a chiropractor for any purpose whatever." [22]

In July 1969, a journalist named Ralph Lee Smith published an exposé called, *At Your Own Risk: The Case Against Chiropractic.* Hundreds of thousands of copies of this anti-chiropractic propaganda were printed and distributed. The AMA purchased some 10,000 copies and distributed them to persons and institutions in key positions, including at least 1,200 copies to the nation's largest libraries. Other copies went to politicians, schools, high school guidance counselors, and the media. Smith was supposedly an "independent" writing a book, but the book was financed and distributed by the AMA and it was based, at least partially, on the AMA's Department of Investigation's files and on Smith's own writings for an AMA magazine. (He also wrote anti-chiropractic articles for *National Enquirer.*)[23]

In 1971, the Committee on Quackery issued a memo to the AMA Board of Trustees stating the following:

Since the AMA Board of Trustees' decision, at its meeting on November 2–3, 1963, to establish a Committee on Quackery, your Committee has considered its prime mission to be, first, the containment of chiropractic and, ultimately the elimination of chiropractic.

Your Committee believes it is well along in its first mission and is, at the same time, moving toward the ultimate goal. This, then might be considered a progress report on developments in the past seven years. The Committee has not previously submitted such a report because it believes that to make public some of its activities would have been and continues to be unwise. Thus, this report is intended only for the information of the Board of Trustees.[24]

Sore Throat Speaks

In 1972, the executive vice president of the International Chiropractors Association (ICA), Dr. Jerome McAndrews, received an interesting package in the mail. The package contained 15 copies of a book entitled, *In the Public Interest*.[25] The book was authored by William Trevor (a pen name), and it detailed the actions the AMA had been taking against the chiropractic profession.

The book's cover depicted the AMA's caduceus superimposed over a Nazi swastika. The tone of the book was sarcastic, but it was well documented. It contained numerous photocopies of internal memoranda and other correspondence that had been smuggled out of the AMA headquarters in Chicago. The information primarily pertained to the Committee on Quackery and its proposed goal of containment and elimination of chiropractic.

Dr. McAndrews later received a phone call from the book's publisher, an underground press called "Scriptures Unlimited," who offered to sell the ICA a truckload of the books and the rights to the copyrighted material. The sellers insisted that they be allowed to arrive unannounced and be paid by cashier's check. The address they gave McAndrews was an already closed post office box in Los Angeles, California. The group was obviously very afraid of what the AMA would do if they were caught distributing these books.

The ICA agreed to the purchase and received 15,000 copies of the book. They then went about distributing them.

Among those receiving the book was Dr. Chester Wilk, a Chicago chiropractor, who coincidentally had been writing his own book around the same time. In 1973, he published, *Chiropractic Speaks Out: A Reply to Medical Propaganda, Bigotry and Ignorance.*[26] Dr. Wilk had seen the effects of the AMA boycott in his own practice, but until he read *In the Public Interest*, he did not realize the full extent of the conspiracy or exactly who was behind it. Upon reading this book, he began to push the chiropractic profession to pursue legal action against the AMA. Neither of the two national chiropractic associations wanted to pursue it, but Wilk didn't give up.

Adding fuel to the fire, in 1975, another AMA informant began sending papers to the press and other interested groups revealing the underhanded activities of the AMA. This individual went by the name "Sore Throat," a play on the "Deep Throat" informant of the Watergate scandal. Many of these documents pertained to the Committee on Quackery and its dealings, and served to throw the issue into the media spotlight.

Just before these documents started showing up in the press, the AMA dismantled the Department of Investigation and the Committee on Quackery, claiming they had succeeded in their mission, despite several significant chiropractic advancements including limited coverage under Medicare and licensure in all fifty states. They then hired a private investigator, a former Secret Service agent, to find the leak within their organization and began shredding documents en masse.[27]

Meanwhile, Wilk had become increasingly frustrated by the apathy of the chiropractic leadership and their unwillingness to go after the AMA for what they had done. So, this rather modest, understated chiropractor took matters into his own hands. On Columbus Day, October 12, 1976, Chester Wilk, D.C., along with three other doctors of chiropractic, filed suit against the AMA and several other medical and osteopathic organizations. It was a huge undertaking—a true David and Goliath story in the making. In Wilk's own words, "It was apparent that we were literally taking on the entire medical establishment." [28]

The Wilk Trial

The group retained George McAndrews, (younger brother of Dr. Jerome McAndrews of the ICA) to try the case. George, an antitrust lawyer from Chicago, was reluctant to be named as counsel, thinking his relationship to the ICA executive vice president could be seen as a conflict and could prejudice the case. However, when no other law firm would take the case, he was forced to accept. With his acceptance of the case, the ICA gave Wilk their support and the American Chiropractic Association (ACA) soon followed suit.

During the pre-trial discovery years of 1977–1980, the AMA tried to clean up its act in an effort to put on a good face. In 1979, they adopted a report stating that not everything chiropractors did was without therapeutic value; however, they reaffirmed that chiropractic theory was unscientific, and that they stood by their ethical code of 1957 prohibiting any association with cultists.[29] In a further attempt to sanitize their records, in 1980 they reluctantly revised their ethical code to no longer ban consultation with unscientific practitioners.[30] This was all done very quietly, however, and they never actually came out and announced that it was acceptable to consult with chiropractors. They also continued to distribute anti-chiropractic material.

The case finally went to trial in December of 1980. During jury instructions, the judge, who was unfamiliar with some of the intricacies of antitrust law, instructed the jury not to find the AMA guilty if its actions were merely designed to inform the public about defects in chiropractic philosophy. The judge also allowed certain irrelevant pieces of evidence into the testimony while disallowing much more relevant pieces, making the case appear to be more about who the better profession was, as opposed to an antitrust case. During the second half of the trial, the incredibly well-funded AMA attorneys applied all sorts of slick legal maneuvering and even had a key witness, Doyl Taylor, conveniently relocated just before he was scheduled to take the stand.

After an eight-week battle, the jury deliberated for just two hours before finding the AMA's anti-chiropractic campaign within legal bounds. Jurors actually apologized to McAndrews in tears after the trial, saying that they felt the AMA was wrong for what they did, but according to the judge's instructions, they were forced to find the AMA not guilty. Mr. McAndrews filed an appeal, stating the judge had mishandled the case, and in 1983 the appeal was granted. In May 1987, U.S. District Judge Susan Getzendanner presided over a non-jury trial, which was, in most other respects, very similar to the first trial.

Highlights from the Trial:

Chester Wilk testified that he was unable to refer patients to the hospital for X-rays, and if a patient he was treating needed medical care, he said, "I turn them over and then I don't see them any more." [31]

Chiropractic patients, many of them medical failures, took the stand and described how chiropractic care had helped with their back and neck pain.

World-renowned medical professor, and orthopedic surgeon, John Mennell, M.D., testified in court on behalf of the chiropractors. Dr. Mennell has taught at eight different medical schools. He's the author of numerous textbooks and articles in medical journals. His credentials are flawless. The following is part of the testimony Dr. Mennell gave while being questioned by one of the AMA's attorneys. Watch how the AMA's attorney tries to corner Dr. Mennell and the tactic backfires:

AMA attorney: "I think you [said that medical residents receive] four or five hours of training in manipulative therapy—is this correct?"

Dr. Mennell: "I think I said zero hours, didn't I, for the most part?"

AMA attorney: "What I'm trying to determine is, when you talk about zero hours' training in manipulation, what particular definition of 'manipulation' were you referring to?"

Dr. Mennell: "I think my testimony was that if you ask a bunch of new residents who come into a hospital for the first time how long they spent in studying the problems of the musculoskeletal system, they would, for the most part, reply, 'Zero to about four hours.' I think that was my testimony."

AMA attorney: "The musculoskeletal system comprises what portion of the body?"

Dr. Mennell: "As a system, about 60 percent of the body."

AMA attorney: "Is your testimony, that the residents to whom you just referred told you they had no training whatsoever relating to problems as to 60 percent of the body?"

Dr Mennell: "That's just about right."

AMA attorney: "Is it your testimony that it is your understanding that the entire medical school curriculum is devoted to about 40 percent of the body?"

Dr. Mennell: "Yes sir." [32]

I often tell my patients that to see an M.D. for a musculoskeletal problem is about like coming to see me for a dental problem. Sure, I could look inside your mouth, tap on your teeth, and fake it a bit, but beyond that, I'm more or less clueless. I've actually had a family practice M.D. admit as much to me. I also had a cardiologist admit that while he could read an EKG strip in nothing flat, a neck X-ray was a bit of a mystery to him. This is nothing against these two fine physicians. I would be equally clueless with an EKG strip at this point. Of course, I wouldn't walk into an ICU, glance at some EKG strips and start prescribing meds either. In practice, one must know one's limitations.

During the trial, AMA lawyer Douglas Carlson admitted that chiropractic had improved as a profession, by becoming more scientific, but then appeared to take credit for the improvement stating, "We suggest that one reason that it changed was because of the criticism of its bizarre methods." [33] Mr. McAndrews likened Carlson's statement to a German U-Boat captain claiming "credit for the American Olympic [swim] team being so good because by sinking their ships, he taught them how to swim." [34]

After a grueling, two-month trial, Judge Getzendanner came to her decision. She ruled that:

[The AMA and its officials] instituted a boycott of chiropractors in the mid-1960's by informing AMA members that chiropractors were unscientific practitioners and that it was unethical for a medical physician to associate with chiropractors. The purpose of the boycott was to contain and eliminate the chiropractic profession. This conduct constituted a conspiracy among the AMA and its members and an unreasonable restraint of trade in violation of Section 1 of the Sherman Act.[35]

She also found the American College of Surgeons, the American College of Radiology, and the American Academy of Orthopaedic Surgeons guilty of being a part of the conspiracy.[36] Several other organizations settled out of court prior to the conclusion of the trial.

She ordered the AMA to admit the "lawlessness of its past conduct" and to alter its official policy on chiropractic. This injunction appeared in the *Journal of the American Medical Association* on January 1, 1988.[37]

The AMA appealed the case, but in February 1990, the Appellate Court upheld the lower court's ruling. The AMA appealed once more, but in November 1990 (fourteen years after the original suit was filed) the U.S. Supreme Court let Judge Getzendanner's ruling stand.[38]

In December 1991, after a year of negotiating, the AMA agreed to pay $3.5 million for the chiropractors' legal expenses and to publish its new ethical opinions, stating that medical doctors and chiropractors could indeed associate professionally.[39]

The Wilk trial has not ended the AMA's war on the competition, of course. If anything, it merely forced the AMA and their allies to go deeper underground in their efforts to suppress anything that does not involve surgery or pharmaceutical medications. This 14-year battle received little to no press in the mainstream media and barely amounted to a slap on the wrist to a medical cartel that is backed by the biggest and most powerful corporations in the world. Yet it *was* a victory.

The AMA's war on the competition has nothing at all to do with safety, because *every* alternative or natural approach to health is considerably safer than even *the safest* of allopathic approaches. So their position is not about *safety*; it's purely about quashing the competition, which is just another way of saying, it's about fear, scarcity, and greed. They're afraid that we have something better to offer. They're afraid that everyone will finally realize that drugs and surgery are no good and that alternative approaches are better and safer, and they're afraid they will lose business (and, therefore, money, power, and prestige) to a bunch of "quacks."

And yet, chiropractic is still being hypocritically attacked on groundless claims of safety issues (as are nutritional supplements and herbs) by a profession that actually *admits* to *knowing* they are killing 280,000 people every year and *confesses* that this is probably only about five percent of the actual total.

Unfortunately, the AMA is not the only enemy in this healthcare revolution of ours, or even the worst. In fact, the AMA could almost be likened to an army of gnats on the battlefield. They buzz around the eyes and ears, and annoy the hell out of you, but never do any *actual* harm, unless of course, it's to distract us from the *real* enemies of health, who we shall discuss next.

For More Information Read:

The Serpent on the Staff, The Unhealthy Politics of the American Medical Association, by Howard Wolinsky & Tom Brune
Medicine, Monopolies, and Malice, How the Medical Establishment Tried To Destroy Chiropractic in the U.S., by Dr. Chester A. Wilk

3

The Drugging & Brainwashing of America

"He's the best physician that knows the
worthlessness of the most medicines."

—Benjamin Franklin

The pharmaceutical industry is the most profitable industry in the world—by far. In 2002, the combined profits for the 10 drug companies in the Fortune 500 amounted to more than the profits for the other 490 companies put together![1] And we in America are doing more than our share to keep those profits high. Americans spent $200 billion on prescription drugs in 2002, not including those that were administered in hospitals, nursing homes, or doctors' offices. (This figure also doesn't include over-the-counter drugs.)[2] This $200 billion accounts for about half of the prescription drug sales in the entire world.[3] In 2008, Joseph Mercola estimated that Americans spent a total of $500 billion on drugs in America.[4] *This* is the healthcare crisis we're facing.

Now if these huge profits were merely the result of good old capitalism in the free marketplace or a good business model, I'd say, "fair enough," but they're not. As I've mentioned before, Big Pharma is a cartel that is not only *allowed* by our government, but one that is endorsed, encouraged, and protected. These companies have so many layers of government protection at this point that our government and Big Pharma are practically business partners.

This "partnership" all but guarantees their continued massive profits—much of which is now at taxpayers' expense. They use these profits to gain ever more government protection, to quash any and all alternatives to drugs, and to continually brainwash us into taking more of their poisons.

We like to think of these multi-national corporations as they depict themselves—benevolent scientists in white coats, forever hunched over petri dishes and microscopes, men and women dedicated to the eradication of suffering and disease. But let's take off the rose-colored glasses for a while and try to look at this from a more objective standpoint if we could. Try to let go of the emotion tied up with disease and suffering and see these businesses for what they really are—businesses. Forget for a moment about the individuals who work for these huge corporations, the people who are *not* on the board of directors, who probably *do* care about you and your health, and focus, if you will, on the corporation as a whole.

Publicly traded corporations like pharmaceutical companies are business entities that exist solely to make money and to make their investors money. They rely on investors' money for growth and to stay solvent. The only way investors can make money is if that corporation's stock prices go up. If stock prices don't go up, it's not a wise investment. The only way stocks go up is if the corporation's profits go up (or show promise of going up). In other words, the company must continue to grow. Even if the company has profits in the billions, if there's no growth, stocks stagnate and investors pull their money. Business CEOs know this. They know that their company must either grow or die. It is their job to keep the profits going and growing—at *any* cost.

The only way a business' profits can go up is if its costs go down, its prices go up, or if its salespeople can somehow manage to sell more product. Therefore, in order to keep their investors happy, pharmaceutical companies must continually sell more and more drugs. There are only two ways to accomplish this: if people are actually *getting* sicker, or if people *think* they're getting sicker. I submit that the drug companies are using both of the above strategies for their benefit.

Injecting Fear

One of the best ways a drug company can sell more drugs is to produce a drug that is "required" by a large segment of the population. Here, we're talking primarily about vaccinations. Vaccinations are mandated by the government, pushed by pediatricians, required by schools, and paid for by insurance companies. Further, if children are injured by these chemical concoctions, the government protects the company that made them from any liability. Though the profit *per dose* on vaccinations is not that high, the sheer volume of sales makes up for it. Millions of children receive these shots every year all across the globe. When the World Health Organization (WHO) says they want to rid the world of polio, and, therefore, need 65 "zillion" doses of polio vaccine, the CEOs of these companies just about wet themselves. So vaccinations, especially those that are mandated and require multiple doses, are practically the Holy Grail for Big Pharma.

Flu shots, which are vaccinations, too, are not far behind. In fact, since they're needed every year, they may even be better. Fear is a great motivator and these companies, with their ingenious marketing tactics, will gladly deal in scare campaigns to sell more drugs, which is precisely why we see a new "killer flu" strain in the news every couple of years. In fact, just the *fear* of widespread disease is enough to give their stock prices a bump. A worldwide pandemic would be a panacea for them, so stories of bird flu, swine flu, SARS, anthrax, or smallpox are just like money in the bank.

In 2005, the WHO stated, "Governments should consider stockpiling vaccine against H5N1 bird flu now, before a pandemic starts." In response to this, the U.S. contracted drug manufacturers to make four million doses of bird flu vaccine. Many other countries followed suit. This caused Roche Pharmaceuticals' sales for the third quarter of 2005 to increase by a whopping 20 percent just from one drug! The stock prices for BioCryst went up 60 percent because of a *potential* avian flu treatment. The revenue generated in response to this announcement was likely several billion dollars for a disease that most experts believed would never become a real health threat, and for drugs that have not been proven to be safe or efficacious. The bird flu mutates very rapidly, so neither a vaccine, nor a flu drug are likely to work well, if at all. All this money was generated out of fear. It was a *complete* waste. And it all came out of your tax dollars! The 2009 swine flu scare was the exact same thing. The only difference was the name.

Stretching the Market

Cholesterol medications (statins) are another panacea for drug companies. Ironically, *they also* fall into the category of "dangerous drugs you really don't need." This is because *high cholesterol is not a disease.* It's almost always a symptom of eating highly processed, sugary, or starchy foods. Furthermore, high cholesterol is *not* a good predictor for heart disease, nor does lowering your cholesterol *prevent* heart disease.

Before cholesterol medications were invented, a total cholesterol count of up to 280 was considered normal. But once they had developed drugs that would lower serum cholesterol, the drug companies decided to expand their market. So, the "normal" was lowered, first to 240, then to 220, then to 200. Now they're actually saying it should be 190 or lower. I've even heard some doctors say, "the lower it is, the better." This is not only ridiculous, it's dangerous. So, is it any wonder that in 2002 Lipitor was the best-selling drug in the world, and Zocor, another statin, was second? [5]

Cholesterol is actually a highly beneficial product that's produced in large quantities by the liver, and in smaller quantities by every cell in your body. That's because every cell in your body needs cholesterol to function. It's needed in high quantities by the brain and other nerves and it's the base molecule for all the steroid and sex hormones in the body. (See Figure 1.) It's also used to repair damaged tissues, much as a painter uses Spackle™ to patch up holes in drywall. (Once again, we see allopathic medicine opposing what the body is trying to do to heal.) This repair mechanism is part of the reason your cholesterol levels go up when you eat nothing but junk food.

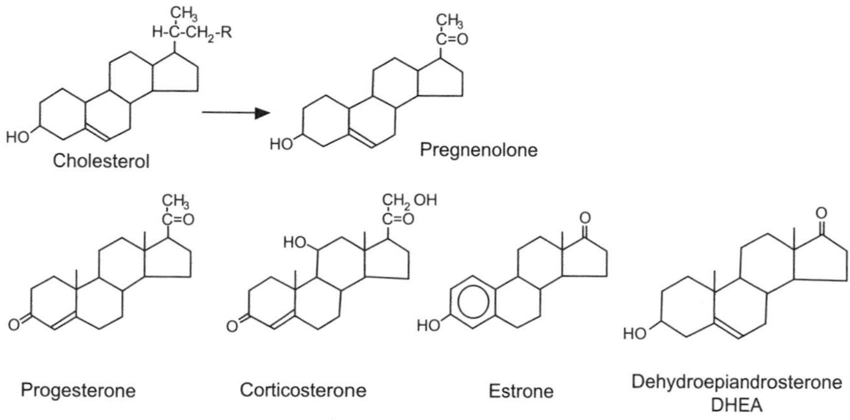

Figure 1. Cholesterol is used to make all the steroid hormones and sex hormones in the body including the estrogens (estrone, estradiol, and estriol), progesterone, testosterone, corticosterone, cortisol, androstenedione, aldosterone, DHEA, pregnenolone, and others. (From *What Your Doctor May Not Tell You About™ Menopause* by John R. Lee, M.D. with Virginia Hopkins. Copyright © 1996 by John R. Lee, M.D. and Virginia Hopkins. By permission of Grand Central Publishing.)

The truth is cholesterol medications do nothing at all that's beneficial, unless, of course, you count making your doctor and the drug companies happy. They *will* lower your cholesterol, but this *won't* unclog your arteries or *prevent* the clogging of your arteries. Therefore, as mentioned, they *don't* prevent heart attacks. They "work" by blocking an enzyme in your liver that produces cholesterol. But this enzyme is also used to produce Coenzyme Q10, a vitamin-like substance that's needed in large quantities, especially by the heart, but also by other muscles, and, in fact, by every cell in the body. This loss of CoQ10 often leads to muscle pain or damage and fatigue. The loss of cholesterol leads to decreased cellular repair, decreased brain function, and a loss of sex hormones. Statins have also been shown to be toxic to the lens of your eye and to cause cancer in animals.[6,7] And in order to get all these worthless or harmful effects, these drugs must damage the liver. Statin drugs are nothing less than a disaster for your body.

Perhaps you're saying to yourself, "But I heard the fatty atherosclerotic plaques in arteries are made of cholesterol." My response is, that's partly true, but does that mean cholesterol is bad? Calcium is often a part of these plaques, which is the reason we get *hardening* of the arteries. Does that mean *calcium* is bad? Platelets are part of these plaques as well, but without them you would bleed to death with just the tiniest of cuts. Please understand, these components (cholesterol, calcium, and platelets) are merely there to *repair* the damage that's been done. They are *not* the bad guys. Just as you don't condemn the cops for being at a crime scene, *don't condemn cholesterol for being at the site of a damaged arterial wall.* Remember there's a big difference between correlation and causation.

If I came up with a drug that lowered your blood calcium to incredibly low levels, would you buy it? Of course not, because you know that your body *needs* calcium, not only for bones but for your heart and other muscles, to maintain the pH of your blood, and for a thousand other functions as well. Well, do you really think your body would *produce* something in large quantities that it doesn't need or that could *harm* it? No, it wouldn't. It's called Innate *Intelligence*, not Innate Stupidness. But, once again, medicine has declared that the body (i.e. nature) is stupid and that they know better. Well, I'm here to tell you, they don't.

I'm sorry to say, you've been sold a bill of goods. Cholesterol is *not* the cause of heart disease. You *need* cholesterol, which is why your liver is producing it in the first place. If it's producing more than the "normal" amount, it's because it's trying to compensate for something *you're* doing. Don't punish your body further for your indiscretions. Look at your diet; look at your stress levels; get the toxins out of your body, including the drugs. Follow the advice and wisdom you gain by reading this book and your numbers should return to normal, which is somewhere between 200 and 280.

What *is* the cause of heart disease? That topic will be covered in a future *Why We're Sick*™ book.

Creating Diagnoses

In an almost Orwellian tactic to sell more product, drug companies have discovered a new slant on that old business model of "find a niche and fill it." The new model is essentially the reverse of the old, where drug companies create new "diseases" in order to fit their drugs. We've seen many of these new diseases of late, such as premenstrual dysphoric disorder (PMDD), social anxiety disorder, attention deficit disorder, erectile dysfunction, and acid reflux disease, a.k.a. gastric esophageal reflux disease (GERD).

Until recently, these were not diseases; they were merely *symptoms.* What's the difference between a symptom and a disease? Not much, as it turns out. The *main* difference is in people's perceptions. Drug companies know that if they can convince you that you're somehow *not normal,* that you actually have a disease or a disorder that can be treated with drugs, their stock prices go up. So these new names are nothing more than marketing tactics. For example, nobody thinks they need a drug for shyness, but for social anxiety disorder—maybe. Suddenly, when they see these commercials, every shy person in the world realizes there's something *wrong* with him/her and starts wondering if maybe s/he needs Paxil, too. (See box below.) A little heartburn after dinner might just call for a Rolaids® or some Pepto-Bismol®, but gastric esophageal reflux disease requires constant medicating, preferably with Prilosec, the purple pill. (Oooh, it's *purple*!? Does it come in dinosaur shapes? By the way, Prilosec, was the *third* best-selling drug in 2002.)[8] A kid with a short attention span sounds fairly normal, whereas attention deficit disorder sounds much more ominous. Suddenly Johnny has a *disorder*—and he *needs* his meds.

> Paxil cut its teeth on "social anxiety disorder," but was later approved for "generalized anxiety disorder" as well. In one of the sleaziest attempts I've ever seen to capitalize on a tragedy, after September 11, 2001, GlaxoSmithKline launched an ad campaign showing images of the World Trade Center towers collapsing, essentially suggesting that everyone take Paxil to help deal with their fears of another terrorist attack.[9]

This new diagnosis tactic is sometimes done in order to extend the "shelf life" of a drug. Such was the case with Prozac, the once very popular antidepressant drug. When the patent on Prozac was about to expire, Eli Lilly, the drug's manufacturer, ran some tests to see how it worked on PMS. It worked (that is, it relieved some of the symptoms), but in order to get a new patent and exclusive marketing rights, it needed to be the only drug approved for the problem. Since there were already drugs approved to treat PMS, they needed a new disorder, or at least a new name—thus Premenstrual Dysphoric Disorder (PMDD) came into being. Next, they gave Prozac a new name, "Sarafem;" gave it a new color, pink and lavender; and finished it off with a bigger price tag. They then began advertising it as a treatment for their newly invented disease. Of course, if it works for PMDD (i.e. PMS with a vengeance), they knew that doctors would prescribe it for regular PMS as well, which was really the intent all along.

By the way, Sarafem now sells for three and a half times the price of generic Prozac (fluoxetine). But then, it *is* pink and lavender, so . . .

There's one more recently invented diagnosis I'd like to discuss. It's called "pre-hypertension." Web MD defines pre-hypertension as blood pressure between 120/80 and 140/90. When I was in school, 120/80 was considered "normal," but it was expected that a person's blood pressure would go up gradually with advancing age and so "normal" could extend all the way up to 140/90, again, depending on age. Now, just as was done with cholesterol, they've lowered the "normal" to *below* 120/80 *regardless* of age. Why? To sell more drugs. So now, doctors are actually being trained to put people on medication for what was previously considered normal blood pressure and they seem to have the ridiculous notion that the lower a patient's blood pressure is, the better. And while a blood pressure of 0/0 will definitely protect you from having a stroke, as well as eliminate every symptom you may have, it will also prevent you from living.

It's as if the doctors have been blinded by "science" (i.e. pharmaceutical research) and completely forsaken anatomy, physiology, and good old common sense. You have to remember that your body is part of nature, and, once again, nature isn't stupid. Nature is *infinitely* smart. So even if your blood pressure *is* high, as in *actual* hypertension, it isn't because your body just one day *forgot* how to regulate your blood pressure. It raised your blood pressure for a reason.

When you run up a flight of stairs, your blood pressure goes up in order to pump more blood and oxygen into your leg muscles. When you see a tiger running toward you, your blood pressure goes up for similar reasons. When you're under constant stress, your blood pressure goes up because your body is trying to prepare you to "run from the tiger" even though the proverbial tiger never actually comes. But your body raises your blood pressure only when the situation calls for it and it does so for a very specific reason— your brain, organs, and muscles need more blood and oxygen. Listen, *you don't want low blood pressure.* What you want is the *appropriate* blood pressure for the situation. Luckily, our bodies have a way of regulating this.

You have an area inside each of your carotid arteries (the main arteries that bring blood to the brain) called the carotid body. The infinite wisdom of Nature/God "placed" it there, between your heart and your brain, for a reason. You see, the carotid body's only job is to constantly monitor the oxygen, carbon dioxide, and pH of the blood that's going to the brain (your body's Central Processing Unit). When it detects a problem in any one of these parameters (called cerebral ischemia), it sends a signal up to the vasomotor center in the brainstem, which then activates the sympathetic (fight or flight) nervous system. That system tells the heart it needs to pump a little harder and/or faster so that the brain can keep functioning. It also causes the arteries to constrict in certain areas (like the digestive organs) and dilate in others (like the muscles). The overall effect of this process is an increase of the person's blood pressure and a brain with plenty of oxygen.

If this was a temporary situation, like running up a flight of stairs, the body will quickly regulate back to normal and soon all will be fine and dandy again. But if it's a chronic condition, as in atherosclerosis or some other process that constricts the arteries like chronic stress, the body will maintain this elevated blood pressure (in spite of the extra stress on the heart, the arteries, the loss of digestive function, etc.) just to keep the brain functioning properly. But this does not make our medical doctor happy. *He* knows that high blood pressure can lead to congestive heart failure and stroke, and he has drugs that can treat it.

Very simplistically, these drugs come in two main varieties—the kind that tell your heart to calm down, chill out, and not work so hard; and the kind that tell your kidneys to start pumping fluids out of your body. (A good blood-letting every week or so would also work.) Either of these courses will cause your blood pressure to drop, but at what expense? Obviously, the brain is no longer going to be happy and neither will any of the other organs. So again, medicine is declaring itself smarter than nature and going directly against what the body was doing to deal with a situation. And once again, it treated a symptom and did nothing about the actual problem.

Actually, they would probably also put the patient on a statin to lower their cholesterol at the same time—whether their cholesterol was high or not. We've just discussed the ineffectuality of *these* drugs. Together these two drugs will force the patient's lab and physical exam findings into the "normal" ranges, but at the same time will play havoc on the patient's body chemistry and physiology. They'll also probably put the patient on an aspirin a day, which will eventually cause a gastric ulcer. This will lead to a prescription for the purple pill, which will prevent the patient from digesting their food. All that undigested food will lead to colon cancer, which will lead to surgery, radiation, and chemotherapy. Or maybe they'll just die from gastric bleeding from the aspirin.

So what happens when you go on blood pressure medication? Well, they *will* prevent you from blowing out an artery in your brain, if that were an issue, but now instead of *that* problem, you have another one. For the rest of your life, or at least as long as you're on the medication, your brain and other body parts (liver, kidneys, genitals, hands, feet, etc.) will not be getting enough blood and oxygen. The "side effects" of these drugs reflect this lack of circulation. The patient becomes depressed, fatigued, swollen, his hands and feet are cold, and he can't maintain an erection. These symptoms lead to *more* drugs such as Viagra, Prozac, a stronger diuretic, and on and on the cycle goes.

When doctors treat true hypertension, at least there is some benefit, but when they treat pre-hypertension, there is literally no upside, unless the patient also happens to own stock in the company that supplies the drug. Fortunately, there *are* natural ways to treat high blood pressure that actually handle the underlying cause.

Annie was 78 years old when she first came to see me. She had never been to a chiropractor before and she was nearly dragged in by one of my other patients. Her main complaint was severe low back pain, which caused her to rely on a walker. She was also quite obese and had significant ankle swelling. Her forearms were black and blue. She frequently had severe nosebleeds and she was anemic. The only medication she was on was one to control her blood pressure. In a few visits I had her walking with just a cane. Within a short time, she no longer needed that either. At that point, I began working with Annie on her blood pressure. I put her on several whole food supplements to help correct the underlying problems that were causing her high blood pressure and one to deal with the bruising and nosebleeds, which were caused by a mild form of scurvy brought on by the medication. In a few months, Annie noticed that her blood pressure was going below normal. I told her that was because her body was actually healing and suggested that she talk with her doctor about lowering her dose of medicine. She decided on her own to start taking half her usual dose, and soon her blood pressure went back within the normal range. Around this time, she went to see her medical doctor for a check-up. When the doctor told her that she had the blood pressure of a teenager, Annie confessed that she had reduced her dose of medication by half. The doctor was shocked and asked Annie what she had been doing. Annie (I think rather reluctantly) told her that her chiropractor had put her on some supplements. Thankfully, the doctor chose to work *with* me instead of *against* me, and told Annie to keep doing what she was doing. Soon, in order to keep her blood pressure from going too low again, Annie had to reduce her dose to half a pill every two days, then half a pill every three or four days. Finally, she stopped taking her medication altogether. She now walks on her own with no cane, she has no bruising on her arms, the nose bleeds have stopped completely, her ankle swelling has dissipated considerably, and her blood pressure remains normal to this day. Amazingly, this was all done without exercise, with no change in diet, and with no herbs.

"Me Too" Drugs

When a drug's patent expires, other companies can begin making and selling that drug. These are called generics. As I'm sure you're aware, generics generally sell for much less than the brand-name drug. This competition takes a serious bite out of the profits on the brand-name drug.

One tactic drug companies use to keep their profits from dropping with the loss of exclusivity on blockbuster drugs is with what are known as "Me Too" drugs. This is where manufacturers slightly alter a drug or perhaps even just alter the *dosage* of a drug, as with "Weekly Prozac," and create a new drug from the old. The drug company is then given a new patent with exclusive marketing rights for their "new drug." Then they get doctors to stop prescribing the old drug (or its generic) and start prescribing the new. This is accomplished by giving M.D.s lots of free samples to try on their patients and by marketing the new drug as an improvement over the old, whether it *is* or not. Of course, they stop the relentless advertising of the old drug at that point too because it's just not good business practice to advertise something you don't have the exclusive rights to sell. The "Me Too" market requires considerably less research and development effort than creating a new drug from scratch. Whether you realize it or not, the bulk of today's "new drugs" are actually just copies of the old. The generics, i.e., old drugs, are usually just as good and in some cases better than the new ones, and as mentioned, they're considerably cheaper.

Nexium is an example of a "Me Too" drug. In this case, when AstraZeneca's patent on Prilosec expired, they stopped pushing Prilosec and started pushing Nexium, the *new* purple pill. (Prilosec is now sold over-the-counter for a fraction of what Nexium costs, which is about $4/pill.) Similarly, Clarinex was Schering-Plough's replacement for Claritin when *its* patent ran out.

Other Games They Play

Drug companies also employ all sorts of tricks in order to extend the patents on their drugs. For example, they are given an extra six months of exclusivity if they test their drugs on children. Therefore, almost all of the major blockbuster drugs are tested on children, including drugs that are designed for treating adult disorders like high blood pressure or PMDD.[10] (Meanwhile, some drugs that *are* prescribed for children have never been tested on them.)

Here's another good one: As the life of a patent is coming to a close and a generic company is getting ready to release the generic version of a drug, the brand-name company can sue the generic company for patent infringement, even if the suit has no merit, and the FDA will automatically delay approval of the generic for 30 additional months.[11] Lawyers use rules like these and many others to tie things up in court, often for years, giving their companies billions of dollars in additional profits. Or, a company may make a deal with a generic company, sometimes paying them not to produce the generic.

Another game drug companies like to play is to convince doctors to prescribe a drug for what are called "off-label" uses. Off-label prescribing refers to using a drug for something that the FDA has not approved it for. It's legal for an M.D. to prescribe any drug for any reason, but it is illegal for a drug company to market a drug for any reason other than those approved by the FDA. What they do to get around this silly law is to run a worthless study that is significantly below the standards of any medical journal worth its weight in paper, *or* the FDA for that matter. The drug companies then pay some doctor to put his or her name on the study. Then, they can legally "educate" doctors as to these novel new uses for their drug. Voilà! They just expanded their market with very little investment and without having to get FDA approval for it. As many as half of all prescriptions are written for off-label uses.[12]

But the most common tactic these companies use to keep their profits growing is their quest to get everyone on earth taking as many of their drugs as possible on a continuous basis, whether they need them or not. In pursuit of this quest, they've become geniuses at marketing, or as I like to call it, brainwashing.

The Brainwashing of America

As was mentioned in the previous chapter, drug companies advertise heavily in the AMA journal. The AMA depends on this money in order to stay solvent. This gives drug companies a great deal of influence over the AMA. The AMA, in turn, has massive political clout. (It's second only to Big Pharma in terms of its lobbying efforts.) Besides its immense political influence, the AMA also has tremendous influence over medical schools, practicing M.D.s, hospitals, nurses, and many other aspects of healthcare.

Drug companies and their major stockholders, like the late J. D. Rockefeller, make major contributions to medical schools, which influences what is taught in those schools *and* what research goes on there. (Please see Appendix A: *How Big Business Took Over Medicine*.) Through their own lobbying efforts and political connections, Big Pharma has major influence over what healthcare research is done in universities, at the National Institutes of Health, The National Cancer Institute, etc. This research dictates what appears in medical journals, which dictates what goes into medical textbooks, which *further* influences what is taught in medical schools. The whole thing is a closed loop system. Nothing but drugs goes in, so nothing but drugs comes out, thereby guaranteeing that M.D.s continue learning the "all for drugs and drugs for all" approach to healthcare.

Practicing M.D.s receive the majority of their education on drugs, not from textbooks or their medical school training, but from pharmaceutical representatives. Of these "reps," only 1 percent has had any formal training in pharmacology. The rest are strictly salespeople with no formal background in science at all. These laypeople are drilled, polished, and trained in what to say and do in order to sell more drugs through doctors. They use free samples, expensive gifts, meals at fancy restaurants, vacations to Hawaii, and all manner of bribes and kickbacks (which are euphemistically called "consulting fees") to influence doctors' prescribing habits. Of course, these reps are given generous salaries and bonuses, which are based on their sales. (Watch the movie "Side Effects" for a humorous, but accurate depiction of the people in this profession. It was actually written and directed by a former drug representative.)

Drug companies also put on lavish seminars at fancy retreats and golf resorts, often with meals and transportation included, to educate doctors about their drugs. The companies pay for all of this and refer to it as "education," but it's really just marketing to doctors. Thanks to some slick lobbying on the part of Big Pharma, these marketing seminars now count toward a doctor's continuing education hours. Whereas other professionals have to pay for their own continuing education, M.D.s have over 60 percent of theirs covered by Big Pharma.[13] Amazingly, drug companies spend a whopping $16 *billion* per year on these "educational expenses" in the U.S. alone. That amounts to $10,000 per M.D. on average.[14]

Besides the $16 billion they spend wooing doctors, drug companies also spend $4 billion per year[15] (that's $11 million a day) advertising their drugs on television, imploring you to, "Ask your doctor if Poisonex is right for you." This "direct-to-consumer" advertising accounts for around one third of all advertising on TV. This means pharmaceutical companies also have massive influence over television *content* and what's reported (or not reported) on those stations' news programs. And in case you're wondering, despite the almost humorous, rapid-fire listing of life-altering side effects these ads often contain, studies have shown that the ads *do* work. Like lemmings, people ask their doctors for drugs, by name, and in the vast majority of cases, the doctors comply. A survey by *Prevention* magazine found that 33 percent of people who have seen these ads have talked to their doctors about one of the drugs. Twenty-eight percent ended up asking for the drug and 80 percent of the doctors complied.

Besides the United States, only New Zealand allows this direct-to-consumer advertising, i.e. brainwashing of her people, and New Zealand is considering repealing the law.

Leaving no stone unturned, the drug companies also advertise relentlessly in magazines and other print media, which means they have a great deal of influence over what stories run (or don't run) in those periodicals as well.

Studies have shown that physicians are actually more influenced by drug *advertising* than they are by scientific evidence. Frighteningly, 34 percent of these advertisements contain misleading or erroneous information.

The High Cost of Drugs

So why are drug prices so high? The perennial excuse drug companies use is the high cost of researching and developing new drugs, in spite of the fact that our government and universities are doing much of this for them now. (See box below.) This would seem to imply that R & D is one of their bigger expenses, but is it? Granted, it's very expensive to bring a new drug to market. But how does the amount they spend researching and developing new drugs compare with the amount they spend marketing them?

Taxol, the best selling cancer drug in history is an excellent example of this. This drug, which is derived from the bark of the Pacific yew tree, was studied for 30 years by the National Cancer Institute (NCI) at a cost to taxpayers of $183 million. In 1991, the NCI signed a cooperative research and development agreement with Bristol-Meyers Squibb. Squibb's part in the deal was merely to supply the NCI with 17 kg of the drug, which Squibb actually obtained from another company, and 0.5 percent in royalties. Squibb was then given five years exclusivity on Taxol, which it parlayed into a 1–2 billion-dollar-a-year industry. The cost for a year's treatment on this drug is $10,000–$20,000. That's a 20-fold markup over manufacturing costs. They also sued and received an additional three years of exclusivity. As of 2003, Squibb had made $9 billion on Taxol.[16]

In 2001, 35 percent of drug company revenues went to what is called "marketing and administration."[17] (Even though they are publicly traded corporations, pharmaceutical companies refuse to give a breakdown of marketing statistics alone and instead insist on lumping them together with administrative costs. This means we must make some estimates here.) Administrative costs include such expenses as the obscene salaries and bonuses of the CEOs and other high-ranking officers. Charles Heimbold, Jr., for example, the former chairman and CEO of Bristol-Meyers Squibb, made $74,890,918 in 2001 not counting his $76,095,611 worth of un-exercised stock options.[18] But getting back to the point, it is estimated that drug companies as a whole spent approximately $9 billion on administration (about 5 percent of total revenues) and nearly $54 billion (30 percent of revenues) for marketing in 2001.[19] Only about 14 percent of their revenues actually went to R & D.[20] This means *they spend more than twice as much on marketing as they spend on research and development.* By the way, Big Pharma's industry-wide profit margin is 17 percent, which is 3 percent more than they spend on R & D.[21] So much for their lame excuse.

Regardless of how things break down, the consumer is paying for all of these expenses (R & D, marketing, "education," free samples, gifts and kickbacks to doctors, lobbying, campaign contributions and other bribes, obscene salaries for CEOs, frivolous lawsuit legal expenses, etc.) all through the cost of their drugs.

> Most people are so caught up in the system that they don't realize they're actually paying these people outrageous sums of money to brainwash them and then drug them—to death. And the CEOs of these companies are just laughing their way to the bank.

The prices for prescription drugs have gone up at four times the rate of inflation for the past 30 years or so. Part of the reason for this is that drug companies have government-protected monopolies, i.e. patents, on their products, which prevent direct competition for 20 years. But also, when two different drugs are competing for the same market, like Paxil and Prozac, the companies have learned not to compete on price. They've learned that price wars lead to lower profits for all sides, and that's just not sustainable in business. In fact, cost is never even *mentioned* in their ads. Instead, they compete on what disease or symptom their drug is proven to treat, how their drugs differ, etc. Also, when a new drug comes on the market sporting a higher price than its competitors, the competing companies take advantage of the price differential and *raise their* prices. The overall result of this is competitive price *escalation*. The truth is, drug companies operate as an oligopoly or a cartel rather than as competitors.

When seniors started complaining that they could no longer afford the drugs they (supposedly) needed, rather than looking at why the drugs were so expensive or putting a cap on drug company profits, Congress passed the mind-numbingly confusing Medicare prescription drug benefit. (The United States is the only developed nation that does *not* regulate drug prices in some way.)[22] The passage of this law was a *huge* boon to Big Pharma. It allows drug companies to continue to charge whatever they want for their toxic, symptom-suppressing products, except that now the *taxpayers* help pay for grandma's drugs. The estimated cost of this law is $55 billion per year, but with no reason for Big Pharma to curtail their costs, it will undoubtedly end up being *much* more. When Congress figures out that they have grossly under funded the program, they will likely begin cutting other Medicare benefits—like chiropractic.

Why would a Republican Congress (which is supposedly "conservative" and against raising taxes and government hand-outs) pass such a bill? Well, part of this is surely Big Pharma's full court press. They have more lobbyists in Washington than there are members of Congress, and in 2002 they spent $91 million in lobbying alone.[23] But the bigger reason is that drug companies are major campaign contributors and have the politicians, especially the Republicans, in their pocket. (See box below.) As further evidence of this fact, Congress also passed a law that prevents Medicare from using its huge purchasing power to bargain with drug companies for lower prices as HMOs, the VA, and other insurance entities can do. There can be no explanation for this other than favoritism.

"PhRMA [the Pharmaceutical Research and Manufacturers of America], this lobby, has a death grip on Congress."

—Senator Richard J. Durbin (D-IL)

In 1999, *The New York Times* reported that Jim Nicholson, who was the chairman of the Republican National Committee at the time, wrote to Charles Heimbold, who was then the CEO of Bristol-Meyers Squibb. Nicholson said, "We must keep the lines of communication open if we want to continue passing legislation that will benefit your industry." Heimbold gave $200,000 worth of "communication" to the Republicans that year (a tiny fraction of his $75 million salary) and convinced others in his company to contribute a total of $2 million.[24] During that same election cycle, drug companies gave a total of $20 million in direct campaign contributions and $65 million in "soft" money. About 80 percent of this money went to Republicans; the rest went to some key Democrats.[25] These wide-open lines of communication got Big Pharma their Medicare legislation. Oh, and Heimbold is now the ambassador to Sweden.

Some people have discovered that the same drugs they were paying through the nose for in the U.S. were much cheaper in Canada or Mexico. Canadians, for example, pay about half to two thirds what we pay here for brand-name drugs.[26] Although they are the *exact* same drugs, often produced in the U.S. then shipped there, the FDA and the Department of Health and Human Services says that these "re-imported drugs" are not safe. Why aren't they safe? For the same reason they're not safe if you buy them here—they're toxic chemicals! But more to the point, because these filthy rich drug companies were upset over losing that *additional* profit, so they cried to their friends in the government who *declared* that they're not safe. There's no other reason than that.

But this brings up another interesting question: Why *are* drugs so much cheaper in other countries? The main reason is that we don't have any sort of cap on their profits as other developed countries do. The only other explanation I've heard is that we (the rich folks in the U.S.) need to help subsidize the cost of drugs in other less fortunate countries—like those poor Canucks up in Canada. But lest you worry about the poor, beleaguered drug companies dealing with unfair price caps, or admire them for their philanthropic ways, they're still making a killing in those other countries as well. They just like to *really* stick it to the people in the good ole' U.S. of A., mostly because our government allows them to.

> Oh, by the way, drug companies pay considerably less in taxes here too. Between 1993 and 1996 the average tax rate for major industries was 27.3 percent. Drug companies only paid 16.2 percent during that same time period—that's 40 percent less than the average.[27]

As you can see, drug companies have a *lot* of control—I would say, *way too much* control—over healthcare research in America, the entire medical field, the media, and our nation's politicians. But they also have major influence over the very government agency that's supposed to regulate them. And that is the subject of the next chapter.

4

Big Pharma & the FDA, An Unhealthy Alliance

"One of the first duties of the physician is to educate the masses not to take medicine."

—William Osler, the Father of Modern Medicine

The Pure Food and Drug Act was passed in 1906, partly in response to Upton Sinclair's novel *The Jungle*. The passage of this long-fought-for act brought into being the Bureau of Chemistry, which was later renamed the Food and Drug Administration (FDA). Dr. Harvey Wiley (1844–1930), a physician and chemist, was the father and architect of this law, and he became the Bureau's first director. While he remained at this post, he worked hard to protect and improve the nation's food supply. During his tenure, he published a series of articles entitled, "Influence of Food Preservatives and Artificial Colors On Digestion and Health" as well as two editions of a book called *Foods and Their Adulteration.* His vision was to eliminate all artificial and processed foods from the market including products containing caffeine, bleached flour, benzoic or sulfurous acid, and saccharin.

In his quest for a healthy food supply, however, Dr. Wiley stepped on too many toes, including those of Coca-Cola (whom he sued in an attempt to prevent the interstate transport of the famous caffeine-containing beverage). Wiley resigned his post in 1912 and went to work at the *Good Housekeeping* magazine where he established the Good Housekeeping Seal of Approval. He later wrote a memoir regarding his life at the Bureau of Chemistry and attempted to have it published. Oddly, his manuscripts kept "disappearing" and despite his high profile on a national level, no publishing house would accept his book. He finally self-published *The History of a Crime Against the Pure Food Law* in 1929. He died the following year and within a matter of weeks all of his books had disappeared from the nation's libraries and bookshops.

Dr. Wiley was replaced at the Bureau of Chemistry by Elmer M. Nelson, M.D., who was a "friend" to industry, and was once quoted as saying, "It is wholly unscientific to state that a well-fed body is more able to resist disease than a less well-fed body." [1] Not only does this statement defy all common sense, it actually defied what the science at that time was saying including the landmark studies performed by Weston A. Price, D.D.S. (who wrote the classic book *Nutrition and Physical Degeneration*), Francis Pottenger M.D. (author of the classic, *Pottenger's Cats: A Study in Nutrition*), and thousands of other references appearing in scientific journals throughout Europe and North America. However, he was able to make this statement "honestly" by simply *ignoring* that science. When one remains ignorant of the truth, one can honestly make false claims. Nelson set a precedent here that the FDA continues to follow to this day—that is, they work very hard at remaining ignorant of any science that does not benefit their benefactors, i.e. Big Pharma and the food industry.

The FDA has been a friend to the food and drug industries ever since Nelson took office. In fact, of late, they've become almost like their government partners, especially to the drug industry. Though they still have authority over the pharmaceutical industry, they rarely use it. They're more like a quality control department for Big Pharma than a government regulating agency. Only when they're *forced* into taking action will they go against their partners in crime and reluctantly do what they were created to do. For example, it has to be blatantly obvious that a drug is seriously harming or killing lots of people before they will even suggest that the company put a "black box" warning label on the drug information sheet. Oooh. Scary. A *black* box? Yes, a **black** box!

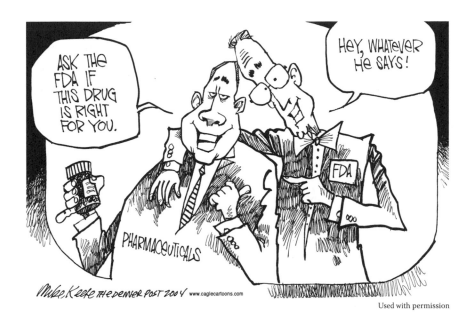

Used with permission

Though it hasn't always been this way, lately, in order for a drug to actually be pulled from the market after its release, several things must happen. First, it has to have killed hundreds or thousands of patients in well-documented, tragic cases. Second, there must be lawsuits against the company. And most importantly, the media has to get involved. It's not until the public starts to wonder how a drug like Vioxx could have possibly gotten through the FDA's "gauntlet" that the good people of the FDA finally get off their well-fed butts and do their job. Of course none of this will happen until the company has already made millions and millions of dollars selling the drug and has more than recouped the cost of developing it.

Basically, only when a drug becomes a liability to the manufacturer rather than a profit will it ever go away for good.

Since I brought it up, let's take a look at Vioxx, as it will serve as a nice example for this discussion. Vioxx is a pain reliever, plain and simple. It's kind of like aspirin, but way more expensive. But since aspirin and other NSAIDs (Non Steroidal Anti-Inflammatory Drugs) can cause GI irritation, which can lead to ulcers, internal bleeding, and death (see box below), Merck created Vioxx. Since Vioxx works differently, it doesn't cause gastric bleeding. Instead, *it causes heart attacks and strokes.*

Conservative estimates in the *New England Journal of Medicine* and the *American Journal of Medicine* state that at least 16,500 people in the U.S. die from gastric bleeding related to NSAID use every year.[2]

During its five years and four months on the market, this one drug caused an estimated 160,000 cases of heart attack and stroke in the U.S. alone.[3] Approximately 55,000 of those patients died. That's over 10,000 Americans *per year* dying just from this one drug.[4] Pretty bad, huh? But what makes this story really interesting is that the good people at Merck and at the FDA *knew* Vioxx would kill people even before it was released.

As you may know, drugs are not tested by the FDA. They're tested by the company that intends to *sell* the drug. The FDA just reviews their research and approves or disapproves. Sounds like an airtight system to *me*. I can't *imagine* any dangerous drugs getting through a system like *that*. Amazingly (and *brashly* I might add), Merck actually reported to the FDA that in clinical trials (that is, before the release of the drug), the low-dose version of Vioxx caused a seven-fold increase in heart attack and stroke. Merck did another test shortly thereafter and found that the *high-dose* version of Vioxx caused a five-fold increase in heart attack and stroke.[5] Sounds backward, I know, but whatever. The point is Vioxx increased the incidence of heart attack and stroke, *a lot.*

Vioxx was marketed as a safer pain reliever than NSAIDs, which meant that it would be used by millions of people around the world. About 30–40 percent of people having a heart attack or stroke die from it. So, if millions of people would be using Vioxx, if they knew that it significantly increased the risk of heart attack and stroke and that about 35 percent of those having a heart attack or stroke die from it, that meant they knew that Vioxx was bound to kill lots of people. Oddly, heart attacks and strokes weren't mentioned as potential side effects in Merck's television ads.

So, Merck and the FDA knew that a lot of people would end up dying from taking Vioxx. What did the FDA do about it—I mean besides approving the murderous drug in the first place? Well, first of all, they waited—for 18 months, presumably just to see if it really *did* kill people. Then, they very quietly added this damning bit of information to the drug's label so they could feign due diligence. But since nobody really reads those labels all the way through, and since they didn't even bother to put the warning in the "Warnings" section of the label, and since the FDA had implied that the drug was safe by approving it in the first place *and* allowed the relentless advertising of it (Merck spent $161 million advertising Vioxx in 2000 making it the most advertised drug in the world that year),[6] this impotent act had absolutely no effect on the drug's sales.

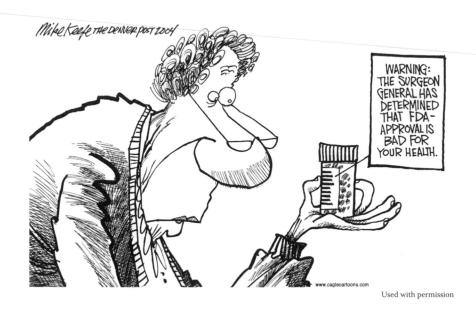

Used with permission

When it finally became *obvious* that the drug was killing people, the FDA's next great act was to deny it—simply pretend that it wasn't happening. After all, they are a responsible and mature organization. It wouldn't *do* for them to be making rash decisions based on just a few thousand cases or so. Likewise, when one whistle-blowing doctor within their ranks (quoted below) tried to actually present a case against Vioxx at an international drug conference, they felt it was their *duty* to put a stop to this and even to threaten him if he didn't change his tune.[7] Apparently, they felt they had already stepped on Merck's toes enough by including that whole heart attack and stroke thing on the label and they didn't want some rogue, whose only interest was the public's safety, pissing their friends off any *more*. So, the FDA never did *anything else* about Vioxx. In fact, they *defended* it right up until a few days before Merck pulled it from the market voluntarily.[8]

On November 18, 2004, David J. Graham, M.D., M.P.H., the Associate Director for Science and Medicine in the FDA's Office of Drug Safety testified before a special Congressional Committee regarding Vioxx. Here are some samples of his speech:

Today, in 2004, you, we, are faced with what may be the single greatest drug safety catastrophe in the history of this country or the history of the world. We are talking about a catastrophe that I strongly believe could have, should have been largely or completely avoided. But it wasn't, and over 100,000 Americans have paid dearly for this failure. In my opinion, the FDA has let the American people down, and sadly, betrayed a public trust... The problem you are confronting today is immense in scope. Vioxx is a terrible tragedy and a profound regulatory failure. I would argue that the FDA, as currently configured, is incapable of protecting America against another Vioxx. We are virtually defenseless. It is important that this Committee and the American people understand that what has happened with Vioxx is really a symptom of something far more dangerous to the safety of the American people. Simply put, FDA and its Center for Drug Evaluation and Research [CDER] are broken... The corporate culture within CDER is also a barrier to effectively protecting the American people from unnecessary harm due to prescription and OTC [over-the-counter] drugs. The culture is dominated by a world-view that believes only randomized clinical trials provide useful and actionable information and that postmarketing safety is an afterthought. This culture also over-values the benefits of the drugs it approves and seriously under-values, disregards, and disrespects drug safety. Finally, the scientific standards CDER applies to drug safety guarantee that unsafe and deadly drugs will remain on the U.S. market.[9]

And now, as if to throw salt on the wound, the FDA has now decided to allow Vioxx back on the market! It's not a new and improved, *safer* version of Vioxx. It's the same catastrophic drug that's killed 55,000 Americans, and by golly, it's back. Why, you ask? Well, since the drug is no more effective at killing pain than NSAIDs and clearly not very safe, the obvious answer is, the money. We'll come back to how exactly that works in just a bit.

Let's now compare the Vioxx story with the story of tryptophan. Tryptophan is a naturally occurring amino acid. In fact, it's considered one of the essential amino acids, which means you *must* get it in your diet if you want to be healthy. It's an important precursor for the neurotransmitter serotonin and the hormone melatonin. It's found in foods like poultry, milk, eggs, red meat, chocolate, and dates, and has a mild relaxing and anti-depressant effect. For years it was used safely as a dietary supplement. But in 1989, when 37 deaths were attributed to some impurities that were left in a bad batch of tryptophan produced by a Japanese manufacturer, the FDA stepped in. That sounds appropriate you say, and I would tend to agree with you; however, they didn't just make *that* company remove *its* tryptophan from the market until they had fixed the problem, or even ban that company from making tryptophan at all. No, they banned *all* tryptophan sales regardless of which company was producing it or how safe it actually was as a supplement. Now, why was *that*? Because Big Pharma and the FDA didn't want something you could get from turkey competing with billion dollar drugs like Prozac, which was about to be released, so tryptophan had to go. All of this, regardless of the fact that Prozac and other SSRI (selective serotonin re-uptake inhibitor) anti-depressant medications frequently cause sexual side-effects, are addictive, and sometimes cause suicidal or homicidal tendencies in teenagers. Turkey almost *never* does that, nor does uncontaminated tryptophan, which finally became available again in 2002.

Do you see the double standard? When a bad batch of Tylenol kills some people, they don't ban all sales of acetaminophen forever. They pull the batch and destroy it, and then Tylenol's back on the shelf in a week. This is a sane and reasonable way to deal with a contamination issue.

Here's another double standard. Ephedra has been used safely in the Orient for 5,000 years for conditions such as asthma, hay fever, and colds. (Note: Ephedra is not used for weight loss in traditional Chinese medicine.) There, they call it ma huang. Among other things, this herb has a stimulatory effect on the body. Knowledgeable herbalists are fully aware of this effect. They account for it, instruct their patients in the safe use of it, and have had no problems for millennia. Herbs, after all, are not supplements or food; they are plant-medicines and must be used with respect. (See box below.) So, when people in the United States started using (abusing?) ephedra to lose weight, and a few well-publicized deaths occurred (about 155 total deaths occurred due to ephedra) the FDA stepped in and banned the herb. It is now illegal to buy or sell ephedra in the United States. The FDA, the champions of public safety, so long as the issue doesn't concern one of their benefactors, has actually said that ephedra is not safe at *any* dose, despite its 5,000-year safety record in the Orient! Sudafed and its generics, pseudo-ephedrine, have essentially the same effects on the body as ephedra, but because *they're* produced by Big Pharma, these drugs are safe from the FDA's wrath. Oddly, if anything, pseudo-ephedrine is *less* safe than ephedra because the molecule is synthetic and the reverse (mirror image) of what nature intended.

It's my belief that herbs, especially powerful herbs like ephedra, *should* be regulated somehow. Again, herbs are not vitamins, nor are they health foods, which means they're not *necessarily* "good for you." Herbs are generally safer than prescription or over-the-counter medicines, but they *are* medicines. Just because they're natural, it does not mean they're as safe as vitamin C. So, yes, access to herbs should be somewhat restricted. The problem is how to *regulate* them without *over*-regulating them. Clearly, the FDA has a strong bias toward pharmaceuticals and I am loath to give them carte-blanche control over the herbs in this country.

The New Inquisition

As you can see, one of the FDA's primary roles now is to serve as *protector* of the drug companies. This means opposing or attacking the sale of anything that might compete with a drug and banning anything that might actually cure disease instead of just treating/managing it. Whenever they catch wind of some "unorthodox" treatment that might endanger one of their partners' drug sales, our friends at the FDA jump into action. They pull on their black jumpsuits, lock and load their .45's, and turn into Pharmafia. And then, they have themselves a little witch-hunt.

The FDA has taken over almost exactly where the Church of old left off. Of course, they don't burn practitioners at the stake anymore—at least not literally; they just burn their *files*, confiscate their computers and equipment, raid their homes, destroy their careers and lifetimes of research, devastate them financially, and throw them in jail. Of course, the media (the drug companies' propaganda puppets) is all too happy to report all of this.

On October 11, 2001, exactly one month after the attacks on the World Trade Center and Pentagon, as anthrax was contaminating Congressional office buildings, and the Bush Administration was gearing up for their war on terrorism, a battle was being waged in another, much older war—the war on quackery. One evening, close to midnight, as nutritionist Joe Di Stafano was leaving his office, he was surprised to find two men wearing rubber gloves digging through his dumpster. He walked up and demanded to know what they were doing. Obviously surprised to see someone at the clinic so late, they replied, "Looking for boxes." Di Stafano knew a liar when he saw one. He told the men to put down the trash and to get off his property. As they drove away Di Stafano wrote down their license plate number. It turned out, the men in his dumpster that night were FDA agents.

The FDA had received numerous complaints about Di Stafano and his group. It seems the rogues had been experimenting with an unapproved cancer treatment on humans. So, a week after the dumpster incident, on October 18th, 120 agents from the FDA, the DEA, Customs, U.S. Marshall's Service, Florida Department of Law Enforcement, and the Hillsborough County Sheriff's Office descended on the clinics of Joe Di Stafano and Dr. Daniel Mayer in Tampa and St. Petersburg, Florida.

Patients receiving treatments that day were shocked and horrified when this throng of agents barged in and took over the place. Some agents began unhooking patients from their IV drips. Others started boxing up the experimental anti-cancer extract. Still others were confiscating the clinic's computers or boxing up patient files and business records.

Across town, agents raided Di Stafano's *home* too, making belittling remarks to both him and his wife as they seized their personal property, including their children's computers.

Simultaneously, in Texas, the clinic of Dr. Ivan Danhoff was raided in a similar manner, as was the pharmacy of Jerry Jackson, who had been preparing the experimental extract being used in the three clinics.

The FDA filed criminal charges against all of those involved for selling a "dangerous, unapproved drug." What *was* this dangerous unapproved drug they were using? It's an intravenous form of aloe vera called Albarin, which Dr. Danhoff had been researching for over 20 years.

Who is this Dr. Danhoff? Well, he's no quack. Ivan Danhoff, M.D., Ph.D., has published more than 80 research papers. He wrote the book *Remarkable Aloe: Aloe Through the Ages*. He's served as a consultant to several pharmaceutical research institutes, and was even a consultant to the FDA for a time.

Dr. Danhoff and his colleagues were in the process of filing the massive amount of paperwork that the FDA requires to conduct a formal study on an experimental substance. They didn't advertise or promote their product. It's a natural product with little or no toxicity. They didn't promise miracles and they didn't charge an outlandish fee for their services. They charged only $1,200 for as many treatments as was needed in order to achieve a remission of the cancer or what could be considered a complete response. If someone could not afford the $1,200, the treatment was given for free. No one was turned away because of an inability to pay. In other words, they were doing everything right—though not necessarily legally. In fact, if they had been treating anything other than cancer, everything they were doing would have been completely legal as well. (As you'll read when we discuss cancer in a future *Why We're Sick*™ book, there's an asinine law in most states that declares *there are only three legal ways of treating cancer: surgery, radiation, and chemotherapy.*)

In the early studies, this non-toxic therapy prolonged survival time, shrunk tumors, reduced pain, increased energy, and patients with advanced cancer were actually achieving remission. They reported about an 80 percent success rate with their patients, which would be an excellent success rate for *any* disease, but for cancer, this is truly remarkable. Because of the results they were achieving, word spread throughout the cancer community that these doctors had something that was far better and *far* more comfortable than the traditional allopathic treatments.

So, how did they get caught performing these illegal treatments? One almost automatically assumes it was some displeased patient or family member of a patient who turned them in, but it wasn't. Not one patient ever complained to the authorities about this unlawful activity. In fact, during the raid on these clinics, one patient pronounced, "We're all adults here making free will choices. Why don't you get out of here and leave us alone?" There is a large faction of patients who are still fighting-mad at the FDA for taking their Albarin away. Many of these cancer patients feel as if the FDA has condemned them to die by taking away the treatment that was working for them and forcing them into the barbaric hands of allopathic medicine.

Who complained then? It was the *oncologists* in the area. Apparently, people so much preferred the IV aloe treatments to being cut upon, burned with radiation, or poisoned with chemotherapy that these cancer specialists were seeing a significant drop in their income. So, they got together and did what any self-respecting, five-year-old would do—they tattled. They called the FDA and complained that someone was infringing on their government-sanctioned monopoly on cancer treatments using an unapproved "drug." And the FDA, "America's Healthcare Police" is always happy to step in and destroy the life's work of a pioneer scientist in order to protect the interests of organized medicine.

Why didn't Danhoff and company just wait until they had FDA approval before starting the treatments if they knew it was illegal to do so without it? Di Stafano swears they were doing everything they possibly could to comply with the FDA's drug approval process. The problem is, the FDA holds all the cards in these situations and with their (unstated) mission of protecting the major drug companies from competition, an individual or a small company invariably finds themselves completely stonewalled in trying to get a drug approved. Oh, it *sounds* like a straightforward process that given the right drug and the proper determination one could get through, but unless you're part of Big Pharma, you would be sadly mistaken.

The FDA says in order to get drug approval you have to first do clinical testing. In order to get approval for the clinical testing, you have to go through the FDA as well. Thus, if the FDA should want to prevent the approval of a particular drug or treatment, for whatever reason, they can do so simply by indefinitely delaying or denying the approval for a clinical study. In cases like this, besides burying the researcher in a mountain of paperwork and continually moving the bar so that it's just out of reach, they are forever adding five more hoops for these researchers to jump through. And they just keep right on doing this until the researcher finally gets the big idea— that they're *never* going to get approval, no matter what they do or how much paperwork they fill out. Eventually, just like a hopeful puppy dog jumping for that ever-elusive biscuit, these pioneers just give up on receiving their coveted prize and mope away.

By stopping things at this early stage, the FDA can, and does, prevent these small groups from acquiring the proof they need in order to show that their experimental drug or treatment is safe and efficacious. This is closely related to the FDA remaining purposely ignorant of the current science as a means of lying about it. In this case, the FDA is going one step further by actually *preventing* the science from happening and then making believe that it's not wholly their doing. This flagrant abuse of power is far more common than you might think, as you'll see in future chapters.

If a group *should* attempt to conduct a study without the blessing of the FDA, as we've seen above, the group is raided, the study is brought to a halt, all of their records and computers are seized, and the doctors are brought up on charges or thrown in jail.

When these cases go to court, the efficacy of the drug is never even in question. The doctors involved are tried for using an "unapproved drug." It doesn't matter in the least if the drug was working or not working or how much better or safer it is than the competing drugs. That's simply not the question—and *that* question never comes up. And since the FDA *steals* all of the drug/extract/treatment in existence, along with all of the computers, research, patient files, etc., no one can build a case *against* the FDA. But lets say someone *did* decide to sue the FDA. They have their own internal court system, so no one can ever hope to win one of these cases either. This is the wall DiStafano and his group was up against. And they are not alone.

The FDA is supposed to be there to protect us from dangerous products, but if researchers are not even allowed to *research* natural products like Albarin, then how can they ever hope to prove that these products work? They say these alternative researchers have no proof their product works, while at the same time *they're* the ones preventing the researchers from proving it. It's not just a *difficult* road for the underdog here; the road is literally impassible. They end up being forced into either abandoning their research altogether, breaking the law, or leaving the country.

The story I've given above, unfortunately, is not unique. There are dozens of similar stories out there and we'll cover more of them when we discuss cancer in earnest. Natural healthcare providers are being raided and summarily put out of business whenever they step too heavily on the toes of organized medicine. This is not about trying to protect the American people from being scammed by charlatans or hurt by dangerous products. This is Mafioso business ethics. This is destroying the competition, and in America that's called "antitrust." There's a reason why monopolies and cartels are not supposed to be allowed to operate in this country. They're unfair to the small businesses. They prevent competition and, therefore, choice. They are, by nature, corrupt.

Our nation was founded on the principal that no one person or one group is allowed to have too much control, lest we find ourselves back in a monarchy or in a dictatorship. A division of power with an ingenious system of checks and balances was devised by our founding fathers to prevent such a takeover. We later developed antitrust laws to prevent similar problems in business. Whereas our Constitution was designed to prevent monarchies or dictatorships, antitrust laws were designed to prevent the formation of monopolies or cartels.

"Unless we put medical freedom into the Constitution, the time will come when medicine will organize into an undercover dictatorship... To restrict the art of healing to one class of men and deny equal privilege to others will constitute the Bastille of medical science. All such laws are un-American and despotic and have no place in a Republic... The Constitution of this Republic should make special privilege for medical freedom as well as religious freedom."

—Dr. Benjamin Rush, America's first Surgeon General and the only doctor to sign of the Declaration of Independence.

Unfortunately, our government, as well as the media, is intimately involved in this powerful cartel, so nothing is being done to stop it. The politicians are involved in several ways, but the most obvious is the hefty campaign contributions they receive from Big Pharma. Another less well-known factor is that politicians often receive advanced word on whether or not a drug is going to be approved by the FDA, and they use this insider information to make a killing on drug stocks. *Oddly, this is completely legal in our system.* The media is also involved in protecting this cartel because of all the advertising dollars spent in this country for pharmaceuticals. With the government and the media each benefiting so greatly from maintaining the status quo, there's really no one with authority left to complain to.

"Now, primarily a marketing machine to sell drugs of dubious benefit, this industry uses its wealth and power to co-opt every institution that might stand in its way, including the U.S. Congress, the Food and Drug Administration, academic medical centers, and the medical profession itself."

—Marcia Angell, M.D., former editor in chief of *The New England Journal of Medicine*[10]

Follow the Money

Perhaps you're still wondering, but how does the FDA benefit from protecting the drug companies? What's in it for them? Well, it's very simple really. The experts who recommend (essentially *decide*) which drugs get approved by the FDA make up what is called the Advisory Board. This Advisory Board is the only branch of government that is allowed to report "incomplete" financial statements. As Congressman Dan Burton said, this is a "violation of the public trust." [11] Why? What are they hiding with these incomplete financial statements? Well, it turns out that *70 percent of the Advisory Board members own stock in drug companies, own patents on drugs, or accept salaries and benefits as employees of the drug companies.*[12] Hmm. Could that be a conflict of interest?

USA Today ran a series back in 2000 that looked into this very topic. They found that *at least 54 percent of these Advisory Board members were being paid by the drug manufacturers.* To quote from the article, *"at 92 percent of the meetings at least one member had a financial conflict of interest...at 55 percent of meetings, half or more of the FDA advisers had conflicts of interest."* [13] [Emphasis added] Between 1998 and 2000, *USA Today* found more than 800 separate conflict of interest waivers issued to the various board members. What do they *do* with these waivers? Nothing. Or perhaps they *file* them in some locked cabinet somewhere, but really, nothing. It's as if they're saying, yes, we know there's a problem here, but we're not going to do anything about it. This is exactly why Vioxx is being allowed back on the market.

There also seems to be a revolving door between the big wigs at the FDA and the fat cats of the pharmaceutical industry. A typical example would go something like this: Someone at the FDA does a food or drug company a big favor (like getting some toxic new drug or food additive approved) and the next thing you know, that person resigns from the FDA and is made a "consultant" for that food or drug company with a million-dollar-a-year salary. This is how the toxic chemical sweetener aspartame, a.k.a. NutraSweet, finally got through the FDA approval process after years of continual denials. (We'll cover this story in a future *Why We're Sick*™ book.)

"The thing that bugs me is that people think the FDA is protecting them. It isn't. What the FDA is doing and what the people think it's doing are as different as night and day." [14]

—Dr. Herbert Ley, Former FDA Commissioner

In order to expedite the passage of new drugs, in 1992, Congress enacted the Prescription Drug User Fee Act. The "user fees" alluded to in the name were to be paid to the FDA by the drug companies. This allowed the expansion of the FDA without raising taxes, but it also turned the drug companies into the FDA's clients. The fees originally amounted to about $310,000 per new drug (it was raised to $576,000 in 2002), which is a paltry sum for a pharmaceutical company, but these fees soon amounted to about half the budget for the FDA's drug evaluation center. That makes the FDA dependent on the industry it supposedly regulates.

But what's more telling is, with the passage of this act, the FDA has gone from being the slowest regulatory drug agency in the industrialized world to being the fastest.[15] They're also slower to remove dangerous drugs. This is what David Graham meant when he said, the "FDA and its Center for Drug Evaluation and Research are broken." We just saw what they did regarding Vioxx. Rezulin is another recent example. Rezulin was a diabetes drug that was taken off the market in Britain in 1997 because it caused liver failure. But in the U.S., the FDA dragged its feet, waiting an additional two and a half years to pull Rezulin from the market. During that time, at least 63 more Americans died from the drug.[16] The FDA used to be slower to approve new drugs, which prevented catastrophes in the U.S., like Thalidomide. Since the passage of the Prescription Drug User Fee Act, a record 13 prescription drugs have had to be pulled from the market after causing thousands of unwarranted deaths. What this amounts to is the drug companies pay the FDA to approve their drugs faster so they can make billions more in profits, and we end up paying the ultimate price with dangerous drugs that kill people.

"...in the past few years the FDA's role has changed. Rather than regulating the drug industry to protect the health of consumers of prescription drugs, the administration has become the industry's partner, rapidly approving drugs for marketing even when medical experts on its own panels raise serious safety questions." [17]

—Dr. Laurence Landow, former Team Leader in the Anesthetic and Critical Care Drug Section for the FDA.

Are you starting to see the picture? You must understand, drug companies are only interested in one thing—profit. They're not *in* business to make people well (though they portray themselves as such). They're in business to make money. If people were well, they wouldn't *need drugs.* The companies' stock prices would fall; there would be massive lay-offs; and these millionaire CEOs would be out of jobs. No, drug companies are not in the healthcare business. They're in the business of selling drugs. In fact, let me go one step further. They're in the business of selling *chemicals for human consumption,* and they're very good at brainwashing people into believing they need them. They have thousands of well-paid, well-dressed, uneducated drug pushers (sales reps—the modern day version of snake oil salesmen), convincing well-educated, even better-paid drug pushers (M.D.s) to force their drugs on you. And sadly, the vast majority of the public is buying this scam. It's making them sick and they don't even realize it. It's like they can't see the forest for the drugs.

If we look at this objectively, we see that health is actually Big Pharma's enemy and that the whole benevolent scientist image is nothing but a dog and pony show. To quote Julian Whitaker, M.D., "Managing disease is a lucrative business. As long as people stay sick, they keep coming back for more." Can you see why these incredibly powerful companies would be so against people eating healthy organic food, having access to things like raw milk, vitamins, minerals, whole food concentrates, and herbs, seeing a chiropractor or acupuncturist, or indeed doing anything at all that might cut into their profits? Can you see why a cure for cancer, heart disease, diabetes, etc., would mean the loss of billions or perhaps *trillions* of dollars for them? Can you see why their version of preventive healthcare is to inject everyone on earth with some attenuated virus particles, toxic chemicals, and heavy metals every October rather than promoting a healthy lifestyle all year and possibly taking some echinacea or some zinc in the winter? Can you see why they would use everything at their disposal, including their friends in the government and the media, to prevent you from knowing all of this and to discredit anyone who tries to expose their scam? And, can you see how following this whole insane program would inevitably lead to more disease?

This is one of the biggest reasons why we're sick. Because we've allowed drug companies to convince us that putting toxic, foreign chemicals into our bodies will make us well instead of the exact opposite. The plain and simple truth is, while drugs may help you to cope with a difficult situation (pain, depression, high blood pressure), they *cannot* make you well, and in the long run, they will only make you sicker.

So What Do We Do?

Obviously, this is a huge problem and I don't intend on coming up with a comprehensive plan to solve it all right here, but I will make a few suggestions. First of all, don't expect the government to fix this without serious pressure from the populace. They're not interested in *fixing* this problem. At most, they're only interested in spreading the burden out in some form or another via a national healthcare system. How will this help the situation? It won't. Taking the responsibility for a person's health away from him rarely does him any good. Only when people take responsibility for their own health will they begin to be healthy. In any case, we certainly can't rely on the government to fix this voluntarily. As Bill Maher said:

"...the government isn't your nanny; they're your <u>dealer</u>, and they subsidize illness in America. They have to—there's too much money in it. You see, there's no money in healthy people; and there's no money in dead people. The money is in the middle—people with one or more chronic conditions that puts them in need of Celebrex or Nasonex or Valtrex or Lunesta... Someone has to stand up and say that the answer isn't another pill; the answer is spinach."

One of the best ways to put pressure on the government is through the media, so the media *has* to get more involved. The best way to get *that* to happen is to do as every other country (besides New Zealand) has done and ban the direct-to-consumer marketing of prescription drugs. With this ban in place, the media will no longer be so beholden to the drug companies and they will actually be free to report on the abuses of Big Pharma. They will also be freer to cover advances in *natural* methods of healthcare as well.

Next, the FDA needs a *major* overhaul. In fact, the FDA is
so screwed up, perhaps it would be easier to just start over from
scratch. But regardless of how it's done, somehow, the conflicts of
interest *must* be eliminated. There is literally no other way to make
the FDA work so that it is actually protecting the public rather than
the food and drug companies.

A survey reported in the January 2003 issue of the *Journal of
the American Medical Association* found that when a drug was
researched by the drug's company, the findings were four times
more likely to be favorable to the drug as when the research was
sponsored by the National Institutes of Health.[18] Logically, clinical
trials on drugs *should* be tested by an independent organization
that's not beholden to any drug company. This could be, as Dr.
Marcia Angell proposes in *The Truth About The Drug Companies*,
an Institute for Prescription Drug Trials. As she says, "It is crucial
that new drugs be shown to be safe and effective as judged by
an impartial agency responsible for the public health and not a
corporation responsible for the value of its shareholders' stock."[19]
This new Institute for Prescription Drug Trials could be part of
the NIH, but could be funded entirely by Big Pharma rather than
by taxpayers. Since these costs would, no doubt, be passed on to
consumers, the Institute would essentially be funded by a drug tax.
Thus, only the drug companies and those who consume their toxic
drugs would be paying for this branch of government. Of course,
the money would go into a general pool rather than going toward
any individual drug, and conflicts of interest (bribes) would have to
be strongly protected against in this organization as well.

New "Me Too" drugs should be compared with older drugs
for the same condition rather than just placebos. (Currently, drug
companies only need to prove that their drug works better than
a sugar pill.) As a reminder, this is important because very often,
newer drugs are merely a ploy to keep people buying expensive
drugs that are still under a patent, rather than older generic drugs,

which are often just as effective or even better. This change alone would cut our country's healthcare expenditures by millions of dollars per year.

There needs to be tighter regulation on what drug companies call "education" for doctors. Ten thousand dollars a year per doctor seems like an awful lot for these companies to be spending on doctor education to me, especially knowing that these costs are often frivolous gifts and are passed on to the consumer through higher drug prices. Going to hear a sales pitch for a new drug at a golf resort should not count toward a doctor's continuing education hours either.

The laws Big Pharma uses to extend their patents and tie things up in court need to be thoroughly reviewed and repealed in some cases. For example, testing drugs on children that are not meant to be used on children seems highly unethical. There is much to this topic that I did not go into in this book because of space and the technical nature of the laws, but these all need to be reviewed for the actual effectiveness of what they were meant to accomplish.

The government must stop protecting drug companies from lawsuits, as is the case with vaccinations. Without accountability to their customers, drug companies have no motivation to be sure their products are truly safe. The government feels compelled to protect Big Pharma in these cases because the government also feels compelled to force vaccinations on schoolchildren, whether the parents want them or not. This issue should be reviewed. At the very least, parents should be given the truth about the risks of vaccination and be made aware of the waivers that are available that allow unvaccinated children to attend public schools.

Drug companies should make the cost for drugs essentially the same for all countries. This would make the re-importation of drugs from Canada and Mexico a non-issue. But since they probably won't do this without major pressure, the U.S. should do like other industrialized countries and impose some sort of cap on drug prices.

Also, if Medicare is going to pay for drugs, they should be allowed to negotiate prices just like any other large insurance carrier.

A law that creates real campaign finance reform needs to be passed. This is the linchpin in getting all these other changes to occur. Until this happens, our legislators will likely just continue to do Big Pharma's bidding. We, the people of this great country, need to make *this issue* the one we are most concerned about during the next election and *every* election until it happens. (This is not only important for healthcare, but for *all* other aspects of our government.) If our current legislators can't or won't pass a good law, we should vote every one of them out and get a brand new Congress. If *they* don't pass the law, we vote them out, too. Eventually, they'll get the idea and we'll finally have the government we deserve instead of the plutocracy we currently have.

To help make this happen, I suggest sending your favorite legislator(s) a copy of this book along with a letter expressing your outrage, demanding that a bill be introduced that insists political campaigns be financed in some way other than by corporate interests. Tell them that your vote depends on it because the only thing politicians need more than campaign money is votes. By the way, if the two major parties don't have a candidate you like, vote for one of the minor party's candidates or write someone in. We *have* to stop choosing the lesser of the two evils if we ever want to have a decent Congress who will do *our* bidding instead of the corporations'. Remember that voting your conscience is not wasting a vote; voting for a semi-evil candidate is.

Finally, stop investing in companies that don't have your (or the earth's) best interests at heart. Pharmaceutical companies may give you a good return on your investment, but remember that when you give them your money, you're investing in the fleecing, brainwashing, and drugging of America. You are basically telling them, "Here's some more money, keep up the good work." There are plenty of good "green" mutual funds or other types of "socially responsible investments" out there that do not include chemical, drug, or oil companies in their portfolios. I have a short list of these "Green" mutual funds on my website www.HealthIsNatural.com. Invest in something that's actually *good* for the earth. Remember, anything we do that improves the environment, will invariably improve our health as a species.

And of course, as long as we're taking money away from Big Pharma, please do everything you can possibly do to get off of all drugs as soon as possible, and make sure everyone you know does the same. Have them read this book and make them understand that drugs are poisons and that they cannot not make you well; they can only make you sicker.

For More Information Read:

The Truth About the Drug Companies, How They Deceive Us and What To Do About It, by Marcia Angell, M.D., former Editor in Chief of *The New England Journal of Medicine.*

Selling Sickness, How the World's Biggest Pharmaceutical Companies Are Turning Us All Into Patients, by Ray Moynihan and Alan Cassels.

On The Take, How Medicine's Complicity with Big Business Can Endanger Your Health, by Jerome P. Kassirer, M.D., another former Editor in Chief of *The New England Journal of Medicine.*

5

Bad Medicine

"If all the medicine in the world were thrown in to the sea,
it would be bad for the fish and good for humanity."

—Oliver Wendell Holmes, M.D., Professor of Medicine, Harvard University

I n 1994, Dr. Lucian L. Leape published a study, which appeared in
the *Journal of the American Medical Association (JAMA)* called
"Error in Medicine."[1] In his research, Dr. Leape found all kinds
of startling statistics on the topic of iatrogenesis or doctor-caused
illness. In his paper, he reported that one researcher had discovered
that 20 percent of hospitalized patients suffered iatrogenic (doctor
caused) injury, and 20 percent of those died. Another researcher
found 36 percent of hospitalized patients suffered an iatrogenic
injury, and that 25 percent of *those* had died. For his own results,
however, Dr. Leape chose to use the much more conservative
estimate, published in 1991 by the Harvard Medical Practice Study,[2]
which found a 4 percent iatrogenic injury rate with a 14 percent
rate of death. Using these very conservative figures, he estimated
that 180,000 people are inadvertently killed by their doctors in U.S.
hospitals each year. (If instead of using the most conservative figures,
Dr. Leape had simply taken an average of the three studies, he would
have come up with the figure of 1,189,576 deaths per year.[3])

Dr. Leape admitted that the information on this topic was
sparse and that his figures represented only the tip of the iceberg.

However, even with these figures, he emphasized that the reported rates are "distressingly high."

Properly Prescribed Medicine

Since the study by Leape, many more studies on iatrogenesis have surfaced. For example, according to a study that appeared in the April 15, 1998 issue of *JAMA, adverse drug reactions to properly prescribed drugs, given in hospital settings, ranks as the fourth leading cause of death* in the U.S.! The authors of this study looked at records dating from 1965–1995 and determined that 2,216,000 *serious* adverse drug reactions (defined as those requiring hospitalization, those that were permanently disabling, or those causing death) occur yearly. Approximately 106,000 of these result in death. Thus, properly prescribed medications account for 4.6 percent of all recorded deaths.

According to the AMA's own flagship journal, here is the breakdown of the four most common causes of death in the U.S.:
1. Heart Disease
2. Cancer
3. Stroke
4. **Properly Prescribed Drugs (in hospitalized patients)** [4]

It's important to note that the *JAMA* study only counted drug reactions from medication that was prescribed in a hospital setting. It did not include those prescribed in an outpatient setting nor those prescribed in nursing homes.

Hospital Induced Infections

Two other studies have focused on "nosocomial infections" or infections people contract while in the hospital. One study found that approximately 5–6 percent of those admitted to a hospital will acquire an infection, resulting in 88,000 deaths per year (that's one person every six minutes).[5] Another study found two million people per year get infections while in the hospital and 100,000 of those patients die because of them.[6] If you combined these nosocomial infections with the *JAMA* study above, you could easily place hospitals as the third leading cause of death in the U.S., well ahead of strokes. But hold on. We're not done with hospitals *yet*.

Medical Negligence/Malpractice

According to a 1993 report by the Harvard Medical Practice Study Group, 80,000 people die every year—that's one person every 7 minutes, and 150,000–300,000 more are injured annually from medical *negligence* in hospitals.[7] According to an article in the February 10, 1992 issue of the *Chicago Sun Times*[8] 155,000 people die as a result of medical malpractice, making it the number one cause of all accidental deaths in the U.S.

Hospital Caused Deaths

Adding the more conservative number of 80,000 deaths caused by negligence to our tally, we see now that doctors kill approximately 286,000 people in hospitals each year. This number corresponds almost exactly with another study, which appeared in July 1995 in *JAMA*. This study reported, *"Over a million patients are injured in U.S. hospitals each year, and approximately 280,000 die annually as a result of these injuries. Therefore, the iatrogenic death rate dwarfs the annual automobile accident mortality rate of 45,000 and accounts for more deaths than all other accidents <u>combined</u>."* [9] [Emphasis added]

Outpatient Medications

Another study looked at the risk of dying from taking *all* prescription drugs, not just those given in the hospital. This study found that 125,000 people die every year from taking properly prescribed prescription medications in the correct dose. This similar, but larger number helps to add credence to the above *JAMA* study, which only looked at hospital drugs. These studies are also supported by one found in the *American Journal of Medicine*, which reported in 2000 that they had found an estimated 350,000 adverse drug reactions in U.S. nursing homes each year.[10] If these studies are correct, that means about 19,000 people die every year from properly prescribed outpatient and nursing home drugs. Add this to our figure above and we have 305,000 people killed by M.D.s per year.

Total Iatrogenic Deaths

The above number corresponds with other studies that have shown medical doctors cause the death of approximately 300,000 people per year. A study done by the Institute of Medicine, estimated that doctors kill 230,000–280,000 people per year.[11] Others have come up with similar figures. This number of around 300,000 iatrogenic deaths is so often quoted that it has basically become the "accepted" number of medical-caused deaths per year.

Before we go on, do you realize how huge these numbers are? Your doctors and hospitals, in all their infinite wisdom, using "scientific" medicine, are killing at least 300,000 people each and every year! That's 25,000 preventable deaths per month or 822 people per day! This is the equivalent of crashing 750 jumbo jets full of people into the ground per year (at 400 people each), or if you prefer, 62.5 jetliners per month, and continuing to do so—forever. Understand, these are not people who just died while they were in a hospital or under a physician's care. These are people who *weren't supposed to die*. These are people who were actually *killed* by their doctors or the drugs their doctors prescribed. But wait, there's more....

Medication Errors

Medication "errors" are the accidents like illegible prescriptions leading to the wrong drug, the doctor prescribing the wrong dose, poor labeling, etc.

A 2002 study appearing in the journal *Pharmacotherapy* surveyed the national pharmacy database and found that medication errors occurred in 5.22 percent of hospitalized patients. The authors concluded from this study that at least 90,895 patients are injured because of medication errors each year.[12] Another study, found in the September 9, 2002 issue of *Archives of Internal Medicine,* found that 20 percent of hospital prescriptions had dosage errors, and that almost 40 percent of those errors were considered potentially harmful.[13] In June of 2003, another study in *Archives of Internal Medicine* reported that pharmacists had intercepted errors on 24 percent of doctors' prescriptions, making the number of patients potentially harmed by their medications as high as 417,908.[14]

Two separate studies, one appearing in *The Lancet*[15] (one of the most prestigious medical journals in the world), and another performed by the Institute of Medicine, a branch of the National Academies of Science,[16] determined that drug errors *kill* 7,000 people per year. Add *these* deaths to our tally and we have 312,000 deaths per year caused by medical doctors.

There are 0–2 deaths per year that are blamed on a massive herb *overdose*. There are probably *no* deaths caused by taking the *proper* dose of any vitamin, mineral, or herb.

Surgical Errors

Surgical errors include: post-operative infections, foreign objects left in wounds, surgical wounds reopening, and post-operative bleeding.

Another study, which was conducted by the U.S. government's Agency for Healthcare Research and Quality, and appeared in the October 2003 issue of *JAMA*,[17] documented 32,000 (mostly) surgical-related deaths. These errors cost an estimated $9 billion and accounted for 2.4 million extra hospital days. As bad as this sounds though, the authors stated in a press release, "The[se] findings greatly underestimate the problem, since many other complications happen that are not listed in hospital administrative data."[18]

Unnecessary Surgery

Surgery, like medicine, can be lifesaving, but each year tens of thousands die and many more are injured as a result of *unnecessary* surgeries. According to Dr. Leape and a U.S. Congressional House Subcommittee Oversight Investigation, in 1974, 2.4 million unnecessary surgeries were performed resulting in 11,900 deaths. This was at a cost of $3.9 billion.[19] In 2001, that number reached 7.5 million unnecessary surgeries, which resulted in 37,136 deaths. This cost $122 billion using 1974 dollars.[20] Another source reports that as many as 50,000 people die each year due to 2.4 million unnecessary surgeries.[21] The large discrepancy in these numbers may be, in part, due to the subjectivity of the term "unnecessary." However, if we take an average of the three studies, we come up with 33,000 deaths per year caused by unnecessary surgeries.

What *are* unnecessary surgeries? Certainly anything that is elective, such as breast enhancement, isn't necessary. Gastrectomy, the so-called stomach stapling surgery for obesity isn't necessary. Many, if not most hysterectomies aren't necessary either. Also approximately 30 percent of cesarean sections, tonsillectomies, and appendectomies aren't necessary.[22] A 1987 *JAMA* study found inappropriate use of the following surgeries: coronary angiography 17 percent; carotid endarterectomy 32 percent; and upper gastrointestinal tract endoscopy 17 percent.[23] As a chiropractor, I can say that most back surgeries aren't necessary either. In December 1994, a large government study done by the Agency for Health Care Policy and Research confirmed this, stating, "Surgery has been found to be helpful in only 1 in 100 cases of low back problems. In some people, surgery can even cause more problems." [24]

According to Julian Whitaker, M.D., 90 percent of angiograms are unnecessary. He states that this alone accounts for 4,500 deaths per year. According to Dr. Whitaker, the angiogram is considered one of the most inaccurate tests in modern medicine. He also reports that two to four percent of angio*plasty* patients die either during the procedure, or within one year. Finally, he says that about five percent of bypass surgery patients die as a result of their surgery, leading to a whopping 14,000–28,000 deaths per year.[25]

Unnecessary Radiation

Dr. John Gofman has studied the effects of radiation on human health for 45 years and has written five well-documented books on the subject. He is a medical doctor with a Ph.D., in nuclear and physical chemistry. He worked on the Manhattan Project; he *discovered* uranium-233 and was the first person to isolate plutonium. In other words, he knows a little bit about radiation. Dr. Gofman's research shows that *X-rays, CT scans, mammography, and fluoroscopy devices are a contributing factor to 75 percent of all new cancers.* In a 700-page report, he shows that the more physicians there are in an area, along with the corresponding increase in the number of radiation-based tests, the higher the rate of cancer and ischemic heart disease in that area.[26] He also states in his book,

Preventing Breast Cancer: The Story of a Major, Proven, Preventable Cause of This Disease that breast tissue is highly sensitive to radiation; therefore, mammograms can actually *cause* cancer.[27]

Angiograms, which we've already mentioned as inaccurate and unnecessary, utilize X-ray almost continuously throughout the procedure. The minimum dosages of ionizing radiation during angiography range from 460–1,580 mrem. As a comparison, the minimum radiation for a routine chest X-ray is only 2 mrem.[28] Similarly, a CT scan exposes patients to 100–250 *times* the radiation of a normal chest X-ray. What's even more frightening is that according to a survey performed at the Yale School of Medicine, most doctors didn't know that the level of radiation for a CT was even close to that high.[29]

Ionizing radiation has a cumulative effect and procedures using radiation have been shown to cause gene mutation. Unfortunately, they are also becoming "routine," such as the "routine mammogram." Doctors are becoming too cavalier about how often they order these harmful tests. Dr. Gofman predicts that ionizing radiation will be responsible for 100 million premature deaths over the next decade. (That's 10 million deaths a year!)

To review, here's the breakdown of annual, doctor-caused (iatrogenic) deaths so far along with some rather credible sources:

	Deaths	Sources
Properly prescribed drugs (hospital)	106,000	*JAMA*
Drug errors	7,000	*Lancet* & IOM
Surgical errors	32,000	*JAMA*
Unnecessary surgery	11,900	U.S. Congress
Hospital infections	100,000	*Emerg. Inf. Dis.*
Negligence (hospitals)	80,000	Harvard
Hospitals (overall) '94	180,000	*JAMA*
Hospitals (overall) '95	280,000	*JAMA*
Iatrogenesis overall	280,000	IOM

As you can see, it's not all that easy to just add these numbers together and come up with a total. Some of these numbers obviously overlap with one another. To make matters worse, each branch of medicine keeps its own records on iatrogenesis. This makes putting the pieces together a daunting task. However, one group of researchers decided to do just that. The group included: Gary Null, Ph.D., Carolyn Dean, M.D., N.D., Martin Feldman, M.D., Debora Rasio, M.D., and Dorothy Smith, Ph.D. They wrote a paper called "Death by Medicine," [30] which appeared in the March 2004 issue of *Life Extension* on the web. The paper includes more than 150 references and an extensive appendix. These researchers analyzed and combined the complete published literature regarding injuries and deaths attributable to medicine. They looked at thousands of studies, put together the pieces, and came up with some rather disturbing numbers.

The study found that, "The total number of deaths caused by conventional medicine is an astounding 783,936 per year." That's the equivalent of 5 ½ completely full 747s falling out of the sky each and every day! (Can you imagine putting your life in the hands of an *airline* with that kind of record?) They went on to say, "It is evident that the American medical system is the leading cause of death and injury in the U.S. By comparison, approximately 699,697 Americans died of heart [disease] in 2001, while 553,251 died of cancer." They projected that the costs associated with deaths caused by medical interventions total approximately $282 billion per year. They also estimate that the costs for unnecessary hospitalization and medical procedures total $122 billion per year. They report, "The number of unnecessary medical and surgical procedures performed annually is 7.5 million. The number of people exposed to unnecessary hospitalization annually is 8.9 million." Every American truly concerned about his/her health and the healthcare crisis we're entrenched in should read this important study.

Burying the Evidence

What makes all of these numbers even more frightening is that according to numerous reports and several sources (among them *JAMA*), only about 5 percent of iatrogenic acts are ever reported.[31] The truth is, doctors very rarely report any iatrogenic injuries as such because they are afraid of being sued.[32] In fact, the AMA strongly opposes the mandatory reporting of medical errors.[33] So, who *is* reporting these medical errors? Usually, it's the patient or the patient's surviving family. If these people haven't reported it, it's probably not included in the statistics given above. As my father has said, M.D.s *bury* their mistakes—*literally.*

Jerry Phillips, associate director of the FDA's Office of Post Marketing Drug Risk Assessment has said, "In the broader area of adverse drug reaction data, the 250,000 reports received annually probably represent only 5 percent of the actual reactions that occur." [34] Dr. Jay Cohen has researched this topic thoroughly, and in his book *Overdose: The Case Against the Drug Companies* he confirms that only about 5 percent of adverse drug reactions are reported and therefore estimates that there are in fact about 5 million medication reactions each year.[35] Another study which appeared in *JAMA* said that if hospitals admitted to the actual number of errors that they are responsible for, which is about 20 times what is reported (i.e., only 5 percent *are* reported), they would come under intense scrutiny. [36]

Are you getting all of this? *JAMA* admitted that doctors are killing around 280,000 people per year and they also admitted that the reported amount of iatrogenic injuries probably only represents about 5 percent of the total problem. If we put those numbers together, that would mean they're killing around six million people per year! (Remember, these numbers came from them. I'm just putting them together for you since you probably don't read *JAMA* in your spare time.) But since the CDC reports that only 2.4 million people died in the U.S. in 2007 from *all* causes, this number cannot be correct. Let's say we give them the benefit of the doubt and say that 280,000 deaths actually represented *15* percent of the actual problem. That would mean there were 1.87 million deaths caused by medicine. This number may be a little high as well, but at least it starts to put Gary Null's estimate of 783,936 deaths into perspective. What are the *real* numbers? At this point, it's anybody's guess since we're using estimation and extrapolation as our constant backdrop, but everyone who's ever studied this problem agrees that medicine is killing far too many of its patients.

Please remember this chapter if/when you hear a medical doctor saying that chiropractic adjustments are dangerous. Ask them for studies in refereed medical journals like *JAMA* showing how many people we kill. They admit to killing more people in a single minute than chiropractors can be blamed for over the course of our entire history since 1895.

Personally, I'm quite sure allopathic medicine is killing far more than *anyone* is admitting to. In addition to all the causes listed above, many people die as a result of their surgeries and medications in less obvious ways. Take, for example, seemingly benign medications such as antacids. By raising the pH of the stomach, antacids prevent the digestion/absorption of protein and calcium, two essential nutrients. Without these nutrients, over time disease *will* happen, and some of these diseases could be fatal. Are these deaths being counted? I sincerely doubt it.

How about the person who has his/her gall bladder removed? If they survive the surgery, it's not counted as an iatrogenic death, but this usually unnecessary surgery is surely the cause of many deaths.

Without a gall bladder, a person has a very difficult time digesting and absorbing fats including fat-soluble vitamins, such as A, E, and D and essential fatty acids like fish oils, which protect the heart. Without these essential fatty acids and fat-soluble vitamins, diseases *will* ensue and many of these diseases could prove to be fatal. Again, are *these* deaths being counted?

In fact, virtually all medications and surgeries (and radiation) interfere with the normal physiology of the body, and, therefore, lead to "dis-ease." In other words, virtually everything that medical doctors can do for you makes you sicker over time, leading you closer and closer to death.

While we're at it, what about all the people the medical system is preventing from getting alternative treatments for cancer? Most cancers can be cured if they are detected early enough and treated properly instead of using the three approved treatments of surgery (which often *spreads* the cancer), radiation (which *causes* cancer), or chemotherapy (which destroys the immune system's ability to *fight* cancer). But medical doctors, along with the AMA and the FDA, are preventing this from happening.

I could literally go on and on, listing injuries and deaths from dozens of individual FDA-approved medications (i.e., Vioxx, Bextra, Celebrex, Rezulin, Premarin) but I think by now you've got the point. Allopathic medicine is dangerous.

The only thing that will turn the tide on this slaughter of innocent lives is for people to learn how to say, "No!" Pharmaceutical companies are not going to read this book and suddenly change their ways, nor are most medical doctors. They're not going to stop producing or prescribing these poisons. Surgeons are not going to stop cutting. CT and mammography centers are not going to suddenly shut down and stop radiating people. It has to start with you. *You* have to take responsibility for your health. When faced with a new diagnosis and offered a prescription for some toxic drug, just say, "No thank you, doctor," and seek out an alternative. If that's too confrontational for you, take the prescription from him/her, but don't fill it. Once you're out of the office, just crumple it up and throw it away. If *this* is too scary for you (or if your condition is life threatening), then go ahead and fill the prescription keeping in mind that it's a toxic drug and will lead to new disease if taken for long, *and* seek out a natural healthcare practitioner who can *co-treat* you. In this way, you'll be dealing with the symptoms *and* the underlying problem at the same time. Whatever you choose to do with your own health, we *must,* as a population, become less reliant on drugs and other medical care. This is *critical*, not just for you, but for our future generations.

In over 10 years of fighting in Vietnam, with camouflaged soldiers shooting bullets, lobbing mortars, throwing grenades, dropping bombs, with all the napalm, Agent Orange, booby traps, and land mines, we lost a total of 58,000 U.S. soldiers. That's less than 6,000 per year on average. (Medication errors alone kill more than that.) People protested in the streets of our nation's capital and all over on college campuses in opposition to all this senseless killing—and rightly so, I believe. But where are the protesters in *this* cause? Why are we not protesting in front of our local hospitals or outside the AMA headquarters at 515 N. State Street in Chicago? Why aren't there protesters carrying signs outside of every pharmaceutical research facility? Why do we continue to make excuses for a profession that kills more people than any other cause in the United States?

I've written this book because my purpose in life is to help improve the state of our health in this world. I want everyone to have the opportunity to experience the vibrant health that I've experienced by living without drugs. If that's ever going to happen, we simply *must* stop using pharmaceuticals except in dire emergencies. The same goes for surgery and radiation.

There are safe and effective alternatives to drugs and surgery, but for this lifestyle to really work for you, you must learn a new paradigm. You cannot wait until you're deathly ill to see a doctor. Prevention and maintenance must become a way of life for you. You must do things that promote health on a regular basis, not just wait until sickness overtakes your body. Natural methods take time to work. Your body doesn't get sick overnight and it won't heal overnight.

Another thing to keep in mind is that symptoms are a sure sign that you're sick, but the absence of symptoms doesn't necessarily mean you're healthy. Don't assume that just because you *feel* fine, that you *are* fine. Many people *feel* fine just seconds before they drop dead of a heart attack or have a stroke. Many people *feel* fine when they're diagnosed with cancer. Be *pro*active, not *re*active.

As I've no doubt drilled into your head by now, drugs *suppress* symptoms. Since symptoms are a sure sign of underlying sickness, if you're taking *any* medication, you *are* sick. The drug is not making you well; it is only making you *feel* well on the surface, while at the same time it's actually making you sicker underneath.

I suggest that we use drugs, surgery, and radiation only when they are *absolutely* called for. If we did just this, hundreds of thousands, if not millions of lives would be saved, millions of serious adverse reactions would be prevented; and millions, if not billions of dollars would not be wasted every year.

Now, imagine what might happen if we took that $122 billion that we spend on unnecessary medical procedures every year, and instead spent it on preventative, natural, holistic healthcare. With no extra money being spent, suddenly, the world would be so much healthier and happier you wouldn't believe it. Each year, people would need fewer and fewer medications and surgeries, which would free up that much more money for other preventative measures, which would circle around again. Pretty soon, the whole country would be riding this wave of health and abounding energy.

Think it can't happen? It *can* happen. All it takes is for you to stop *thinking* that it's impossible. Change *yourself* and become an inspiration to others! Decide that from now on, you will only take the medications that you absolutely *have* to have, and do whatever you have to do to get off of those as soon as possible. Then, make sure that everyone you care about follows this "rule," too. Show them the facts in this chapter if they won't listen to you. *Make* them understand. Their health depends on it.

For More Information Read:

"Death by Medicine," by Gary Null, et al. *Life Extension*
     www.lef.org/magazine/mag2004/mar2004_awsi_death_01.html.

PART II

Germs & Worms:
Paranoia May Destroy Ya

"At the heart of science lies discovery which involves a change in worldview. Discovery in science is possible only in societies which accord their citizens the freedom to pursue the truth where it may lead and which therefore have respect for different paths to that truth."

—John Polanyi, Nobel Laureate in Chemistry

6

A New Germ Theory

"Disease is born of us and in us."

—Antoine Béchamp, M.D.

As we discussed back in Chapter 1, in the days before the Renaissance and the advent of modern science, diseases were blamed on all sorts of ill-defined sources. Anything from bad humors to a punishment from God could have received the blame for a person's infirmity. Then along came a fellow named Louis Pasteur.

Now Louis Pasteur was not a doctor of any sort and not really much of a scientist either as it turns out, but he *is* given credit for what is now known as The Germ Theory of Disease. He was *not* the original discoverer of bacteria or germs, though he often receives credit for it, nor was he the first to hypothesize their involvement in human disease. In reality, Louis Pasteur *should* have gone down in history as "Louis the Impostor" because he stole most of his important "discoveries" from smarter colleagues of his and then claimed them as his own. Not only that, but it's obvious from Pasteur's writings that he often didn't even understand the science behind what he was reporting. In 1995, on the centennial of his death, the *New York Times* ran an article entitled, "Pasteur's Deceptions" which described how he had given a misleading account of his experiments on the anthrax vaccine. In this case, Louis lied about the method he used to weaken the anthrax in his vaccine, claiming he had discovered a new way, while in reality he had merely used a rival's method. (See box below.) He was also known to falsify data to make it fit his needs. For example, he lied about the success of his animal studies on the rabies vaccine, which allowed him to experiment on a human boy. In short, Louis Pasteur was nothing short of a fraudulent, plagiarizing scumbag. But because of his aggressive personality and incredible knack for self-promotion (his two biggest attributes, or character flaws, depending on how you look at it), he turned out to be a much better PR man than his rivals. A charlatan and a salesman who took credit where it was not due, Pasteur rose to the top of his field riding on the backs of other people's discoveries. But despite all this, or rather *because* of it, Pasteur became the champion of the germ theory cause.

Many of Pasteur's deceptions are revealed in his handwritten laboratory notebooks, which are now on display in Paris. In his will, Pasteur ordered that these notebooks be kept from outsiders, but when his grandson died, he left them to the Bibliotheque Nationale, where they are now available to scholars. Dr. Gerald L. Geison, a medical historian from Princeton University spent 15 years of his life reading these and writing the book, *The Private Science of Louis Pasteur* which was released in 1995. In it, he details many accounts of what would today be considered scientific fraud.

The Germ Theory

The germ theory basically says this: We get sick because microscopic germs enter our bodies from the air or the bodily fluids of other sick people and cause disease. Furthermore, certain germs cause certain diseases. Streptococcal bacteria cause strep throat; staphylococcal bacteria cause staph infections; influenza viruses cause the flu, etc. These germs take on one form and remain in that form throughout their lives. In other words, a bacterium does not change from being round one day to rod shaped the next. Also, bacteria, viruses, and fungi are all completely different types of organisms.

Another original assumption of the germ theory was that a healthy human body is completely sterile, i.e. it contains no germs. Even Western medicine now accepts that this part of the germ theory is completely false. We now know that just as healthy soil requires lots and lots of microorganisms, the human body also requires lots of microorganisms, which we call "normal flora," to be healthy. These include the beneficial bacteria, such as acidophilus, as well as some good probiotic yeasts. In fact, far from being sterile, a healthy human body actually has about ten times more bacteria than it has cells (there should be around 100 trillion bacteria, or about three pounds worth, just in your guts)[1] and these germs make up a significant portion of a strong, healthy immune system.

We all *assume* the germ theory is true, don't we? After all, it is seemingly confirmed whenever we get sick after being around someone else who was sick. Then we go to the doctor for an antibiotic and are miraculously cured. It's further "confirmed" when a doctor takes a throat culture and finds streptococcal bacteria on our swollen, inflamed tonsils.

The germ theory is so widely accepted that it's rarely even called a theory anymore and is more or less accepted as fact. However, just because you've heard something over and over again, even if it makes sense on the surface, doesn't necessarily mean it's true. And whenever a theory has holes in it that cannot be explained, the theory is either incomplete, or it's just plain wrong. And the germ theory has gaping holes in it.

But there *is* another theory having to do with germs and disease, and *this* theory doesn't leave any unanswered questions. It will also change how you think about germs forever.

A Revelation in Fermentation

Like any good story, this one has a hero and a nemesis. Louis the Impostor's counterpart was a man by the name of Antoine Béchamp. Béchamp (1816–1908, *that's 91 years old!*) was a medical doctor, a doctor of science in chemistry, a master of pharmacy, and a university professor of physics, toxicology, medical chemistry, and biochemistry. He was also the author of several medical textbooks on blood and disease. In short, he was not only a genius, he was a very well respected scientist. Pasteur, by comparison, was a simpleton. But since Béchamp's only passion was science, and Pasteur's main motivation was improving his status in life, it is Pasteur's name we all know today.

Today, the idea of germs is known even to kindergarteners, but in the mid-1800s the idea of living creatures so small that they cannot be seen with the naked eye was a foreign one. Indeed, the notion received a fair amount of ridicule from non-believers—as do all major discoveries at first. The discovery of germs was also more of a slow realization than a sudden, "aha!" and it actually had nothing at all to do with the study of disease, but with something much more important—the production of beer and wine.

For thousands of years, people all over the world had used fermentation to their benefit, but no one really knew how or why it worked. People also wondered about why meat putrefied and why the dead decomposed. What invisible forces caused these processes to occur? Were they related? These questions led to deeper questions having to do with the origins of life, and "spirited" debates ensued (pun *fully* intended).

Scientists found themselves divided into two distinct groups around this argument. One side believed that complex life forms could arise spontaneously from decaying organic matter. This theory was known as "spontaneous generation." For example, these people believed that mice spontaneously appeared in stored grain or that maggots just grew out of meat that had been left out. For decades, spontaneous generation was the prevailing theory in the world. In fact, even Aristotle, philosopher and teacher of science and logic, was a believer in spontaneous generation. He believed that aphids arose out of the dew that fell on plants; that crocodiles grew out of logs at the bottom of lakes; that mice came from dirty hay, and that fleas came from putrid matter.[2] The other side of the argument (which can be termed *omne vivum ex ovo*, or "everything from an egg") firmly believed that life could only come from other life.

Much like the battle between Creationists and Evolutionists today, this battle raged on for generations with a religious fervor. In his early career, like most scientists of his day, Pasteur was an enthusiastic advocate of spontaneous generation, and performed many poorly designed experiments that supposedly "proved it."

Antoine Béchamp on the other hand, was not one to accept things based on conjecture. Being a pure scientist, he set out to discover what mysterious force was behind the process of fermentation and set up rigid experiments with no presuppositions in mind. After performing a series of these, he discovered that he could prevent fermentation simply by preventing the concoction from making contact with the air. This led him to formulate the theory that it must be tiny organisms (germs) in the air that were eating the sugars, and through the process of metabolizing it and excreting of their waste, converting it into alcohol. This was the first accurate and complete description of fermentation, but what was more, it was also a serious blow to the die-hard believers in spontaneous generation—including Mr. Pasteur.

Béchamp reported his findings to the Academy of Science, but the idea was just so preposterous that very few believed it. Spontaneous generation, after all, was the prevailing theory at the time.

Perhaps Pasteur was jealous of Béchamp's genius. Perhaps he couldn't stand to be proven wrong. Whatever the cause or motivation, a bitter rivalry soon began between the two men. To Pasteur's credit, he *was* smart enough to recognize genius when he saw it; but he was also just ruthless enough to exploit it. He realized at that point that he was on the wrong side of the spontaneous generation argument, so he took Béchamp's new theory and attempted to reproduce his experiments. Being a rather bumbling scientist, he didn't do it correctly, but he *was* able to come up with something that looked reasonably close to what Béchamp had done. He then published his results and claimed he had figured it out first, even though he obviously didn't fully understand Béchamp's findings.

Suddenly the world knew that sugar did not spontaneously ferment—that living creatures were needed for the process to work and Louis Pasteur had given them the answer. In one fell swoop, Pasteur claimed credit for figuring out how fermentation worked, the discovery of germs, and dispelling the myth of spontaneous generation, and in the process, he made himself out to be the savior. Soon, he was famous. He was respected by the world—scientists, businessmen, authors, noblemen, French royalty. He was even dining with the Emperor on occasion. Meanwhile, Béchamp had simply moved on to his next set of experiments.

"More secrets of knowledge have been discovered by plain and neglected men than by men of popular fame. And this is so with good reason. For the men of popular fame are busy on popular matters."

—Roger Bacon, English theologian, philosopher, and Franciscan Friar

Pasteur's fame led to his receipt of several assignments from France's Emperor at the time, Napoleon III. He was charged with figuring out what the problem was with France's wine crop, and also the problem with its silk worms. On both of these occasions, Béchamp donated some of his time to the problems facing his country and quickly figured out not only the problem, but how to fix it. He reported his answers to the Academy of Sciences, but no one would listen to him. Years would go by, but always the world seemed deaf to the cries of Antoine Béchamp. "No, no," they'd say. "Our man Louis is on the case and we will not accept anyone's word but his."

Finally though, Pasteur would succumb to pressure. Having been unable to figure out the problem on his own, he would find out what Béchamp had said, quickly throw together some experiments to give the illusion that he was on the right track, and then report Béchamp's discovery as his own. "Hooray," the world would say. "Pasteur has done it again!"

Pleomorphism: The "Other" Germ Theory

Though he was not a doctor, Pasteur was eventually called to look at the cause of human disease. Meanwhile, Béchamp's discovery of germs had led him to do the same. Pasteur, by now completely obsessed with the idea of germs in the air, set out to prove that they were the cause of human disease.

"The greatest derangement of the mind is to believe things because one wishes them to be so."

—Louis Pasteur, Academy of Sciences, 1875

Béchamp came at the issue of disease from a completely different angle than Pasteur. Around 1870, using a powerful microscope, Béchamp discovered what he called "little bodies," or microzymas—tiny, motile granules, which he found present in every living thing. He theorized that these microzymas organize and nourish cells at the molecular level and that they, not the cells, are the elementary units of all living things.

He found that when he changed their conditions, these microzymas changed in an effort to adapt to their environment. And here's the kicker: *Under toxic conditions, microzymas would change into what we think of as disease-causing microorganisms, i.e. viruses, bacteria, fungi, and parasites.* This phenomenon, he called "pleomorphism."

The theory of pleomorphism says that germs go through many different stages of development during their lives, always starting out as microzymas, but as their environment, or the "milieu" becomes more and more toxic, they become progressively more pathogenic. As the milieu becomes healthier, or less toxic, they become less pathogenic, eventually becoming normal microzymas again.

According to *Dorland's Medical Dictionary*, pleomorphism literally means, "the assumption of various distinct forms by a single organism or species." So, when a caterpillar becomes a butterfly, or a tadpole becomes a frog, these are common examples of pleomorphism. When you think about it, humans are pleomorphic, too. We start out as a sperm and an egg. Those two distinct forms come together to form a zygote (a fertilized egg). The zygote goes through several series of cell divisions to form a tiny ball of identical cells. Those cells eventually take on different characteristics, forming specialized cells with symbiotic relationships to each other. The specialized cells go on to form separate, individual organs, and little by little, *you* start to take shape. But on the way, you go through many different non-human looking stages. Thus, the human animal (the one we're used to seeing, that is) is really just the final stage in our development.

Béchamp and his contemporaries said it was the "terrain" that mattered most and that germs are merely *opportunistic* creatures. Much as a tomato seed won't germinate as long as it's sitting on your desk, but will grow and produce many more tomato seeds when it's put in fertile soil, germs need the right environment to live and reproduce. Béchamp felt that disease-causing germs could only survive and proliferate in a body that was already sick.

> *"Serious illness doesn't bother me for long because I am too inhospitable a host."*
>
> —Dr. Albert Schweitzer

But Béchamp actually went considerably further than that. He boldly declared that, **"Disease is born of us and in us."** In other words, he felt that through pleomorphism, a sick body actually *created* the germs we associate with causing disease. He is not alone in this sentiment, as you'll soon learn.

Out of this beautiful theory, Pasteur only understood the tiniest fraction. He knew that there were germs in the air and theorized that if they could ferment beer, they could certainly cause disease as well. Béchamp wrote papers and books and tried his best to get the world to listen to his elegant theory on pleomorphism, but the world already had its spokesman for germs.

Pasteur developed a much simpler germ theory that once again removed all responsibility for health from the person and placed it somewhere "out there." His theory also had one more major advantage over Béchamp's. It lent itself to an entire industry of germ hunters (microbiologists) and germ killers (antibiotics, antibacterial soaps, vaccinations, antiviral medications), which meant that money could be made. Because of these factors and others, the world was quick to embrace it.

In 1895, Louis Pasteur was buried at the Institute that still bears his name (The Institute Pasteur). His name is further memorialized on nearly every milk and juice container in the world. He is by all accounts one of the most famous men in all of medicine. Tragically, the true hero and genius of our story, Antoine Béchamp, is virtually unknown.

Pleomorphism Returns

In 1933, an optical engineer named Royal Raymond Rife (1888–1971) invented (among other things) a microscope that allowed him to see *living* bacteria. With the exception of Béchamp, this had never been done before. (See box below.) The best microscopes of his day could magnify, at best, to 2,000 diameters. But Rife's "Universal Microscope" could magnify 50,000–60,000 diameters with sharp resolution. This was *so* unheard of that many scientists of his time could not and simply *did* not believe it, even when actually looking through the eyepiece of the huge microscope.

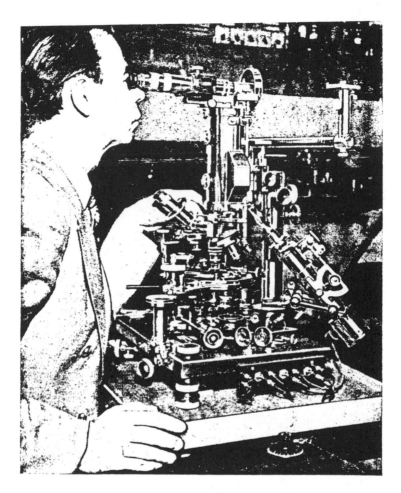

Giant Microscope Explores New Worlds

REPORTED to be so powerful that it reveals disease organisms never seen before, the giant microscope pictured above has just been completed by Royal R. Rife, of San Diego, Calif., whose home-built instruments have long been ranked among the finest in the world. To eliminate distortion, the image produced by the new two-foot-tall apparatus does not pass through the usual air-filled tube, but along an optical path of quartz blocks and prisms. Weighing 200 pounds, the microscope has 5,682 parts.

OCTOBER, 1940

Using regular light microscopes, (no matter how powerful) you have to fix and stain bacteria in order to see them. This means you have to kill them. Electron microscopes, likewise, only allow one to see germ *carcasses*. Since 99.9 percent of the world still uses either regular light, or electron microscopes, and since dead bugs don't change size or shape, it stands to reason that they would be ignorant of the pleomorphic nature of germs.

Through years of experimentation, Rife discovered that every organism vibrates at a certain frequency and that each species has its own particular frequency range. Others, including Dr. Hulda Clark, have since confirmed this. Quantum physicists would also concur. So instead of staining the bugs, Rife used plane-polarized light to visualize his subjects. This meant he didn't have to kill them to see them and thus could actually watch the little buggers in action. When the correct frequency of light was shined up through the specimen, the germs would vibrate and glow, literally giving off their own particular colored light, which allowed him to see things that could not otherwise have been seen, even at these high magnifications.

What he saw was amazing, and though Rife didn't know it, it confirmed exactly what Antoine Béchamp had declared years earlier. Rife watched and studied as living germs morphed into completely different forms with a simple change of the environment. They would morph from the familiar round, or "cocci" form of bacteria, to the long, rod-shaped "bacillus" form, to the corkscrew shape of a "spirochete" with what amounted to a change in the food supply. He could also make them transform from a virus to bacteria, to fungus, to parasite, and then all the way back again.

Rife knew that this flew directly in the face of what conventional knowledge said (both then and now), but the evidence was incontrovertible. There it was, right before his eyes. And since everyone else in the world was merely studying germ *carcasses*, he knew he was on to something big.

It seemed that the simple structure of microorganisms allowed for much more rapid "evolution" than we 10 trillion-celled beings could even fathom. Among the many forms these microorganisms took was something Rife did not recognize. Because he did not know what they were called, and because of the color with which they resonated, he decided to simply call them "turquoise bodies." These turquoise bodies were Béchamp's microzymas.

After years of experimentation with both lab animals and humans, Rife, like Béchamp, said that germs arose from within the body and that they were not the *cause* of disease, but rather, the result.

Rife knew this information had to be disseminated to the world, so he did what any reasonable person would do—he reached out to the medical profession. He found several doctors who were very interested in his work and who tried to help him, but before he had gained much momentum, Dr. Morris Fishbein, chief henchman of the AMA, got wind of this new information and did what he did best. He suppressed the damning evidence in the most expedient way possible.

The idea of pleomorphism was earth shattering to the medical profession. Rife's discovery threatened to nullify their precious germ theory of disease, the very foundation of their existence since Louis Pasteur got it wrong back in the 1870s. But rather than accepting this startling new evidence and giving Rife the Nobel Prize for Medicine, Rife was arrested, his lab was broken into, and his microscope was destroyed. All of his records were stolen as well. Thus, the AMA succeeded in destroying the instrument, as well as the man, which proved the germ theory was incorrect. The entire life's work of this genius disappeared in the blink of an eye because his discovery did not fit in with the medical dogma.

Royal Rife also developed a machine that was able to cure cancer in every single case that he attempted including over 400 animals and dozens of humans. Fishbein had every one of these machines destroyed as well. This will be discussed further in a future *Why We're Sick*™ book. (For even more information on this topic, read *The Cancer Cure That Worked!* by Barry Lynes.)

Rife's arrest and trial led him to a nervous breakdown. He died a depressed alcoholic and is virtually unknown in the scientific community today, despite his amazing *re*-discovery of pleomorphism and these two incredible inventions. To my knowledge, nobody has been able to reproduce Rife's microscope to this day.

As an interesting side-note, Dr. Milbank Johnson, Rife's most ardent supporter, died under very suspicious conditions. It appears he was poisoned to death.

Pleomorphism III: The Theory That Wouldn't Die

There have been many other renegade scientists who have independently discovered these tiny microzymas and the phenomenon of pleomorphism. Guenther Enderlein (1872–1968) saw these granules and called them "protits." Wilhelm Reich (1897–1957) saw them and called them "bions." More recently, there is Gaston Naessens (1924–present) who is currently alive and still doing research in Canada. Each of these scientists studied *living* bacteria instead of simply looking at their stained, dead bodies and trying to formulate theories based on that.

It now appears that these tiny creatures have finally been discovered by someone who actually matters. In 1982, while studying the spongiform encephalopathy diseases (diseases similar to "mad cow") Creutzfeldt-Jakob ("mad human" disease) and scrapie ("mad sheep and goat" disease), Stanley B. Prusiner of the University of California at San Francisco announced that he had isolated the "hypothetical infectious agent" which he implicated in these diseases. He named these agents "prions," a term he coined by combining the words *proteinaceous* (because they only contain protein, i.e. no DNA or RNA), *infectious and viron*. He was awarded the Nobel Prize in Physiology or Medicine in 1997 for his discovery.

Suspiciously, however, not all prions cause disease. There are apparently two different kinds, though they both contain the exact same amino acids. According to the most current knowledge in Western medicine, there are normal prions (which they designate PrP^C) and there are abnormal or infectious prions (currently designated PrP^{Sc}). In addition to the above-mentioned diseases, bovine spongiform encephalopathy (BSE), or "mad cow disease," is also associated with these abnormal prions, though there are many within Western medicine who believe that prions are not infectious at all and are merely present in these diseases by association.

Normal prions, which we know as microzymas, et al., are found on the surface of all cells including those of plants, animals, and fungi. So far their function is officially listed as "unknown," but they have been associated with aiding in long-term memory and acting as a copper-dependant antioxidant. In 2006, it was also reported that they were necessary for producing new bone marrow cells from hematopoietic stem cells.

All prions, whether normal or abnormal, are notoriously hard to kill.[3]

Gaston Naessens, much like Royal Rife, invented a very powerful microscope, which because of its design also allows incredible resolution. Once again though, the important difference between his microscope and others is not just its power or resolution, but the fact that it allows him to see *living* bacteria.

Naessens' "Somatoscope" magnifies to an amazing 30,000 diameters with a resolution of 150 angstroms. Conventional microscopes only magnify to 2,500 diameters. There *are* microscopes in the world that can achieve up to 25,000 diameters of magnification, but their resolution (1,000 angstroms) is several orders of magnitude less than Naessens' Somatoscope. In fact, Naessens' scope actually defies all currently known optical laws in its abilities. Because he cannot explain how he is able to achieve this, he cannot get a patent and, therefore, cannot reproduce his scope for others. (Remember, Rife's Universal microscope could magnify 50,000–60,000 diameters!)

Like Rife, Reich, and Enderlein before him, Naessens too saw what Béchamp called microzymas and what are now called prions. But being unfamiliar with these other scientists' work, he called these ultramicroscopic, sub-cellular, living and reproducing granules "somatids."

Naessens is probably the top scientist in the world on this subject and has dedicated much of his life to studying these tiny creatures. He has found that somatids are essentially indestructible or "immortal." They can survive temperatures of more than 200° C (392° F). They survive exposure to 50,000 rems of nuclear radiation (far more than enough to kill any living thing). They cannot be killed by any known acid, and they can't be cut with a diamond knife. Ironically, one of the only ways he's found to kill them is to bombard them with electrons. This is exactly what electron microscopes do, so they cannot be seen in their living state using electron microscopy. According to Christopher Bird, who has interviewed Naessens extensively, "At the death of their hosts, such as ourselves, they [somatids] return to the earth, where they live on for thousands or millions, perhaps billions, of years!" [4] (Antoine Béchamp actually found microzymas in limestone dating back 60 million years ago, to a time when mammals first began to appear on earth. Another French researcher, this one a paleontologist, has found similar forms in sections of rock that are over three billion years old.)[5]

Since they contain no DNA or RNA, Naessens believes that somatids are the precursors of DNA and the previously unknown factor between the living and nonliving. Put another way, he theorizes that somatids are able to transform energy into living matter. Thus, they are essential to life—that is, without them, there would be no life. He's found that their activity is not restricted to bone marrow stem cells, but that all cells require the presence of somatids in order to divide.

On December 9, 1977, Gaston Naessens took a dismembered chunk of rabbit meat about the size of his fingertip, injected it with cultured rabbit somatids, put it in a vacuum-sealed quart jar, and placed it in the sunlight. Amazingly, the meat did not rot, but to the contrary, *grew*— enough in fact to fill the entire bottom of the jar, about three inches thick! According to Ralph Moss, Ph.D. the rabbit meat was still "alive" in 1994. Naessens has removed the meat and examined it under microscope on several occasions and states that it has all the characteristics of normal rabbit tissue. He theorizes that the somatids he injected back in 1977 convert the energy of sunlight into matter and that that's what keeps the meat looking pink, fresh, and apparently alive.[6]

Somatids are found in the cells of all living beings (including plants) and also among the remains of the previously living. In hundreds of years, if they were to dig up your bones, they would find living somatids there. It is felt that these somatids help to form the cells when they are "born" and help them to decompose when they die. Naessens feels he has stumbled upon nothing less than "...a brand new understanding of the basis of life," and "...an entirely new biology."[7] His theory threatens to destroy what is known as the "central dogma of molecular biology," which states that all living things require nucleic acids (DNA or RNA) to reproduce and that the genes on these nucleic acids control life.

Naessens found that somatids go through three stages of life in a healthy organism: somatid, spore, and double spore, after which they return to the somatid form. In the *unhealthy* organism, however, they have 13 additional stages, including bacterial, mycobacterial, and yeast or fungal stages.

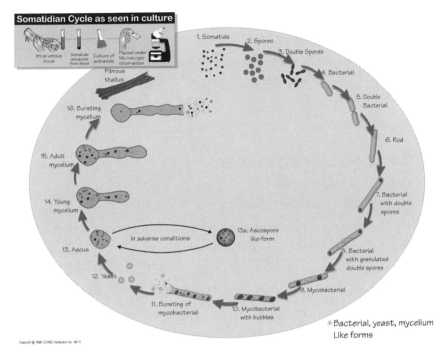

Used with the permission of Gaston Naessens

Naessens has also found that the factors that cause somatids to enter these abnormal life stages are the very same factors that are the root cause of all human disease. Those factors are: nutritional deficiencies, chemical and heavy metal toxicity, accidents/physical trauma, shock, chronic distress, and psychological depression or emotional factors. In other words, these factors cause susceptible tissue to become diseased; and the presence of diseased tissue triggers somatids to morph into some new life form (bacteria, virus, fungus, etc.).

The above factors also form the backbone of this entire book series and constitute the entirety of why we're *really* sick.

"Microzymas can become disease entities as a result of what we eat, think, say, do, and feel. They can also become toxic because of chemicals in the air, water, soil, food, and many other factors of our lifestyle."

—Nancy Appleton, Ph.D., *The Curse of Louis Pasteur*

To understand why this happens, you must take a completely new look at germs and see them not as your enemy, but as your partners in life. Germs are absolutely *essential* to life on this planet.

One of the many things germs do for us is eat diseased or dead flesh in order to return unviable tissue back into soil. This is how dead plants and animals decompose. When you die, your somatids will become bacteria, which will then eat your flesh and turn you back into soil. When you are sick, this same exact process happens, but on a smaller scale. Somatids are the ultimate recyclers on the planet.

In the process of eating this diseased tissue, germs create waste products that cause the symptoms we associate with being sick. (Rife and his colleagues performed experiments where they took the toxic waste products of certain germs and injected them into animals and reproduced the symptoms of disease without ever exposing the animals to the germs themselves.[8]) These symptoms often cause people to go to the doctor. If the patient has a sore throat, the doctor may swab the throat and find bacteria there. Much like the cholesterol we discussed a couple chapters back, the doctor then assumes that the presence of these germs means they are *causing* the disease, when, in fact, the germs are merely there to clean up the mess. He then prescribes an antibiotic to kill the germs. With the germs dead, the symptoms stop and the patient thinks the drug worked. But until the actual cause of the diseased tissue has been resolved and the dead tissue is removed, the disease remains and the symptoms will likely return.

Béchamp saw from his experiments that life was adaptive. He said that even death is a necessary part of life. White blood cells will destroy themselves when they become engorged with bacteria in a heroic effort to save the whole organism. Skin cells, as they venture ever closer to the surface are on a collision course with their own death. So, too, are we, from the very moment we are conceived. These microzymas, somatids, or prions are a part of that process. Béchamp wrote:

> After death, it is essential that matter is restored to its primitive condition, for it has only been lent for a time to the living organized being... The living being, filled with microzymas, carries in itself the elements essential for life, disease, death, and destruction.[9]

When abuses are piled on top of abuses, disease can become chronic and degenerative. When this happens, the body can find itself in a vicious cycle. As one or more of the above abuses cause tissues to degenerate, abnormal somatids (i.e., bacteria, viruses, fungi) proliferate to the point that they're out of control. The eventual outcome is a body with multiple diseased tissues and a severely compromised immune system that's completely overrun with bugs. Other systems then begin to break down and eventually the patient is diagnosed with a disease like AIDS, lupus, chronic fatigue syndrome, multiple sclerosis, or cancer. Very often in these cases, the bugs are held to blame.

Like Royal Rife, Gaston Naessens has developed a cure for cancer, which also works for other immune system problems such as AIDS. His is called 714-X. This is a natural medicine made from camphor that is injected directly into the lymph nodes. Naessens' 714-X helps return the immune system to its normal function, thereby ridding the body of cancer and returning somatids to their normal cycle. Doctors wishing to use this formula can order it directly from Naessens' lab along with an instruction video on how to inject it. Patients can actually be taught how to inject themselves as well. The address and phone number where you can order these products is listed at the end of this chapter.

Also like Rife, Naessens has been persecuted for his contributions to science. He has been arrested for practicing medicine without a license and forced to go to court to defend himself over his 714-X formula. He has spent most of his life trying to get the powers-that-be in cancer research and in Western medicine to look at his amazing work to little avail. Christopher Bird covers this story fully in the book, *The Persecution and Trial of Gaston Naessens*.

By the way, if you'd like to *see* these tiny microzymas/somatids that we've been discussing throughout this chapter, you can contact Naessens' laboratory and get a copy of a videotape that actually shows them in action. It was recorded right from Naessens' microscope. (The information for ordering these is listed at the end of this chapter as well.) I've seen the video myself and was amazed to see these tiny somatids/microzymas dancing around huge cells like hundreds of tiny servants. The video also shows bacteria morphing from rod shaped to round. These videos can be found on the Internet as well.

Pleomorphism IV: The Final Chapter

Nowadays, we have something called "dark field microscopy," which allows doctors to do live blood cell analysis and to see living bacteria. Thus, a whole new generation of scientists and doctors have now seen what Béchamp, Rife, Reich, Enderlein, Naessens, and others have seen—albeit, not quite so clearly. Among these scientists, pleomorphism is an established fact and Pasteur's germ theory has long since fallen from grace. You, too, now have a choice on which germ theory you choose to believe in—the one you've heard all of your life, which is based on the study of germ carcasses and incomplete information; or the one you've just read about, which is based on the independent discoveries of many amazing, yet unsung, scientists who have spent their entire lives studying living germs.

To help further illustrate the differences between the two competing theories (i.e. the germ theory, a.k.a. monomorphism vs. pleomorphism), there is yet another theory you may not have heard of. It's called "The Rat Theory of Garbage." It says that wherever you find lots of garbage, you'll find rats. Louis Pasteur and his camp would have you believe that the rats (germs) *caused* the garbage (diseased tissue). Béchamp's camp would say that the garbage created the perfect environment for rats, and so they came in, made it their home, and had lots of baby rats. Pasteur's camp (Western medicine) would use harsh chemicals to kill the rats, leaving the garbage and the lasting effects of the chemicals behind. Of course, once the chemicals are gone, the rats will probably return. Although it may take a little longer before the effects are seen, Béchamp's camp would address the cause of the problem. First, they would clean up the garbage that was already there. Then they would set up recycling centers, compost heaps, and the like, (clean up the liver, kidneys, colon, etc.) to prevent the problem from cropping up again. With this done, the rats will eventually just go away on their own. These processes are referred to as detoxification and drainage in the world of holistic healthcare.

If you think about it, this new germ theory (pleomorphism) explains an awful lot of questions that the old germ theory left unanswered. For example:

1. Why do some people get sick and others seem to be immune even though they are exposed to the same germs? Aren't germs equal opportunity attackers, or do they just collectively decide to all gang up on certain people?
2. If germs are the cause of disease and germs are always in the air, why aren't we always sick?
3. Why do people who eat unhealthy diets and don't take care of themselves get sick more often?
4. Why do people get sick more often when they are under lots of stress?
5. Why do people tend to get sick more in the cold, winter months?

"I desired to know why one person was ailing and his associate, eating at the same table, working in the same shop...was not. Why? What difference was there in the two persons that cause one to have [disease] while his partner...escaped? Why?"

—D. D. Palmer, Founder of Chiropractic

I'm sure you've noticed how many people are sick around the holidays. It's almost "normal" to be sick at this time, isn't it? It seems everyone is coughing and has a runny nose at the very least. Have you ever stopped to think about why that is? Do germs just really love the cold weather? Does the joy of the holiday season make them so randy that they breed like little rabbits? (Actually, germs are asexual so I doubt they get randy at all.)

Well, perhaps the cold weather somehow makes them divide more rapidly then, could that be it? Actually, no. Viruses need other cells in order to reproduce, so as long as they're out in the cold, they're as good as impotent. Bacteria much prefer the warmth of a body, too. In fact, many bacteria can only survive in the open air for a short time. So, what is it that makes so many people sick during the cold, winter months, especially around the holidays?

While the holiday time of year is a joyous one for many of us, it's also a time when we tend to indulge in more sweets and alcohol than we should. There is also inevitably more stress than usual with the shopping, the spending, the traveling, the company, dealing with family, etc. And then, as mentioned, in many parts of the northern hemisphere, the weather is cold. We also get less sunlight, especially on exposed skin, and, therefore, produce considerably less vitamin D as well as other health-promoting hormones in the winter. All of these things stress the immune system. When the immune system is weak and the body is toxic, the body breeds more bugs. *This* is the reason for all the sickness at holiday time. So cold weather doesn't breed more bugs. Sick and toxic bodies breed more bugs. The cold weather is just one of the stressors to the immune system.

Does this mean germs are never passed from one person or animal to another? No. Germs *can* live in the air for a short time. If someone coughs or sneezes in your face, you *could* catch their cold or flu, but only if your immune system is weak and can't handle the attack. You can also get diseases from mosquito bites, tick bites, rabid animal bites, stepping on rusty nails, being injected with infected blood, or drinking polluted water. I'm not denying any of these things, but this is not the whole picture.

In many diseases, especially chronic diseases like chronic fatigue syndrome, peptic ulcers, cancer, and as you'll read later, quite possibly AIDS, there are germs present that do not *cause* the disease, but are merely there for opportunistic reasons. Béchamp's theory, unlike Pasteur's, says that you could live in a completely sterile, germ-free environment and still find germs running rampant throughout your body. In fact, scientists who live in the arctic regions of the world attest to this. The weather there is so cold that germs cannot survive in the environment, and yet the people living there definitely get sick. Where do the germs come from in this instance? In all of these cases, treating the disease with bug killers of various sorts does nothing at all to help the patient and can often be very detrimental to him.

It took over 50 years for Béchamp's discovery to be confirmed by Rife. By then, Pasteur's bogus germ theory was so entrenched in the medical textbooks and education, *and* in the public mindset, that it was nearly impossible to extract. Morris Fishbein's suppression of the truth and the early success of antibiotics only helped to entrench the theory that much further. People have always been anxious to blame some outside source for their problems—be it germs, bad humors, God, the devil, or their parents—rather than looking inward where most problems really begin.

Pasteur, on his deathbed, finally recanted and admitted that his competitors had been right all along. "The microbe is nothing," he said, "the terrain is everything." Also, in 1914, Madame Victor Henry of the Pasteur Institute stated that Béchamp was correct and Pasteur was wrong.[10]

Royal Rife, Gaston Naessens, and many others have proven that pleomorphism is a fact of life. It has been compared with evolution and symbiosis, two theories with which it is intimately tied. The evidence for it is, for all practical purposes, incontrovertible, but the medical world has yet to embrace it. Why? Perhaps they're afraid that if they let this cat out of the bag, they would see their stranglehold on healthcare start to loosen.

Western medicine has been built on the overly simplistic foundation of the germ theory of disease—a theory with many, many holes. They say that for every disease, there is one pathogenic organism. The pharmaceutical industry has fully embraced this theory and taken it on as their purpose in life to find a drug or chemical to kill every disease-causing organism on the face of the planet, no matter what the cost. It must be frightening for them to realize that their entire foundation is actually nothing but a house of cards built on quicksand. Take away the germ theory of disease and the whole reason for their existence practically disappears.

For More Information Read:

The Curse of Louis Pasteur, by Nancy Appleton, Ph.D.
Béchamp or Pasteur: A Lost Chapter in the History of Biology, by
    E. Douglas Hume
The Private Science of Louis Pasteur, by Gerald L. Geison
The Dream & Lie of Louis Pasteur, by R. B. Pearson (available online)
The Blood and its Third Element, by Antoine Béchamp
The Cancer Cure that Worked, by Barry Lynes
The Persecution and Trial of Gaston Naessens, by Christopher Bird

To order a videotape showing somatids, or to purchase 714-X, contact: The Center for Experimental Biological Research, 520 Rue Fontaine, Rock Forest, Quebec, Canada, J1NB6. Phone: (819) 564-7883

7

Antibiotics & the Yeast Connection

"For new ideas to be accepted, one has to wait for a generation of scientists to die off and a new one to replace it."

—Max Planck, Nobel Laureate in physics, 1918

In light of what you've just learned about iatrogenic illness, drugs, and the germ theory, hopefully you're well on your way to making this paradigm shift with me to a life where medications are a last resort, only to be used in the direst of emergencies and only for a very short duration. If you're not there yet, the next few chapters should help to take you the rest of the way. As a reminder, throughout the rest of this book, and whenever germs are discussed elsewhere, always remember that pleomorphism is real and that germs are good or bad only because of the environment you've set up for them.

On September 3rd 1928, the Scottish physician, Sir Alexander Fleming, discovered a ring of blue-green mold (penicillium notatum) growing on a culture of *Staphylococcus aureus* (the bacteria involved in Staph infections). He noticed that the area around the mold did not have any bacteria growing on it. Curious, he then grew a pure culture of the mold and found that it produced a substance, which he named penicillin. He experimented with the substance, using it on small animals and found that it was able to kill a number of pathogenic bacteria with no side effects. In 1929,

Fleming wrote a paper detailing his research, stating that penicillin may have therapeutic value if it could be produced in large enough quantities. This proved to be easier said than done.

> Fleming wasn't the first to discover penicillin. In fact, it had been "discovered" at least 140 times by other scientists, most notably by France's Ernest Duchesne in 1897. But instead of seeing the usefulness of this mold, most merely saw it as a contamination of their experiment and threw it away.

Ten years after Fleming's paper, Dr. Howard Florey and Ernst Chain, of Oxford University, began serious investigation into penicillin's antibacterial properties. With World War II underway, Britain was desperate for a way to stop the biggest wartime killer—infected wounds. It wasn't until they teamed up with scientists from the United States that they were able to find a way of producing penicillin in large enough quantities to make mass production feasible. Once they had overcome that hurdle, however, the group began clinical trials. Penicillin was the most effective antibacterial medicine anyone had discovered to date. They quickly scaled up production and penicillin was available to treat soldiers wounded on D-Day. It was immediately hailed as a "Wonder Drug."

Within four years, the first penicillin-resistant bacteria had appeared.

The amazing thing about penicillin and other antibiotics is how they work. Many antibiotics kill bacteria by destroying their cell walls (or to be technically correct, by inhibiting cell wall synthesis).

Now despite what you may have heard in the common vernacular, only plant cells have *walls*. Animal cells have *membranes*. These two things are vastly different. And while you may think of bacteria as being tiny little bugs belonging to the animal kingdom, bacteria have cell walls, so technically, they belong in the plant kingdom. Therefore, antibiotics only kill bacteria and have no effect on human or animal cells. **Please Note: Viruses do *not* have cell walls. Therefore, *antibiotics will not kill viruses*.** Antibiotics also do nothing for yeast, fungi, or parasitic infections.

This is a very important point, and it bears repeating: **Antibiotics only kill bacteria.** Colds and flus are viral infections. Many other infections, including ear, throat, upper respiratory, and urinary tract infections can also be viral, fungal, or parasitic in origin. Antibiotics will do nothing for these types of infections.

Penicillin was an amazing shot in the arm for allopathic medicine. After more than a century of their cures being worse than the disease, they finally had a safe and effective medicine that actually *saved* lives instead of took them. But as we've just learned, penicillin comes directly from nature. It's an extract of a mold. Isn't penicillin then essentially an herbal remedy that allopathy has taken monopolistic control over?

Superbugs

So if antibiotics don't affect animal cells, what's wrong with taking them just to be on the safe side? That's a very good question, and I'm sure this line of reasoning is exactly what has led to their overuse. There are actually two major problems with that idea. One, I'll discuss here. The other will be covered very shortly.

When antibiotics are used, especially when used indiscriminately or improperly, bacteria build up a resistance to them. It's like the old saying, "What doesn't kill you, just makes you stronger." The way it works is like this: Invariably, some bacteria are exposed to the antibiotic and are not killed by it. These stronger strains of bacteria go on to reproduce. (It has been estimated that a single bacterium can multiply into 16,777,220 bacteria within 24 hours.) Their offspring are genetically immune to that antibiotic. Therefore, the more we rely on antibiotics, the more we kill off the weaker strains, leaving the stronger mutant strains to survive and reproduce. Not only that, but just as a nursing mother can pass on antibodies to protect her children from the germs she's been exposed to, it's been discovered that these stronger breeds of bugs can actually pass on their antibiotic immunity through mere contact with other bugs and "teach" *them* how to become immune as well. These antibiotic-resistant bacteria have been dubbed "superbugs."

We now have superbugs that can resist virtually any antibiotic. Thus, we may already be coming to the end of the antibiotic era. We may very well see in our lifetimes a return to a time where bacterial infections kill thousands of people every year. It's already happening on a smaller scale. People are now dying from infections (including *Staphylococcus aureus* and tuberculosis) that were easily treated by penicillin a decade or two ago.

How did this happen? How could we have squandered one of the most important medical breakthroughs in history in the course of a single lifespan? The biggest reason is our unfaltering over-confidence in a flawed and incomplete germ theory. People were too quick to embrace a theory with an outside agent as the cause of disease. Pasteur had found the cause of disease and Fleming had found the cure—end of story. All of our medical woes were over—or so we thought.

Strange as it may sound, perhaps antibiotics worked *too* well. Medicine's discovery of this highly useful herbal extract (penicillin) caused us to become overly confident in their abilities to keep us healthy, and, thus, we became lazy. Our health was not something we needed to work at. After all, what could we do? Medicine had ingrained in us the idea that sickness was a result of our being haphazardly attacked by an unseen foe, hardly different from being a punishment from God or bad humors, except that now, they had the cure. So, we put our faith in doctors and in medicine and handed them the responsibility for our health. And that was a big mistake.

"The optimism of a relatively few years ago that many of these diseases could be brought under control has led to a fatal complacency. This complacency is now costing millions of lives."

—Dr. Hiroshi Nakajima, Director-General of the World Health Organization

It was all just too easy, though. If you get sick, just run to the doctor for a pill or an injection and you'll be right as rain in no time. We definitely took the easy route, and now we're paying for it.

If instead of running to the doctor for every sniffle or sneeze, we had focused on building up our immune systems, and only used antibiotics as a last resort, they would have lasted much longer— perhaps forever. In other words, if we had taken a holistic approach to healthcare, to include the use of antibiotics when absolutely necessary, instead of the antibiotics-for-everything approach, we'd be much better off right now.

We've become obsessed with killing germs in our culture. We use antibacterial soaps and cleansers in our homes; we pasteurize our milk, cheese, and juice to kill the bacteria in them; and we use antibiotics in agriculture—big time. Cows, chickens, and pigs are actually fed antibiotics as part of their diet. Good ole' vitamin A, right? (Wink, wink, nudge, nudge.) Makes 'em *healthy*! In fact, according to some estimates, more than 70 percent of all antibiotics are given to feed animals that have no disease.[1] All of these things add up to the breeding of superbugs.

What can you do to protect yourself from these antibiotic-resistant bacteria? The only *real* way to protect yourself from germs of any kind is to have a strong immune system. How does one achieve that? Following the advice given throughout this book and the remaining books in this series will result in a healthy body and a strong immune system, but for now, here are a few tips: Get off of all medications that aren't absolutely necessary. (Ideally, you'll want to work with your doctor on this.) Eat only real food. What *is real* food? Fruits, vegetables, nuts and seeds, eggs, raw milk, fermented foods like yogurt and sauerkraut, and meats of all kinds including the smaller fishes all constitute real food. Avoid all processed, pre-packaged junk food. Any grains in your diet should be whole grains or sprouted grains and these should be kept to a minimum. The meat, eggs, and dairy you eat should be free range and organic. This guarantees the animals are free from hormones and antibiotics, able to move about freely, and they're fed their natural diet. The produce you eat should also be organic and as much of it as possible should be raw. It should also be in season and the more locally grown it is the better. You should drink lots of water. How much? Drink half your body weight in ounces per day (e.g. a 200 pound person should drink 100 ounces of water). Detoxify your body, concentrating most of your effort on cleaning out your liver, kidneys, and colon, at least once or twice a year. Take essential fatty acids (one tablespoon of raw flax seed oil per day is a good start). Take a good probiotic supplement. (This will be explained later in this chapter.) Avoid sugar, fake sugar, and trans fats (like fake butter) like the plague. Exercise. The more you exercise, the better. Do something to help you handle your stress (meditate, dance, jog, walk, punch a bag, make love). Have some sort of bodywork done on a regular basis (chiropractic, massage, craniosacral therapy, etc.). Take whole food nutritional supplements. Avoid all toxins as much as possible. Laugh, sing, have fun, take vacations, nurture your spirit, listen to your intuition. All of these things will help strengthen your immune system, making you virtually impervious to infection.

RESEARCH ON ANTIBIOTICS

Sinuses, Sore Throats & Bronchitis

The most common reasons adults go to the doctor and receive antibiotics are for non-specific upper respiratory tract infections such as colds and flus, sore throats, sinus infections, and acute bronchitis. As we've discussed, colds and flues are caused by viruses, so antibiotics simply don't work for them. But what about these other problems?

A study in the March 8, 1997 issue of the *British Medical Journal* concluded that antibiotics were of no value in fighting common forms of tonsillitis and pharyngitis (sore throats). The study looked at more than 700 patients with sore throats and found that most patients were better in three to five days whether they took the antibiotic or not. Those who *did* take the medication were, of course, likely to believe that it was responsible for their cure, and were more inclined to come back for more if they became ill again.[2]

A study in the *Archives of Internal Medicine* also found that adults suffering from acute sinusitis were no better off with amoxicillin than they were with a placebo. The amoxicillin group also suffered from more side effects such as diarrhea.[3]

In March 2008, the BBC reported on a study appearing in *The Lancet* that looked at nine separate trials on antibiotic use for sinusitis. They concluded that even if the patient had been ill for a week to 10 days (which supposedly indicates a greater chance that the problem is bacterial rather than viral), only one patient in 15 would be helped by antibiotics. Co-author Dr. Ian Williamson was quoted as saying, "Antibiotics really don't look as if they work. We have found that antibiotics aren't effective for sore throats and ear infections, but sinusitis, which is similar, is the one that people are slightly more die hard about."[4] This study led the National Institute for Clinical and Health Excellence (NICE) to publish draft guidance advising doctors to not prescribe antibiotics for these conditions nor to issue delayed prescriptions which patients can use if they don't get better.

Many educated patients today know that antibiotics don't work for a cold, but once a cold has progressed to bronchitis, they feel justified, indeed they often feel as if there's nothing left to do but go in for the drugs. Before doing the research for this chapter, I tended to agree with them, but now that I've read through the research, it seems these patients would have actually been better off just taking a placebo, too. This is because, as should be assumed with the general progression from cold to bronchitis, that the vast majority (more than 90 percent) of bronchitis cases are viral in origin.

The journal *Chest* states that fewer than 10 percent of acute bronchitis cases are bacterial in origin. (Those few that *are* bacterial are almost always due to pertussis, or whooping cough, and this is found in adults who were vaccinated for it multiple times as children.) The article goes on to say, "For patients with the putative diagnosis of acute bronchitis, routine treatment with antibiotics is not justified and should not be offered."[5] Another journal suggests that doctors refrain from even calling it bronchitis and instead refer to it as a "chest cold" to help appease the patient and keep them from expecting an antibiotic.[6]

According to research in the *Annals of Internal Medicine*, randomized, placebo-controlled trials do not support the use of antibiotics in uncomplicated acute bronchitis (in other words, when there's no pneumonia or whooping cough). Further, this study also shows that when a doctor does *not* prescribe an antibiotic, it doesn't cause a rash of return visits to the doctor, nor does it lead to a dissatisfied patient, as many doctors fear.[7] Another article in the *Annals of Internal Medicine* goes on to advise doctors that if they *do* suspect pneumonia or whooping cough, that they perform the proper tests to make the diagnosis rather than simply prescribing an antibiotic for what is usually just a viral infection that will resolve on its own.[8] In other words, start being a doctor instead of just a drug dispensary. Educate your patients that this is not a condition for which antibiotics are likely help and that to prescribe them would be irresponsible and would actually do them harm.

Imagine how valued you'd feel as a patient if your doctor took a moment out of his/her busy day to briefly explain all this to you instead of simply reaching for his/her prescription pad.

WHAT TO DO FOR A COLD OR FLU:

At the <u>very</u> first sign of a cold or flu, that uneasy twinge in your throat or sinuses that doesn't feel quite right and makes you wonder if you <u>might</u> be coming down with something, do what your mother taught you: Stay warm, drink lots of fluids, and get plenty of rest. Herbs such as echinacea and goldenseal help increase the number of circulating white blood cells. Chiropractic adjustments do the same. Real whole vitamin C (not just ascorbic acid), either from food or whole food concentrates has also been proven effective in recovering from colds. I recommend

Cataplex AC, Immuplex, Congaplex, and Thymex from Standard Process. Yin Chiao works well for some people, as does the herbal supplement Airborne. Colloidal Silver is also an excellent anti-microbial remedy, as is garlic. The earlier you implement these treatments, the more effective they will be. The trick is to recognize when you're getting sick, rather than waiting until you're already there. Preventing all illness using the steps given earlier in this chapter is even better.

Ear Infections

The most common reason for kids to go to the doctor and, in fact, the most frequent (medical) use for antibiotics in the United States is for otitis media or middle ear infections. Each year, approximately 30 percent of British children under the age of three see their doctor for an ear infection and 97 percent of those children are given antibiotics.[9] The numbers are similar for most other industrialized nations as well (except for the Netherlands and Iceland where antibiotics are not used so routinely). Yet, as was mentioned above, antibiotics don't seem to work any better than a placebo for *these* infections either.

An article in the *Journal of the American Medical Association*, which reviewed a series of studies including seven randomized, placebo-controlled trials over the past 30 years, stated, "Given the lack of evidence for benefit and the potential for adverse effects, including altering normal respiratory flora and developing resistant organisms, routine treatment using ten days of antimicrobials [antibiotics] for all cases of acute otitis media is not warranted." The authors went on to write, "Following treatment of otitis media, pneumococci [a type of bacteria] with multi-drug resistance have developed and spread in day care centers and to surrounding communities... *Deaths from meningitis resulting from resistant organisms have occurred in patients previously treated for uncomplicated otitis media.*[10] [Emphasis added]

A study appearing in the July 12, 1997 issue of the *British Medical Journal* echoed the above study. The authors state, "...we conclude that existing research offers no compelling evidence that children with acute otitis media routinely given antimicrobials have a shorter duration of symptoms, fewer recurrences, or better long term outcomes than those who do not receive them. It is also not clear that routine compared with selective use of antimicrobials prevents complications. Thus, it is prudent to reconsider routine use of antimicrobials for otitis media and to consider other approaches."[11] This study also compared the antibiotic resistance of bacteria in the Netherlands (who don't use antibiotics so cavalierly in these cases) versus the countries who *do* overprescribe and found that the Netherlands have less of a problem with superbugs. (Oh, and the outcome of their ear infection cases are essentially identical to ours, too.) Iceland has adopted a program similar to the Netherlands and in fact doctors in *all* countries have been urged to be more conservative in their prescribing of antibiotics by the Institute of Medicine, the Centers for Disease Control, and the World Health Organization. However, this has been slow in coming.

Another study on otitis media, involving 3,660 children in nine countries, and again appearing in the *British Medical Journal*, stated, "Antibiotic treatment did not improve the rate of recovery of patients in this study." In fact, the authors stated, *"Patients who did not take antibiotics had a higher rate of recovery than those who did..."*[12] [Emphasis added]

A medical doctor in Canada performed a review of the literature regarding antibiotic use for otitis media from 1939–1991. His study also showed "poor evidence supporting the routine use of antibiotic therapy."[13]

When antibiotic therapy is unsuccessful in treating chronic ear infections, tympanostomy tubes are often recommended. Unfortunately, most children who have this procedure have recurrent effusion (fluid in the ears) within two months,[14] and up to 25 percent may have total hearing loss.[15]

While we're on the subject of kids receiving antibiotics, you should know that a small, seven-year study performed at Henry Ford Hospital in Detroit involving 448 children showed that children who received antibiotics in their first six months of life were 1.5 times more likely to develop allergies to pets, ragweed, dust mites, etc., and 2.5 times more likely to develop asthma.[16]

The National Institutes of Health (NIH) has found that low birth weight babies are increasingly contracting *E. coli* infections instead of the relatively benign *streptococcal* infections, apparently because of antibiotic use. It is thought that antibiotics given to women in labor are killing friendly bacteria that would normally have inhibited *E. coli* growth. This allows *E. coli* growth to go unchecked, which leads to systemic infection or "sepsis." This is troublesome because *E. coli* can be much more dangerous than *streptococcal* infections. This study was reported in the *New England Journal of Medicine*.[17]

Antibiotics in Dentistry

Since 1955, patients with heart conditions such as mitral valve prolapse, rheumatic heart disease, bicuspid valve disease, calcified aortic stenosis, and certain congenital heart conditions have been prescribed antibiotics prior to and shortly after any dental procedure, including cleanings. The reason given for this was that during these procedures, bacteria in the mouth could conceivably be released into the bloodstream and settle in the heart causing what has been called bacterial or infective endocarditis. This meant that people with benign heart murmurs who followed their dentist's recommendations required a short course of antibiotics at least twice a year—for their entire lives. This chronic use of antibiotics causes undeniable damage to the gut flora and by extension the gut itself. For many of these patients, this loss of gut flora sets the stage for chronic, systemic yeast overgrowth, leaky gut syndrome, allergies, autoimmune diseases, a compromised immune system, and all the other things that come along with these issues. As it turns out, all those antibiotics that were given "just in case" (for 52 years) and caused many thousands (if not millions) of patients irreparable harm, were unnecessary and a complete waste of money.

In 2007, the American Heart Association (AHA) released new guidelines that no longer recommend giving these patients antibiotics prior to dental procedures. These guidelines were immediately adopted by the American Dental Association and were also reported in the journal *Circulation* as well as endorsed by the Infectious Diseases Society of America and the Pediatric Infectious Disease Society. Walter Wilson, M.D., the chairman of the AHA writing group and a Mayo Clinic Professor said, "We've concluded that if giving prophylactic antibiotics prior to a dental procedure works at all—and there's no evidence that it does work—we should reserve that preventive treatment only for those people who would have the worst outcomes if they get IE [Infective Endocarditis]." [18]

But be warned. There may be some lag time before every dentist catches on to these new guidelines, so be prepared to fight for your right to say no. If your dentist gives you any hassles, the American Dental Association lists these guidelines on their website www.ada. org. Print them out and bring them to your dentist. He or she may need some re-educating as well.

Patients who *are* still recommended prophylactic antibiotics prior to dentistry include those with artificial heart valves, a history of infective endocarditis, a heart transplant that develops a problem in a heart valve, and certain serious congenital heart conditions.[19] Of course, there's no evidence that antibiotics help *these* patients either, but we mustn't admit to too much all at once.

Global Issues

In 1996, the World Health Organization (WHO) warned that the spread of devastating diseases, including AIDS and Ebola, may be blamed in great part on the overuse of antibiotics throughout the world. In a report given in Geneva, they singled out "the uncontrolled and inappropriate use of antibiotics," as one of the primary reasons for the outbreak of drug-resistant strains of infectious diseases. "They are used by too many people to treat the wrong kind of infections at the wrong dosage and for the wrong period of time," the report states. [20]

This was not surprising news, however, because the May 1971 issue of *Drug Notes,* contained an article that stated, "The general prophylactic value of antibiotic therapy has been questioned by informed clinicians; its effectiveness in warding off infections in most clinical situations has never been proved. Conversely, *there is a growing body of evidence to suggest that the incidence of serious infection is greater in patients treated prophylactically with broad-spectrum antibiotics than in those not so treated."* [21] [Emphasis added]

The article mentions a study done in a hospital in Glasgow, where after 10 weeks of (reluctantly) using no antibiotics, they actually saw a *reduction* in the number of infections. The respiratory infection rate fell from 45 percent to 15 percent, and the urinary tract infection rate fell from 21 percent to eight percent. The article went on to say, "This experience and other reports relating to antibiotic overuse suggest the age of antibiotic miracles may be over. *There is little question that many infections resolve in spite of rather than because of antibiotic therapy; conversely, the primary etiologic factor in many infections attributed to other causes is the misuse or overuse of broad-spectrum antibiotics.*" [Emphasis added]

The CDC has estimated that each year, one third of the antibiotics that are prescribed in a doctor's office are prescribed inappropriately and unnecessarily.[22] According to Richard Besser, M.D. (director of the CDC's Coordinating Office for Terrorism Preparedness and Emergency Response, and director of *Get Smart: Know When Antibiotics Work*, the CDC's national campaign to promote appropriate antibiotic use in the community), this amounts to *tens of millions of antibiotics being prescribed annually and unnecessarily for viral infections.*[23] And this doesn't even touch on the huge amount of antibiotics being fed to cows, chickens, and other livestock (almost all of which could be stopped if the animals were simply allowed to graze outside of a cramped cage or stall and to eat their natural diet).

Please notice: These are not stories written up in the *National Enquirer*, nor are they chiropractic journals or even health magazines I'm quoting from. These are studies found in the most prestigious *medical* journals in the world. These are recommendations issued to doctors around the world by the World Health Organization, the Centers for Disease Control, and the National Institute of Health. (And this is just a taste of the research that's out there on this topic. If you want more proof, you can find dozens of free abstracts to read on www.Pubmed.gov)

Obviously, medical doctors are ignoring the very science that they claim to revere. Perhaps they feel satisfied merely that the studies are being done, regardless of whether or not they actually follow what the studies say. I guess this makes them the more scientific profession. At any rate, they must be much smarter than I am because try as I might, I can't figure this one out.

Assuming they actually attended microbiology class while in medical school *or* that they attend conferences, read their own journals, or even read the newspaper or other popular media where this topic has been discussed, one is left with only a handful of possibilities as to why M.D.s would continue prescribing antibiotics for viral infections like colds, flus, bronchitis, etc. Here are the only excuses I can come up with for them:

1. To appease a sick patient. Many doctors feel the need to give the patient *something*, even if they know it won't help, and apparently, even if they know it will *hurt* the patient. Many patients will actually request antibiotics, and some doctors will rationalize that if they refuse the request, the patient will simply go to another doctor and get them anyway.* This translates into a loss of business. (*Research has disproven this.*)

2. The placebo effect. This ties in with appeasing the patient, but with the caveat that it may actually help them by psychologically fooling the body into becoming well on its own. This seems highly unlikely, and with the danger of creating superbugs and the certainty of throwing off the body's delicate ecology, leading frequently to systemic or vaginal yeast infections (see next section), very irresponsible.

3. To prevent a secondary bacterial infection. This excuse is really born out of laziness. The doctor is too lazy (or the doctor is assuming the patient is too lazy) to have the patient return if the infection hasn't cleared up in a week or so or if it's gotten worse. They're also too lazy to simply culture the microbe to see if it's viral or bacterial. Secondary

bacterial infections *can* happen, but as their journals state very clearly, the prophylactic use of antibiotics for every infection is not warranted. In fact, the journals give strong recommendations *against* it.

4. Despite the fact that studies appearing in highly respected, peer reviewed medical journals have repeatedly shown this to be ineffective and irresponsible, they either don't understand the science or they don't believe the studies are true. This also seems highly unlikely.

5. Or perhaps they are (knowingly or unknowingly) part of a vast conspiracy, in cahoots with the pharmaceutical industry, the AMA, and the FDA that's trying to keep the public sick and reliant on drugs and medical care their whole life, so that they can all make more money.

To summarize, according to the top medical journals in the world, antibiotics are not effective for colds, flues, or other viral infections. They're no better than a placebo for ear infections, sinus infections, throat infections, or bronchitis. They don't need to be used (except in the rarest instances) in dentistry either.

HOW ANTIBIOTICS SHOULD BE USED
(IF YOU REALLY, *REALLY* MUST)

At the first sign of infection, you go to your doctor or healthcare provider. S/He will take a culture of the infection and send it to the lab for what is known as a culture and sensitivity test. Here, they grow the microbe on a petri dish and then, if it's bacterial, they see what antibiotic it's sensitive to. In the meantime, you're at home, staying warm, getting lots of rest, drinking lots of fluids, taking echinacea, and doing everything you possibly can to help your immune system fight off this attack. When the doctor gets the lab results, he calls you to see how you're doing. If you're still sick, and the bug is bacterial, and you deem that you just might die if you don't get something to help your immune system fight this off, the doctor calls in the exact prescription for you. You stay home and have someone go to the pharmacy to pick it up for you. Then, you take the full prescription (i.e. you don't just take it until you feel better and save the rest for the next time you come down with something). I know this is a little more involved than what you're used to, but this reduces the speed at which bacteria become superbugs.

Candida and the Yeast Infection Connection

Nature is a beautiful thing. Everything in nature is provided for in perfect balance and even the evil bacteria serve a purpose in this ongoing circle of life. As mentioned in the previous chapter, death and decay are a necessary part of life. Without them, there would be no room for renewal. Our bodies are made from the earth and to the earth they must return. Bacteria help this to happen.

Microzyma/somatids (which can be accurately thought of as immature bacteria), if you remember, are thought to be the immortal link between life and death. When you're healthy, they help your cells to grow, mature, and divide. When your body becomes sick and toxic, they become pathogenic bacteria to help clean up the toxic waste. And when you die, they become bacteria again to help your body decompose. When the job is done, they go back to being microzyma/somatids and await their next assignment.

Just as our bodies need these normal flora, so too does the soil. Bacteria help decompose dead bugs and animals and the remnants of plants after harvesting by eating and excreting these things. This decomposed matter becomes useful fertilizer for the soil and the circle of life continues. Therefore, plants need bacteria in order to be healthy, too.

There are at least a few other very important things that bacteria do for us while we're living as well. In fact, we are in a total symbiotic relationship with bacteria, whether you realize it or not. We actually need them to survive as much (or more) as they need us. Beneficial bacteria, which we call normal flora, help us to metabolize vitamins B and K, but more importantly, they help keep yeasts like *Candida albicans*, and harmful bacteria like *E. coli* in check. Because there is limited space and also a limited food supply in your colon, along with the rest of your digestive tract, these different organisms are in constant competition with one another. The idea here is we'd like to maintain a healthy balance down there, so as to not allow any one group to become too strong. (Sounds like a good foreign policy tactic as well, doesn't it?) Antibiotics, as we've mentioned, kill bacteria and do nothing at all against yeast or fungal infections. Also, antibiotics cannot distinguish between the good bacteria and the bad—all are affected equally. So when we kill off the good bacteria (and the "bad" bacteria) and leave the yeasts, the yeasts become the dominant group and the delicate ecology of your inner world is lost. Yeasts become all-powerful and their evil empire spreads to all parts of the body. Over time, this leads to a chronic condition known as candidiasis, or systemic yeast infection. And every dose of antibiotics only helps to strengthen their empire.

Please keep in mind, everything I'm describing here about humans who take antibiotics on occasion is happening *in spades* in the livestock that are fed antibiotics as a part of their normal diet.

THE YEAST CONNECTION...A VICIOUS CYCLE

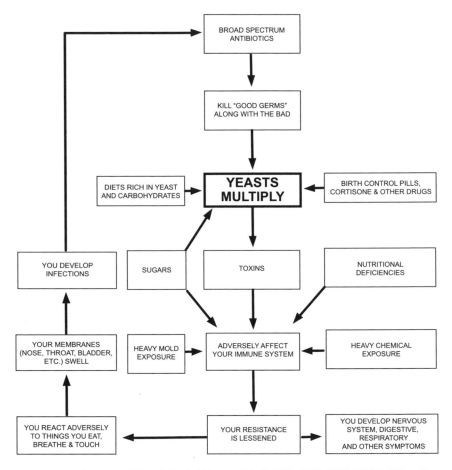

From *The Yeast Connection*, William G. Crook, M.D., copyright © 1983, 1984, 1985, 1986 by William G. Crook, M.D. Used by permission of Random House, Inc.

This can be a very difficult problem to treat and can cause symptoms including fatigue, lethargy, PMS, digestive disorders, vaginitis, skin problems, impotence, hyperactivity, depression, learning difficulty, short attention span, memory loss, irritability, muscle pain, headache, and hypoglycemia. Patients with systemic candidiasis often feel sick all over and many are labeled with chronic fatigue syndrome. Some go from doctor to doctor only to be told it's all in their head. Many medical doctors actually prescribe more antibiotics for these people, ignorantly making the problem worse. I've heard it said that by the time a woman starts getting vaginal yeast infections, she may have had a systemic yeast problem for up to 20 years. Any of this sound like anyone you know? Perhaps *everyone* you know?

Testing for Candida

There are no blood or urine tests for yeasts, so your M.D. probably won't know how to test for them. I test people using muscle testing, but there are also stool tests that can pick up *Candida*. There's also a home test that you can do for free though. What you do is, first thing in the morning, before you brush your teeth or drink anything, spit into a clear glass of water. You may want to spit several times so you have enough to cover the top layer of water. Then, periodically (about every 15 minutes), for the next hour, check on your spit to see what it's doing. If you notice it starting to travel down into the glass, with stringy little legs, or if it sinks, or the water becomes cloudy, you can bet your bottom dollar you have *Candida*. (See illustration on next page.) If your spit remains floating on top, you're okay. A majority of people will find they have *Candida*. Getting rid of your yeast will require discipline, but it will also have a huge impact on your health.

How to Get Rid of Candida

The first thing you must do to get rid of your yeast is avoid antibiotics. Many of the patients I see with systemic yeast have been on a constant merry-go-round of antibiotics for years. As mentioned, this only makes them sicker. They may have chronic sinusitis or other infections (especially of the ear, throat, and bladder), which leads their M.D. to continually prescribe more antibiotics, thus prolonging and compounding the problem.

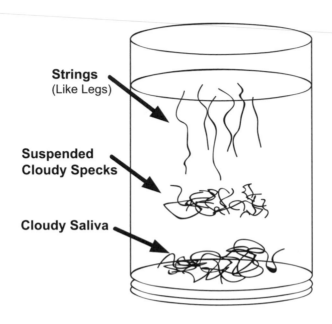

Strings (Like Legs)

Suspended Cloudy Specks

Cloudy Saliva

Bi-annual antibiotics for dental cleanings also fall into this category. You *must* break out of this vicious cycle.

Remember, we also get antibiotics from non-organic meat, chicken, eggs, milk, etc. If you want to get rid of your yeast for good, you will need to start buying organic, free-range foods that have not been raised on a steady diet of antibiotics.

The next thing you'll need to do is get all the sugar and refined carbohydrates out of your diet. Sugars are the primary source of fuel for yeasts and we want to starve those little buggers out. The problem is, yeasts often cause you to *crave* sugar. (Inositol from Standard Process and the herb gymnema can help with these cravings.) Of course, you may not crave *refined* sugar; you may crave other things like beer, or wine, or pretzels, or any other simple, refined carbohydrate, which turns into sugar once it's digested. These things all promote yeast overgrowth and must be avoided.

Other things to avoid include coffee and tea, cheese, fruit juice (unless it's freshly made), melons, mushrooms, processed foods, breads, pastries, and other baked goods, all alcohol products, cereals, honey, molasses, maple syrup, processed or smoked meats, dried and candied fruits, and leftovers. Also, avoid any foods you are allergic to.

Other foods fall into a gray area, which may be acceptable for some, but not for others such as fruit, nuts, and milk. These should be avoided for at least the first three weeks of the diet when trying to rid your body of yeast.

So what are you left with? Meat, Eggs, Vegetables, and Yogurt are all safe foods. They call it the MEVY diet. The meats should obviously be free of hormones and antibiotics. The vegetables should be organically grown. The yogurt should be plain, with no sugar or fruit added.

After the first three weeks on the diet, you can add almonds, Brazil nuts, cashews, hazel nuts, pecans, and pumpkin seeds. You can use butter or sunflower seed oil, too. You can eat the following whole grains on occasion—barley, corn, millet, oats, rice, and wheat, but remember, no yeast!

You may need to stay on this diet for a long time. You should try to stick as closely to this diet as you can until your spit floats with no strings. The time it will take will depend on how closely you follow this program and how bad your problem is.

The next step in the process is to re-establish your normal flora. Our bodies are very much analogous to the ecology of the earth. Amazingly, one teaspoon of healthy soil contains more microorganisms than there are people on the earth. Similarly, a healthy body contains three to four pounds of beneficial bacteria, and as I mentioned in the previous chapter, you should have ten times more bacteria in your body than you have cells! That's a *lot* of bacteria. If you've ever been on antibiotics, eaten food that contains antibiotics, or used other drugs that help promote yeasts like the birth control pill or steroids (like cortisone), you probably have a yeast issue and you will need to be on a probiotic for a long time. How long? Until your spit stays on top of the water with no strings. (The same holds for the rest of these suggestions.)

A probiotic is basically the opposite of an antibiotic. Instead of killing bacteria, it promotes good bacteria growth. (Antibiotic literally means anti-life; therefore probiotic means pro-life.)

A good probiotic will contain at least *Lactobacillus acidophilus* and bifidobacteria. These are actual living bacteria in a powder, capsule, or liquid form. There are many other strains of bacteria that may be beneficial as well, but these two are the main staples. A good probiotic may also contain fructooligosaccharides (FOS), which is food for the bacteria to eat while they're all cooped up inside the bottle. These are sometimes referred to as *pre*biotics. There are also probiotic yeasts that can help. These are good yeasts that help fight the bad yeasts and can be likened to the "soil" of the intestines. They provide the right environment for the flora (the "seed") to live. In many cases, I find these probiotic yeasts are more important to the case than the acidophilus and bifidus are. Standard Process makes two great probiotic yeast products—Zymex and Lactic Acid Yeast. Most probiotic supplements need to be refrigerated, and since these are living bacteria, they *do* expire.

Plain yogurt can also help to maintain healthy flora levels, but I don't believe yogurt by itself is sufficient to treat *Candida*. Acidophilus milk and fermented foods like sauerkraut may help as well.

If your body is overrun with yeast, I also recommend two other products by Standard Process—Spanish Black Radish and Cal Amo. In addition, there are several herbs that can help fight off yeasts. Caprylic acid, pau d'arco, garlic, barberry, ginger, cinnamon, thyme, rosemary, and goldthread are a few I recommend. Taking digestive enzymes and hydrochloric acid with your meals is also important in killing off yeasts, as is supporting the liver.

Getting rid of yeast will have tremendous impact on your life, so please stick with it. When done in combination with the other important steps to health, you won't believe all the nagging problems that will go away.

I also suggest you kill your yeast off slowly. Yeast act as natural chelators of heavy metals. In other words, they attract and hold on to them. When you kill off lots of yeast all at once, your body not only has the dead yeast to deal with but the newly released heavy metals as well. This combination can cause what is called a "healing crisis" or a "yeast die-off reaction." The symptoms can be rather unpleasant and can include anything from itchy skin rashes to flu-like symptoms. To minimize this, make sure your body's "exit channels" are all working well, i.e. that you're not constipated, and that your liver and gall bladder are working well. Start with low doses of any anti-yeast herbs, as well as probiotic yeasts such as Zymex or Lactic Acid Yeast, and go high on doses of those supplements that get yeast and toxins out of the body, such as Spanish Black Radish and garlic.

What to Do After Taking Antibiotics

I suggest that at a bare minimum you take a good probiotic supplement for *at least* six months following any course of antibiotics. Two years would probably be better.

I would also recommend you check yourself for yeast using the spit test as described above. It *may* not show up immediately (as it will take some time for the yeasts to engulf your intestines, move into your bloodstream, and take over your body), so check yourself weekly for a month or so just to make sure.

I can almost guarantee, though, that you *will* have yeast overgrowth following any antibiotic regimen. In fact, unless you've done the *Candida* treatment faithfully for years, never take antibiotics, and never go to restaurants or eat foods that have been treated with antibiotics, I can almost guarantee you have yeast running rampant through your body right now. If you *do* have yeast overgrowth, you'll need to follow the recommendations above for treating *Candida*.

This will need to be done *every time* you take antibiotics. Now, I know what you're thinking..."Jeez, what a pain in the *arse!*" I understand. Sorta makes you want to avoid taking them altogether, doesn't it?

For More Information Read:

Beyond Antibiotics, by Michael A. Schmidt, D.C., Lendon H. Smith, M.D., and Keith W. Sehnert, M.D.

The Yeast Connection, by William Crook, M.D.

The Yeast Syndrome, by John Parks Trowbridge, M.D. and Morton Walker, D.P.M.

Complete Candida Yeast Guidebook, by Jeanne Marie Martin, with Zolton Rona, M.D.

8

Parasites—Look Who Came To Dinner

"Your genes brought you the good things about your ancestors,
not the bad things. Parasites and pollution
brought you the bad things."

—Hulda Clark, Ph.D., N.D.

Patients don't like to hear they have parasites and it's no wonder. They're disgusting and scary creatures who live off of us or off of our food. In fact, parasites can actually cause us to crave the foods that *serve* them but *harm* us. It gives *me* the willies just reading about them, but I feel we must cover this topic because, like it or not, they are one of the reasons we get sick, and most likely (unless you fit into a certain set of classical signs, symptoms, and history) your M.D. won't check for them.

I find parasites fairly regularly in my testing of patients—perhaps 30–40 percent show positive signs for a parasite. Fortunately, the ones I usually find are the protozoan types, which are single-celled organisms and easier to get rid of than the worms, which can lay hundreds of thousands of eggs in a day.

Parasites can take months to get rid of and re-infection is common, especially if someone else in your family or a pet has parasites. For this reason, you may want to just treat everyone in your family and your pets if *any* of you are discovered to have parasites. Many parasites are shed in the feces, so washing your hands thoroughly after petting or being licked by your dog or cat, after cleaning the litter box, changing diapers, picking up after your dog, or any other way you could get fecal matter on your hands is of major importance. But parasites can be acquired in any number of ways including eating fish, sushi, pork, beef, potatoes, fruits, vegetables, or even walking around barefoot in your backyard.

Parasites *can* be in the intestines, in which case they can be found with stool testing, but they can also be in virtually any organ in your body including your brain, liver, lungs, pancreas, and eyes. When they're in these other organs, stool testing won't find them. In these cases, other testing methods must be used.

A few years ago, I heard of a woman in our area who had been diagnosed with a brain tumor. The CT scan showed the very clear outline of a tumor, but when the doctors went in to operate, instead of finding a malignancy, as they suspected, they found a three-foot-long parasite. Ewww! They removed the worm and the woman recovered completely. Apparently, this is fairly common.

The symptoms of parasite infestation can range from none at all, to mild, non-specific symptoms such as anemia, allergies, asthma, appendicitis, or arthritis. Some parasites can even kill you, as can happen with malaria.

Technically, anything that lives off of you can be considered a parasite, which means we could consider bacteria, yeast, fungi, viruses, and teenage children all to be parasites. However, typically, these types of infections are not included when we discuss parasites.

The invaders we typically think of as "parasites" can be divided into two broad categories: the single-celled protozoa (such as *Giardia*) and the worms. The worms can be further divided into flatworms and roundworms. Flatworms include tapeworms, which tend to live in the intestines, and flukes, which can invade virtually any organ. The roundworms include threadworms, pinworms, and hookworms (the only worm with teeth). Included in this family are the worms that cause trichinosis and heart worm. Then, there's a special category of invaders, which is sometimes discussed under the parasite umbrella, called the spirochetes. These corkscrew-shaped bugs are grouped sort of somewhere in between the bacteria and the protozoa, but they tend to lean a bit more toward the bacterial side. For this reason, they are often treated with antibiotics. The spirochete *Treponema pallidum* causes syphilis; the spirochete *Borellia burgdorferi* causes Lyme disease.

Most parasite infections will respond to herbal formulas. My choice for the larger (non-protozoan) parasites is usually either wormwood or black walnut. Garlic is also helpful. Whenever we're dealing with worms that lay eggs, we have patients take the remedy for 10 days, then take five days off. Patients then continue cycling 10 days on and five days off until the worms are all gone and they no longer test for needing the herb.

I also use digestive enzymes to kill parasites. Standard Process makes a great proteolytic enzyme supplement called Zymex II that works well, especially on the protozoa, but it will often work on the bigger parasites as well. In order for it to work best, it needs to be taken away from food—the idea being that we're using the enzymes to "digest" the parasites rather than your food.

If you happen to be lucky enough to have worms in your intestines, sitting in a warm milk bath for an hour or so will sometimes draw the worms out. (Of course, then you're sitting in a bath full of worms, which is not so nice.) Pinworms may also respond to a garlic and milk enema. To do this, you take two cloves of garlic, mash them thoroughly, boil them in six ounces of milk, let it cool, and then strain the garlic out. Then you inject four ounces of this milk into the rectum three nights in a row. After that, wait seven days, and repeat the process. Good luck getting your seven-year-old to agree to this.

Another treatment for parasites is to use something called a Zapper, invented by Hulda Clark, Ph.D., N.D. A Zapper is a battery-operated device that uses a direct current in a certain frequency range to "zap" the parasites. The patient simply holds two brass rods for certain prescribed time periods, and the electricity travels through them killing the worms wherever they may be. (Dr. Clark does claim, however, that if the parasites are in a hollow organ like the intestines, that the electricity may just travel along the outside of the organ and, therefore, miss the worm. For these infections, she recommends going with the herbal remedies.)

Dr. Clark has written several books, each of which discusses her theory that "parasites and pollution," (i.e., chemical toxicity) are the major causes of human disease. She claims that certain chemicals (found in everyday foods and household cleaners), when present in your body, allow parasites to set up permanent housekeeping in your organs much more readily than if you were free of those chemicals. Most, if not all of her books, give instructions on how to build your own Zapper, as well as many suggestions on how to get rid of and prevent parasites.

Whereas Dr. Clark feels that chemical toxicity is behind most of the parasitic infections she finds, other researchers have found that parasites thrive in a body suffering from nutritional deficiencies. One such researcher was Dr. Francis Pottenger. Dr. Pottenger ran a series of experiments between 1932 and 1942 using cats, where he gave one group of cats raw milk, raw meat, and cod liver oil, and the other group of cats cooked (i.e., pasteurized) milk, cooked meat, and cod liver oil.

Cooking any food destroys the enzymes that are naturally present in that food and certain vitamin complexes as well. What

Pottenger found was that the cats receiving the cooked food would always develop degenerative diseases similar to the problems we humans have, such as arthritis, diabetes, vision problems, sexual and fertility problems, etc., and they would often develop parasites. Somewhat counter-intuitively, the cats receiving the raw food *didn't* get parasites, even though they were subjected to the exact same living environment as the other cats! Because they were better nourished, their bodies either didn't make suitable hosts for the parasites to set up camp, or their bodies didn't *produce* the parasites through pleomorphism. If we combine what Dr. Clark tells us with what we've learned from Dr. Pottenger, once again, we can see that the terrain is most important and that the germ (or in this case, *worm*) is nothing.

While living free from toxins and having the perfect diet may very well *prevent* parasites, once you have them, it's wise to go ahead and work both ends of the equation. That means you want to get the proper nutrients into your body, get the chemicals out, and kill the parasites, too. This holistic approach is the best way to make sure you kill the invaders and keep them from coming back.

Muscle Testing and Electrodermal Testing

Though we'll be covering this topic in more detail in a future book, for those of you unfamiliar with muscle testing, I wanted to at least give you a brief description here because it is one of the best and only ways I know of to find parasites, especially when stool testing won't work. Muscle testing (sometimes referred to as Applied Kinesiology, a system that *uses* muscle testing) is a method of combining the body's own intuitive and innate healing abilities with energy medicine.

Let me preface the explanation of this technique by saying that to someone who's never seen or felt this kind of testing, it often sounds a bit like voodoo or something that just can't possibly work.

In fact, I thought that way myself until I actually felt it and saw the incredible results people were getting using this testing method. And though it's used by thousands of practitioners around the globe, the truth is, we really don't know exactly how it works— much like acupuncture. But the fact is, a trained practitioner can use muscle testing to find out virtually anything that's going on in the body.

The way it works is thus: The doctor finds a muscle or muscle group on the patient (typically the deltoid muscle is used) that will hold strong to direct pressure. In other words, the patient holds an arm out and the doctor tries to push it down. If the arm is able to hold strong or "lock" in that position, that's a good muscle to use. Muscles can either be strong or weak, so this is basically a binary testing method. We're looking for a change in the strength of the muscle. More accurately, we're looking for the muscle to either lock, i.e. remain strong, or not to lock, i.e. be weak.

Remembering from your science classes, our bodies (as well as everything else in the universe) are entirely made of energy (protons, neutrons, and electrons whirling around in space) and that energy doesn't stop where our physical bodies stop—it extends out a ways. Furthermore, if I touch you, my energy and your energy are now interacting with each other. Likewise, if you hold a supplement or a food in your hand, the different energies are interacting. Those interactions can be positive, negative, or neutral.

In my office, I test every organ and gland in a patient's body using muscle testing. The patient simply holds his/her arm straight out, I touch over the organ or gland on certain "reflex points" and push down on the outstretched arm. If the arm stays strong, the indication is that the organ is healthy. If the arm goes weak, this indicates that the organ is having some difficulty. We then use test kits, which contain the energetic signatures (similar to homeopathic remedies) of various substances to see if they elicit a change in the testing. For example, if I touch over your heart and your arm goes weak, we would say you have some sort of problem with your heart. If placing a vial containing the energetic signature of a parasite in your hand or on your body makes your arm strong again, we've seen a change in the test, indicating that a parasite is at least part of the problem. We can then remove the parasite vial from your body and look for an anti-parasitic remedy, like wormwood, that also makes your arm go strong again, indicating that that remedy will help the heart by killing the parasite.

Again, I realize that to those unfamiliar with this sort of medicine, muscle testing may sound like something that could never work. The reality is, it works beautifully. Because we're using your body's own innate intelligence rather than some relatively ignorant outside source (like mine) to determine both diagnosis and treatment, it tends to hit the nail right on the head rather than the typical course of trying something for a while, then when that doesn't work trying something else, until finally a cure is (hopefully) stumbled upon. Muscle testing basically takes all the guesswork out of the equation. It also tends to be much safer for the patient because a food, herb, or supplement that's going to cause a problem for a patient will almost always test poorly. Therefore, it will not be given to the patient, thus virtually eliminating any side effects or allergic reactions.

Dorothy is an incredible patient of mine. As I write this, she is currently 84 years old. She's also one of the most active patients I have. I see Dorothy once every four weeks for her monthly chiropractic adjustment. Every time I see her, she tells me about the retaining wall she just built; the transmission she just overhauled; the chicken coop or back porch she just built; or some other such heroic feat. This incredibly upbeat woman basically never sits still. She came to me a few months ago after having had some blood work done by her M.D.—she went in complaining of fatigue and dizziness whenever she bent over. Her doctor told her that she was *severely* anemic and that she would need to have five units of blood pumped into her veins right away. Dorothy didn't like the idea of someone else's blood coursing through her veins, so she came to see me, her "natural doctor." I told her that we needed to find out *why* she was anemic instead of just putting a Band-Aid on the problem and she agreed with this philosophy. I did some muscle testing on her and within a few minutes, found that she had a parasite. I put her on Zymex II and Ferrofood (an iron supplement) and the following month, she reported that her symptoms of dizziness were completely gone and that her blood tests now showed she was only *two* units low. On her next checkup, Dorothy's doctor informed her that she was no longer anemic at all. I fully expected this, as I had found the cause of her problem and knew what to do about it. One of the wonderful side effects of natural corrections like this is that it gives the patient a renewed sense of confidence in his/her body—a *knowing* that it can heal itself of anything once the obstacles to healing are removed.

Electrodermal testing works using a similar philosophy in that we're once again testing energy. Instead of using a muscle test, however, we use a very sensitive ohmmeter to measure the skin's resistance at different acupuncture points. The amount of resistance at these points is directly correlated with the amount of energy or chi present at that point. Through years of testing, we know how much chi *should* be present in these points, and the whole basis of acupuncture is that whenever there is too much or too little chi, the body has a problem. By introducing different substances or energetic signatures into the "circuit," we can see their effect on that acupuncture point. Some things may raise the chi; others may lower it; still others may have no effect. Thus, we can use the readings on these items to make a proper diagnosis and then to help balance the chi in those points and thus in the whole body. So if we find a low reading in your liver meridian and putting the energetic signature for a particular parasite into the circuit changes that reading, we know that that parasite is at least part of the problem. If we then introduce an herb into the circuit and it balances that meridian, we've found the cure for that particular parasitic infection. Thus, we've discovered the way to heal that meridian and by extension, that organ, and eventually the entire body.

Both muscle testing and electrodermal testing can be used to determine hundreds of different problems in patients from allergies, to emotional problems, to nutritional deficiency and toxicity issues, to areas of spinal misalignment, or even dental problems. Parasite testing is but one tiny aspect of these techniques. I only bring them up here because they are among the best ways to find parasites, figure out what will kill them, and to know when they're gone.

For More Information On Parasites, Read:
The Cure For All Diseases, by Hulda Clark, Ph.D., N.D.
Parasites: The Enemy Within, by Hanna Kroeger
Pottenger's Cats: A Study In Nutrition, by Francis Pottenger, M.D.

9

Vaccines: Are They Safe? Do They Work?

"When once an error is accepted by a profession
corporately and endowed by Government,
to uproot it becomes a Herculean task."

—Walter Hadwen, M.D.

There are few issues in all of healthcare that inspire more passionate viewpoints than that of vaccination. This is no doubt because of the age at which we vaccinate. Vaccination is an issue about children's lives and their health.

At the root of this issue is, once again, the germ theory of disease. For those who continue to accept that microscopic invaders are the cause of disease, the theory behind vaccination seems plausible. And of course we've all heard the notion that vaccination has virtually wiped polio and smallpox off of the earth. It seems this "fact" has been pounded into our heads so much that we all accept it without question and then use this to justify subjecting our kids to "routine" vaccinations, with total faith in the so-called science behind them. Once again though, let me remind you that no matter how many times you've heard something, it doesn't necessarily mean it's true.

Vaccinations are a built-in part of every child's "well-baby" visits to his or her pediatrician. Schools, of course, insist that every child be immunized prior to entering—or so they would have you believe. There are also vaccinations to prevent illnesses when we travel and vaccinations to protect our military from bio-weapons. The flu shot is another vaccination that many people subject themselves to every year. In fact, for virtually every malady known, there is either a vaccination already in place, or someone somewhere is working on one. This is a huge issue, so let's jump in.

Before we do, I need to add a short disclaimer. I am assuming you've already read the chapter on the germ theory. As you read this chapter, please keep in mind that all of the information you just learned on pleomorphism and the terrain mattering more than the germs still applies. However, for simplicity's sake, the language I'll be using in this chapter will be worded according to the old germ theory (i.e., such and such a virus causes such and such disease). Just remember, the "terrain" is still, and always has been, the key to avoiding illness. Okay, with that understanding, let's begin.

Vaccines: A Primer

The theory behind vaccination is that vaccines offer protection to the inoculated by artificially stimulating the immune system to produce antibodies against a disease. This antibody response is one way our immune system protects us when we are exposed to a disease. However, vaccines do not affect the body in the same way natural diseases do.

For one thing, by being injected into the body, they bypass many of the immune system's components such as those in the skin, lungs, mouth, digestive tract, nasal passages, etc. These are our body's frontline defense and play a role not only in blocking invading pathogens, but also in activating other immune system components against these tiny invaders should they get through.

Also, vaccines are composed of lab-altered live viruses or killed bacteria. Because they are weakened/altered or dead germs, our immune systems do not mount a full response to them. This partial response means we only get partial immunity—at best.

Vaccines also contain additives such as aluminum, mercury, formaldehyde, sodium chloride, gelatin, antibiotics, sorbitol, phenoxyethanol, yeast protein, phosphate, and glutamate. Many of these components are very toxic to the body as will be discussed throughout this chapter.

So, at best, vaccines offer partial, temporary, artificial immunity rather than the permanent, cell-mediated immunity, which we get from recovering from natural infection. But as you'll read in this chapter, often even this artificial, temporary immunity is elusive. Despite a high rate of vaccination in the population, outbreaks of measles, mumps, chickenpox, pertussis, hemophilus influenza, and the flu still occur among vaccinated individuals.

Another concern is that just as antibiotics have led to stronger bacteria that are immune to all but the strongest of our bug killers, many believe that the vaccination movement has helped to push viruses to mutate faster and cause more virulent diseases. All living organisms adapt to stress: "What doesn't kill us just makes us stronger." Viruses are quite adept at adapting to stress, and trying to weaken or attenuate a virus is definitely a form of stress. Thus, by trying to eliminate all forms of disease through antibiotics and vaccination we are actually helping these germs to evolve, which is leading to even worse forms of disease!

In the past two decades, we've seen the number of doses of vaccines more than double. At the time of this writing, the average American child receives a total of 36 doses of 13 different vaccines by the time he or she is 18 months of age. If s/he takes the yearly flu shot, s/he will receive another 32 by the time s/he graduates from high school for a total of 68 vaccines.[1] And these numbers are still growing. No other country has a vaccination schedule like this. (See the CDC's immunization schedule at the end of this chapter.) At the same time, the number of children suffering from asthma, autism, ADD/ADHD, diabetes, and learning disabilities has *more* than doubled. Other diseases are also on the rise. Look at multiple sclerosis, Alzheimer's disease, chronic fatigue, fibromyalgia, ALS or Lou Gehrig's disease, lupus, Crohn's disease, ulcerative colitis, and other autoimmune disorders.

As you'll see, many people today are blaming vaccines for much of this, and with good reason. Horrifically, more and more parents are reporting that their once healthy children have regressed into autism following vaccination. Doctors, hospitals, schools, healthcare workers, and the government all laud vaccinations as the be all, end all—the Holy Grail of preventive medicine. Is it possible that vaccines could be harming our children? Let's take a closer look.

SMALLPOX

Smallpox is an infectious disease caused by the virus *Orthopox variola*, however before isolating the disease to this agent, smallpox was regarded as divine punishment for crimes unknown. Sometime in the late 1700s, a superstition emerged which said that milkmaids who contracted a mild disease known as cowpox were immune to smallpox. Based on that superstition, an English "physician" named Edward Jenner developed the theory that *cow*pox was actually *small*pox in cows. He further theorized that if you gave a person cowpox (supposedly a mild, non-infectious form of smallpox), it would prevent them from getting full-blown smallpox.

While this may sound like a third grader's approach to healthcare, during the 2001 "smallpox scare" shortly after 9/11, we were *still* using *Orthopox vaccinia*, the virus that causes *cowpox*, to vaccinate against smallpox (*Orthopox variola*).[2] These two viruses have different sizes, shapes, genetic sequences, and characteristics, but most importantly, they cause completely different diseases.[3] This is what is known as "entrenched medical error," and if you look for it, you'll see it everywhere. The term "vaccination" actually comes from the word *vaccinia*, which is Latin for cow. *Sanctus vaccinia! (Holy cow!)* Interestingly, vaccines have *become* the sacred cow of medicine.

In 1796, with nothing more than this superstition to back him, and perhaps the fact that the two diseases have similar names, Jenner withdrew some pus from an infected cowpox pustule, which he got from a milkmaid, and injected it into a healthy 8-year-old boy named James Phipps. With no testing whatsoever, he immediately declared that he had given the boy lifetime immunity against smallpox and went about vaccinating others.

Most people don't know however that James Phipps died at the age of 20, having been vaccinated for smallpox *over 20* times. Jenner's own son died at 21, also having been vaccinated over and over.[4]

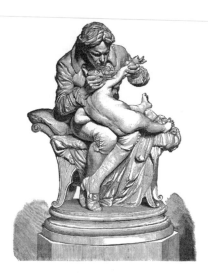

EDWARD JENNER

Like Pasteur, Jenner was not a physician, although both were regarded as such. They were also both amazingly adept at convincing people in high places that their theories were sound enough to make sweeping doctrines based upon them. Jenner, however, saw the value in *having* a medical degree, just not in *earning* one. So, he *bought* one from St. Andrew's College in Scotland for 15 pounds. He never attended the school.[5]

Jenner's colleagues disputed his claim, stating that they knew of dairymaids who had had cowpox, and afterwards had contracted smallpox. Soon thereafter, Jenner admitted that he too had seen many cases of smallpox in milkmaids who had been exposed to cowpox.

Not to be dissuaded, in 1798 Jenner declared that he knew of men who milked cows soon after dressing the heels of horses afflicted with "grease" (a disease distinguished by a disgusting, oily, pus that oozed from the heels of infected horses) and that *these* men were immune to smallpox. Therefore, he theorized, if he were to infect a cow with the rancid horse grease, and then inject children with this new horse grease cowpox, that *they* would have lifetime immunity. At that point, he acknowledged that plain cowpox clearly had no protective virtue.

As it turns out, cowpox is not a natural disease in cows. It is a disease of the udder, which came about after farmers milked their cows with filthy hands—often having just cleaned infections behind horse hooves. Syphilis and tuberculosis were also commonly present in the cowpox lesions from which the vaccine was extracted and many people contracted these diseases from the vaccine.

The public was appalled and wanted nothing to do with this new detestable horse grease vaccination. So, Jenner, very scientifically, bowed to public pressure and went back to using plain cowpox, ignoring the fact that he had only just recently admitted to its worthlessness.

In 1802 and again in 1807, he petitioned the House of Commons for large sums of money claiming that plain cowpox had "the singularly beneficial effect of rendering through life the person so inoculated perfectly secure from the infection of smallpox." [6] Parliament was apparently so impressed with his flowery language, or perhaps so confused by his sentence syntax, that they awarded him £30,000[7] and soon began passing laws to make this untested vaccine compulsory throughout the British Empire. Other European countries soon followed suit.

Soon thereafter, the first cases of smallpox appeared in those who had been vaccinated. At first, Jenner simply denied it. When it became glaringly obvious, he insisted that they had contracted a milder form of the disease. When vaccinated people began dying of smallpox, he claimed these were a result of what he called "spurious" smallpox. He said that when the vaccinated *recovered* from the disease, it was normal smallpox; when they *died*, it was spurious.[8, 9] Sounds scientific.

After Jenner's death in 1823, the vaccine advocates continued making excuses for the failure of the vaccine to protect against smallpox. At one point, they said that one injection site was incomplete and ineffective and advocated giving two or more injections. (The current standard is 15 punctures with a double pointed needle, after which a scab forms, followed by a vesicle.) One source recommended giving the shots in at least four different sites. (Keep in mind that the needles of the time were made of ivory and probably not that sharp.) When that was seen to be ineffective, they said that, "Vaccine prophylaxy is only real and complete when periodically renewed." Thus, the birth of the "booster" shot. They said that patients should be vaccinated again and again "until vesicles cease to respond to the insertion of virus." [10] A vesicle is considered "proof" that the vaccine "took." The theory was and still is: If no vesicle forms, the patient is immune.[11] There is no scientific basis for this theory whatsoever.

When even *this* failed to protect patients, they tried a new tactic—falsifying legal documents. Vaccinated patients who died of smallpox were listed as *un*vaccinated on their death certificates.[12] Another ploy was to use creative diagnoses. When the unvaccinated came down with smallpox, it was labeled as such, but when a vaccinated patient came down with smallpox, it was listed as "pustular eczema" or anything besides smallpox.[13] Other names used included "varioloid" and "monkeypox." In this way, they improved their statistics greatly.

Before England began its mandatory vaccination campaign in 1853, no more than 2,000 people ever died of smallpox in any two-year period.[14] In the period of 1857–1859, 14,244 people died of smallpox. In the period of 1863–1865, 20,059 people died of smallpox. In response to the increasing epidemic, in 1867, Parliament enacted even stricter vaccination laws. So what happened then, with a full 97 percent of the British population vaccinated? In the year 1868 alone, 44,840 people died of smallpox.[15] Pretty effective vaccine, huh?

Germany, Italy, France, Japan, the Philippines, and other countries saw similar statistics.[16, 17] Prussia passed a mandatory vaccination law in 1834. Every infant was vaccinated for smallpox. They were revaccinated upon entering school, again upon graduation, and every male was vaccinated yet again when they entered the army (and all men went into the army). After 35 years of nearly 100 percent vaccination, Prussia saw nearly 125,000 of its people die of smallpox in a single year.[18] In fact, all of the statistics show that the more people were vaccinated, the more people died of smallpox. (See below.)

Ten-Year Period Ending:	Percent of Babies Vaccinated:	Smallpox Deaths (per million):
1881	96.5	3,708
1891	82.1	933
1901	67.9	437
1911	67.6	395
1921	42.3	12
1931	43.1	25
1941	39.9	1

(Figures represent official statistics from England and Wales)[19]

It seems obvious from the statistics that as the governments of these countries persuaded more and more people to be vaccinated, more people died of smallpox. As the people realized what was happening and fewer and fewer people accepted the shots, fewer people died of smallpox. Also, improvements in sanitation and other improvements in people's way of life helped boost their natural immunity until eventually the disease was completely wiped out. At that point, the vaccine advocates took full credit for ridding the world of this deadly disease.

The U.S. didn't begin vaccinating for smallpox until 1902. England finally got wise and stopped compulsory vaccinations in 1907. Australia quit in 1925. Holland quit in 1928.[20] The U.S. continued until 1971. We were the last holdout in the world, and for 30 years, the only source of death from smallpox in the U.S. was the vaccine itself.[21] Although we had only begun vaccinating in 1902, by 1929 almost every state had decided against compulsory vaccinations because there were just too many complications.[22]

More people died from the smallpox vaccine than any other vaccine in history.[23]

POLIO

Poliomyelitis is a disease that affects the gray matter of the spinal cord and brain stem. Its main symptoms are paralysis and atrophy of the arms and legs. Early symptoms include sore throat, nausea, and fever. Later, victims become weak and have abnormal sensations in the arms or legs. If it attacks the part of the brainstem that controls breathing, it can be deadly.

The official story is that polio is caused by the poliovirus. However, 90 percent of those who carry the poliovirus never have any symptoms at all.[24] Another five percent have only mild symptoms and fully recover with no permanent damage.[25] The only way to catch the "wild" virus (there are actually three polio viruses) is from an infected person. The virus is found in soil and the stools and enters through the mouth, which is why infants and small children are the ones most at risk for catching it. The virus proliferates in the gut, then makes its way to the spinal cord or brain stem and begins destroying motor neurons, which can lead to paralysis.

People who lived through the polio epidemic in the first half of the twentieth century had fear instilled in their hearts and are still haunted by memories of children in leg braces and pictures of row after row of children in "iron lungs." Most people know President FDR was afflicted with the disease and bound to a wheelchair or forced to use leg braces much of his life.

Polio has been around for centuries, perhaps millennia, but it had never been epidemic until the late 1800s. Prior to that, polio had been associated largely with metal workers, but in the epidemic of which we speak, it struck middle-class, American children, mostly in the summer and autumn—odd behaviors for a virus. Other countries, even where there was poor sanitation, starvation, and overcrowding (conditions most often associated with the spread of infectious diseases), were much less affected by polio.

When the epidemic started, with the electron microscope not having been invented yet, viruses were not much more than a theory. In fact, the germ theory itself was still in its early phases, having been refined somewhat from Pasteur's day by Robert Koch and others. And while many at the time believed that polio was caused by a toxin of some sort, quite possibly a heavy metal (why else would it have been associated with metal workers?), those who blindly put their faith in the germ theory concluded that polio *must* be caused by a virus because try as they might, they could not find a bacterium in the diseased tissues. So, the search for the poliovirus was on.

As you'll see later in Chapter 12, it was precisely this same sort of tunnel vision thinking that led to the HIV theory of AIDS overtaking the toxicity theory, despite the latter having better science and several doctors reporting *cures* simply by having their patients abstain from drugs (both the prescribed kind *and* the illegal kind).

Much like the story of smallpox, the science behind finding the poliovirus and creating the vaccine was rather crude. One of the first "breakthrough experiments" on polio came in 1909, when Carl Landsteiner and Erwin Popper ground up the spinal cord of a nine-year-old boy who had died of the disease, made a solution of that tissue, passed it through filters that would extract anything bacteria-sized and larger (on the overly simplistic assumption that viruses would be all that's left), then injected the solution into two monkeys' brains. One of the monkeys died immediately. The other was slowly paralyzed and developed lesions on its spinal cord that appeared "similar to polio." This experiment was considered "proof" that polio was caused by a virus, and is still celebrated by the World Health Organization as the first isolation of the poliovirus. (See box below.) But when Landsteiner and Popper ground up these monkeys' spinal cords and injected them into other monkeys, they failed to pass on the paralysis.

Virologists apparently have a different definition of the word "isolate" than the rest of us. When I think of isolating something, I tend to think of it as being all by itself, but when they say they *isolated a virus*, it simply means they think they *found* it; *not* that they've created a pure culture of it. Remember this while reading the rest of this book.

In 1910, Simon Flexner and Paul Lewis performed a similar experiment, but rather than grinding up the monkeys' spinal cords, they simply extracted some fluid from their brains and injected that into the next set of monkeys. This experiment *did* successfully pass on the paralysis, and continued to do so for several series of monkeys. However, they found that the mixture had to be injected directly into the monkey's brain and that if it were drunk or injected elsewhere, that it had no effect on the monkeys.

The two experiments described above are celebrated as the first time a virus was proven to be the cause of a disease. Yet as Janine Roberts says in her outstanding book *Fear of the Invisible*, "How could a scientist credibly claim that injecting cellular debris into the skull of a monkey proves a virus to cause polio?" [26] After all, there are many things that will pass through these filters besides viruses, including broken up cell bits, neurotransmitters, enzymes, DNA fragments, toxins, and prions/somatids. Also, *this is foreign material being injected directly into the brain.* This is hardly a normal route of infection.

In 1913, Henry Fauntleroy Harris injected filtered tissue from pellagra patients into monkeys and observed that they developed something similar to pellagra. He concluded from this experiment that pellagra was caused by a virus. If we had restricted our search for the cause of pellagra to viruses (as we did with polio, and now AIDS), we might never have discovered that it was easily cured with B vitamins. [27]

Other experiments performed in the 1920s and 1930s also involved grinding up spinal cords and brains as well as many other things, including fecal matter and flies, and injecting them into the brains of monkeys, none of which proved much of anything.

In 1932, the electron microscope was invented, and in 1933, FDR was elected president. Roosevelt started the March of Dimes and pumped all kinds of money into finding the cure for the disease that had crippled him as a child. But even with this advanced technology, tons of money, the support of the federal government, and a vast public outcry, by 1945 (37 years after the virus had supposedly been isolated and five *decades* into the epidemic) the virus hunters were still unable to find a virus in the nervous tissue of polio victims. Rather than accept defeat or consider possibilities other than germs (like toxins), they tried another tack.

In 1948, Gilbert Dalldorf and Grace Sickles diluted the feces of polio victims, treated it with ether to kill the bacteria, centrifuged out the big particles (cells, bacteria, etc.), and then injected the remaining material (toxins, proteins, prions, enzymes, viruses, broken fragments of cells, DNA, and who knows what else) into the brains of three-to seven-day-old mice. Amazingly, when the tiny, suckling mice became paralyzed and the researchers subsequently found a (scapegoat?) virus under the electron microscope, they claimed to have isolated the virus that causes polio. Again, this is incredibly shoddy science. Injecting poop soup into a mouse pup's noodle and producing paralysis proves positively nothing, especially knowing that the "poliovirus" was probably produced by pleomorphism (see box below). It's preposterous! And yet, this experiment led to the current theory, which is that the poliovirus somehow makes its way from the digestive tract to the spinal cord of its victims and begins destroying cells there. How this supposedly happens has never been adequately described, much less demonstrated, nor have they ever to this day found the virus anywhere in the vicinity of the spinal cord destruction!

It is now known that the poliovirus is produced by cells in the human intestine, meaning it's not an invader at all. It has recently been re-classified as a human enterovirus.

These feces-derived suspensions, which they referred to as "viral isolates," were much cheaper to work with and more easily accessible than ground up human spinal cords and monkey brains. In addition, they had the added benefit that one could actually find and demonstrate viruses in fecal matter, whereas they seemed to be totally absent in the actual diseased tissue. (Reminds me of the old joke where the guy is looking for his keys under the streetlight because the light is better there than where he actually dropped them.) These same suspensions were also used as the seed lots for the upcoming vaccine experiments. In fact, the Salk vaccine actually came from the feces of three *healthy* (i.e., they didn't have polio) children. Before I go on to describe the vaccine, let's first go back to the *other* theory of polio—the one that suspected toxins as being the cause.

The Toxin Theory of Polio

In one of the earliest medical reports on polio written in 1894, Dr. Charles Caverly, the Government Inspector of Vermont, noted that the families who were affected by polio usually did not know each other and that it did not seem to spread within families, even when there was no attempt to isolate the victim. He, therefore, ruled it out as being a contagious disease. He also noted that it often struck after the child had eaten some fruit. He concluded that polio was probably caused by a toxin rather than a germ.

What toxin? Well, it just so happens that around that same time in Vermont (1892 to be exact), the apple farmers had begun spraying their crops, up to 12 times each summer, with a new pesticide that contained lead and arsenic. This was done to kill the codling moths. The timing of this lead arsenate spraying tied in well with the facts that the polio epidemic always struck in the summer and fall; that its victims often became ill after eating fruit; and that it struck first in orchard-rich New England. It also tied in with the fact that metal workers who worked with lead and arsenic had also been frequent victims of polio. The toxin theory also explained why farmyard chickens and other animals would often be paralyzed at the same time as the children. (As viruses don't usually jump species, the poliovirus, a human enterovirus, should not have affected these animals, unless it was injected into their brains, that is.) In fact, *the pesticides used on the apple trees actually worked by paralyzing the moths so that they eventually suffocated!* (Remember, this is also how the victims of polio died and why they were put in iron lungs.) So, it was really not a big leap to suspect that this pesticide may cause similar problems in children, especially since toxins (even in minute amounts) can accumulate over time in nervous tissue. They say hindsight is 20/20, but you have to wonder sometimes how they could have been so blind to have missed this connection.

The United Kingdom banned apples from the U.S. during that era because of the lead arsenate issue. Perhaps not surprisingly, they also had far fewer cases of polio than we had. Also, many former apple orchards in the U.S. are now listed as health hazards. Building is not allowed to take place there without first removing all of the poisoned soil.

In 1824, the English scientist, John Cooke, observed, "The fumes of these metals [lead and arsenic], or the receptance of them in solution into the stomach, often causes paralysis." [28] In 1878, Alfred Vulpian discovered that lead damages the motor neurons of dogs, and in 1883, Russian scientists found that arsenic does the same thing.[29] Again, this is the very part of the nervous system that's affected by polio—the part where they just can't seem to find the virus, even with today's technology.

In 1907, calcium arsenate was introduced for use on cotton crops. A year later, a Massachusetts town claiming three cotton mills *and* apple orchards, was struck with 69 cases of paralytic polio.[30]

Some cases of polio were associated with drinking milk. And wouldn't you know it, at that time, lead arsenate was also used in the cow dip. Formaldehyde (embalming fluid) was also added to milk back then in order to prolong its shelf life. In 1897, the *Australian Gazette* reported several cases of paralysis caused by formaldehyde in milk.[31]

The DPT vaccine, introduced in the mid-1940s, also corresponded with a vast increase in the number of polio cases seen. Coincidentally, the paralysis almost invariably occurred in the vaccinated arm.[32] As you'll read later, the DPT shot contained formaldehyde, mercury, and aluminum.

Also in the mid-1940s, the organochlorine pesticide known as DDT was introduced. The National Institutes of Health reported in 1944 that DDT worked by damaging the anterior horn cells (motor neurons) of the spinal cord, thus causing paralysis.[33] But since flies and household pests were often blamed for the spread of polio, DDT was used and promoted as a way of *preventing* polio. (Something very similar to this is now happening with the paralysis currently being blamed on the West Nile Virus, as you'll read in Chapter 13.) Though DDT was known to be highly toxic and deadly to *other* animals, people were told that it was harmless to humans.

Thus, it was sprayed in kitchen cabinets, directly on the skin, on bedding, and clothing. Children's rooms were even covered in wallpaper soaked in DDT.

At the end of WWII, Americans stationed in the Philippines were often afflicted with polio, and yet the Filipinos in the neighboring settlements were not.[34] The main difference seemed to be that the U.S. military camps were sprayed daily with DDT to kill mosquitoes, while the surrounding areas were not.

DDT was also linked to an outbreak of polio in the United Kingdom town of Broadstairs, Kent where the cows from a certain dairy were washed down with the chemical. When milk from the dairy was stopped, the outbreak ended.[35]

In 1949, Endocrinologist Dr. Morton Biskind found that DDT caused "lesions in the spinal cord resembling those in human polio." [36] Biskind believed that polio was caused by pesticides and presented evidence of this to Congress in 1950.[37] This evidence was ignored, however, most likely because we had already invested so much time and effort into proving that polio was caused by a virus.

That same year in Germany, Daniel Dresden found that acute DDT poisoning produced "degeneration in the central nervous system" just like those found in infantile paralysis (a.k.a. polio).[38] Dr. Ralph Scobey found clear evidence of poisoning in the blood and urine of polio victims. He discovered a chemical called porphyrin in the urine (we'll be discussing this lab finding in a future book when we talk about dental toxins) and guanidine in the blood, both of which indicate poisoning has taken place.[39] A more recent study also reported that organophosphate insecticides impede nerve messages to muscles through their anti-cholinesterase effect, thus causing weakness and paralysis.[40]

Perhaps even more convincingly, many people were cured of polio and post polio syndrome using detoxification methods. Dr. Biskind found that simply eliminating the offending toxin from the person's diet often did the trick—especially contaminated milk and butter products.[41] In 1951, Dr. Irwin Eskwith reported curing a child who had been paralyzed by polio using the anti-toxin dimercaprol.[42] Dr. F. R. Klenner reported in the *Journal of Southern Medicine and Surgery* in 1949, that he had cured 17 cases of acute polio using high doses of ascorbic acid. These cures all took place after only *72 hours* of such treatment![43]

By 1951, health authorities were starting to see the light—sort of. They finally realized that DDT and other pesticides could cause health issues in humans. Though they didn't admit to its link with polio, the U.S. Public Health Service reported, "DDT is excreted in the milk of cows and of nursing mothers after exposure to DDT sprays and after consuming food contaminated with this poison. Children and infants especially are much more susceptible to poisoning than adults." [44]

This led to a phasing out of DDT and other persistent organochlorides in this country, with a concomitant *increase* of them in Third-World countries (which is probably why polio is still so prevalent there despite all our vaccination efforts). In the U.S. and other industrialized countries, DDT was replaced with safer, less persistent chemicals. Thus, by 1955, when the Salk vaccine was finally introduced, the number of infantile paralysis cases in the U.S. was less than half of what it had been in 1952—just three years prior. (The DDT years, between its inception in the mid-1940s and its phasing out, beginning in 1952, were the worst years of the polio epidemic since 1916. The number of polio cases *tripled* in that time.[45] In the U.K., cases of infantile paralysis dropped by more than 82 percent between 1950 and the first administration of the vaccine in 1957.)[46]

Many doctors and scientists of the time (those who were not completely entranced by the germ theory) believed pesticides and other paralysis-inducing toxins were the cause of polio, not some magical, mysterious virus. But despite all the evidence for this, the authorities (who *were* and still *are* entranced by the germ theory) chose to believe that polio was caused by a virus that was found in the stools of *some* polio victims but not others, was found in the stools of many patients who did *not* have polio, and was *never* found in the diseased spinal cords of said victims.

The viral theory of polio is based on very dubious and illogical science—if one can *call* such a thing "science." It offers no explanation for the summer/fall timing of the epidemic, nor does it even offer a *theory* as to how the virus can affect the spinal cord without actually being present there. It also ignores several other facts, offering no explanation for how metalworkers are apparently more prone to catching the virus, or how *insects and animals* are paralyzed by DDT, but *humans* aren't. Et cetera. By contrast, the toxin theory answers all these questions and more.

In science, when two theories are competing with one another, generally the more elegant theory, that is, the one that answers the most questions without having to invent radical new theories to fill in holes is viewed as the correct theory until proven otherwise. In this case, the toxin theory wins hands down. But, thanks to Pasteur and all his germ theory cronies, any theory regarding toxicity, especially *chronic* or long-term exposure as a cause of human suffering, is relegated to the field of quackery. So, science was thrown aside, and polio was blamed on a poop virus.

As you'll see in Chapter 13, this same pattern of blaming viruses rather than toxins continues to plague Western medicine today. It seems we still have not heeded Pasteur's final warning that "The germ is nothing; the terrain is everything."

The Polio Vaccine

Once the poliovirus was "isolated" (as described above), the race to discover an effective vaccine was on. But the science that went into producing *this* vaccine was really not much better than the cowpox pus and horse grease injections Jenner and his cronies had used with their dangerous and ineffective smallpox vaccines. Since the so-called poliovirus is a human pathogen (that is, it's only found naturally in humans), the vaccine researchers decided that chimps and monkeys would be the best animals to use for experimentation and the actual production of vaccine.

In order to make a vaccine, especially when one wants to vaccinate the entire population multiple times, one needs *lots* of viruses. This presents a bit of a problem. Not only are viruses incredibly tiny and hard to find (and probably *impossible* to actually isolate), they cannot grow in a pure culture because by themselves they don't have the machinery to reproduce. The current understanding (i.e., official story) is that viruses reproduce by invading a cell and then using that cell's machinery to make copies of itself. That meant vaccine researchers needed a huge supply of living cells to grow polioviruses on.

So, what they did was basically this: They caught monkeys in the wild, shipped them to labs in the U.S., anesthetized the monkeys, surgically removed their kidneys (and sometimes their testicles), then killed the monkeys. Then they ground up the kidneys and introduced their poliovirus "isolates" (poop soup) to the mashed up organs (mutilated monkey meat) and allowed the viruses to reproduce.

One doctor, Hilary Koprowski, rather than using the fecal matter "isolates," used the ground up spinal cord of a polio victim to produce his vaccine, assuming the virus *must* be there, even though it's never been found there. He then injected this human spinal cord/monkey kidney mash into the brain of a mouse, waited a few days, then took some fluid from the mouse's brain and injected this into another mouse's brain. He repeated this process until he had "infected" seven series of mice. From the final mouse, he removed the brain fluid and injected this into the brains of *monkeys*. When the monkeys survived, he assumed his vaccine was safe, but just to be sure, before trying it on humans, he "passaged" his vaccine through one more species—a series of three cotton rats. At that point, he finally deemed his concoction was safe enough to inject back into humans.[47]

> Jonas Salk admitted to killing 17,000 monkeys and chimps just in *developing* his vaccine. Albert Sabin admitted to killing 9,000 monkeys in developing *his* vaccine. All told, many millions of monkeys have been killed in our quest to rid the world of polio.

This "passaging" of a vaccine through other animals is referred to as attenuating a virus. An attenuated virus is supposedly weakened to the point where it won't cause the actual disease, but just stimulate the immune system to produce antibodies. This process supposedly makes the virus weaker because it forces it to mutate many times. There are at least two problems with this theory: One, nobody knows what this mutated virus is really capable of when they finally try the vaccine on humans. It could be weaker or it could be stronger, but one thing is for sure, it's *different* from anything found in nature. And two, since it's no longer the same virus and antibodies are very specific, how can our immune system possibly be primed to fight the real one if and when it shows up?

> *"In point of fact, we [are practicing] biological engineering*
> *on a rather large scale by use of live viruses*
> *in mass immunization campaigns."*
>
> —Joshua Lederberg, Department of Genetics, Stanford Medical School [48]

Albert Sabin's oral sugar cube vaccine was similarly attenuated by passaging the virus through many different species of animals.

Jonas Salk, however, *killed* the poliovirus for his vaccine, or at least, he tried. He killed it by simply mixing in some formaldehyde just prior to use, but there were no tests to *make sure* the viruses were all dead; it was just assumed. (See box below.) Then, they added sodium bisulfate to "neutralize" the formaldehyde. Again, no tests were run to make sure it was all neutralized. This concoction of "dead" viruses and trace amounts of formaldehyde was then injected into the patient. But wait. Didn't someone prove that formaldehyde could cause paralysis? Yes. Glad you've been paying attention.

In reality, viruses are not considered living organisms, so the idea of "killing" them is actually a misnomer. As you'll read in later chapters, viruses are nothing more than tiny bits of DNA or RNA encapsulated in a protein shell. Therefore, "inactivated" is probably a more accurate term.

In 1951, several vaccine researchers reported that they had not been able to find the poliovirus in many of the polio patients they had been working with. In some cases, they found *other* viruses and the discoverers proposed that *these* viruses might cause polio as well. But a multiple virus theory seemed to indicate that a vaccine would either be more expensive, less effective, or both. It also didn't follow one of the main change to tenets of the germ theory—that one bug is responsible for each disease—and so the theory was discarded as a possibility and these findings were quietly swept under the carpet. Again, you can see how scientific this all is.

Safety of the Vaccine

Testing of the various polio vaccines took place on prisoners, the mentally retarded, and on children in foreign countries, including Ireland, Poland, tens of millions of Russian children, and more than a quarter million in the Congo area of Africa.[49]

Whether attenuated (altered) or killed (inactivated), both polio vaccines (Sabin and Salk) are grown on monkey kidneys. Even today, these vaccines are *far* from the pure cultures of isolated poliovirus that you might have imagined (had you ever given it a second thought, that is). As mentioned, this degree of isolation is probably impossible (and certainly cost prohibitive) even with today's technology.

You must understand that most of what we "know" about viruses is merely theoretical because they're just so damn small—*much* smaller than bacteria. So, you can't just pop your sample under a microscope and determine whether or not it's pure. You have to run complex tests, and even then, you can only test for things we're aware of and have tests for.

The result of all of this is that between 1955 and 1963, 98 million Americans were injected with polio vaccines that were contaminated with a virus called SV40 (Simian Virus #40).[50–54] By 1961, more than 90 percent of U.S. children, and many millions of adults had received the vaccine. SV40 is a monkey virus that has been linked with cancer in humans and rodents. Researchers like Dr. Michele Carbone of Loyola University, and Dr. Joseph Testa, a molecular geneticist, consider SV40 a cancer-causing virus. Its distinctive DNA pattern has been found in previously rare brain tumors (ependymomas), bone tumors (osteosarcomas), lung tumors (mesotheliomas), leukemia, non-Hodgkins Lymphoma, and other human cancers.[55, 56] All of these tumors are on the rise, not only in adults who received SV40 in their polio vaccines, but in their children as well.

Mesothelioma (a malignant tumor of the lining in the chest and abdomen) had previously been thought to be caused solely by chronic exposure to asbestos, but 20–50 percent of people diagnosed with the condition have not had long-term exposure to the substance. Dr. Carbone has found SV40 in 60 percent of those with mesothelioma and he states that, "clearly, it [SV40] is a risk factor in developing this disease." Nearly 3,000 people die of mesothelioma every year in the U.S. alone.[57]

It appears that SV40 may be transmitted from mother to child through the placenta and may also be passed through blood transfusions and sexual contact. It's been detected in human semen and in tumors of children who've never received the contaminated vaccine.[58] It's feared that the virus may have integrated itself into the human genome and can now be passed on to the offspring of those who received the virus via the polio vaccine. In other words, *the polio vaccine very likely caused at least one wild monkey virus to enter human cells and thereby permanently altered the human genome!* As Cecil Fox, a senior scientist with the National Institutes of Health from 1973–1991 says, "When you inject ground-up monkey guts into children, all kinds of things can happen." [59]

"Great," you say. "When did they find out about this virus?" Well, Dr. Bernice Eddy, the scientist in charge of safety testing the vaccine at the National Institutes of Health (NIH), reported *something* (she called it a toxic substance) in the Salk vaccine was paralyzing monkeys as early as 1954. (These "safety tests" on monkeys were being done *at the same time* millions of U.S. children were being injected with the vaccine.) Dr. Eddy's report was ignored, however. In fact, she was sharply reprimanded by her boss and ordered to stop all work on the polio vaccine. Thankfully, she ignored that order and continued working on the Salk vaccine in secret. In 1959, she injected 154 hamsters with the vaccine and found that within 18 months 70 percent of the hamsters had grown tumors.[60] She reported this to her boss, and again was severely reprimanded, this time for doing unauthorized research. In October 1960, she gave a talk to a New York Cancer Society and mentioned that something in the polio vaccine was causing cancer. Eddy returned to an even harsher scolding, had her lab taken away, was prevented from attending professional meetings, and soon found that none of her research would be accepted anywhere. Bernice Eddy had been blackballed.[61] SV40 was *officially discovered* that same year. "What did they do about it?" you ask. Well, they didn't want to worry you, so they just kept their mouths shut and kept on infecting, I mean, injecting you.

"The discovery in 1960 that a DNA tumor virus, designated simian virus 40 (SV40) was an inadvertent contaminant of rhesus monkey cells, and consequently of the poliovirus and adenovirus vaccines made in these cells, was a watershed event in vaccine development..."

—FDA, 1997

Dr. Maurice Hilleman was Merck's top vaccine researcher at that time and was in charge of the Salk Vaccine. His job was to find a way to outperform/out-market Albert Sabin's oral sugar cube vaccine, which was then being tested on millions of Russian children. Sabin's vaccine was said to be cheaper, easier to administer, and more effective than the Salk, so the competition was fierce. Hilleman thought the SV40 angle could possibly give his employer a nice edge. He thought, since the Salk vaccine used formaldehyde to kill the poliovirus, this should inactivate the SV40 virus as well. So, he went to work.

As suspected, SV40 *was* detected in Sabin's vaccine and when it was injected into hamsters (remember, this was the competitor's *oral* vaccine), it caused them to grow tumors. Scientists working on the project joked that the U.S. would beat the Russians in a future Olympics because the Russians would be so loaded down with tumors, they wouldn't be able to run. In June 1960, Hilleman announced to the Second International Conference on the Polio Vaccine that he had found SV40 in every sample of Sabin's vaccine he tested.[62] (See box below.) He also stated that the virus was ubiquitous, i.e., it was found in *all* monkey kidney samples. This announcement backfired, however, because another researcher soon found that SV40 survived for *30 days* in formaldehyde, indicating the Salk Vaccine would also contain live SV40 as well.[63] Hilleman then reproduced Bernice Eddy's hamster experiment, finding that his employer's vaccine also caused hamsters to grow tumors.

When Sabin heard Hilleman's report, he said, "This is just another obfuscation that is going to upset vaccines." Years later, when questioned about it again, Sabin said, "I think to release certain information prematurely is not a public service. There's too much scaring the public unnecessarily. Oh, your children were injected with a cancer virus and all that. That's not very good." Regarding the secrecy surrounding this issue, Hilleman himself said, "It was important not to convey to the public [this] information, because you could start a panic. They already had production problems with people getting polio [from the shots]. If you added to that the fact that they found live [monkey] virus in the vaccine, there would have been hysteria." [64]

At that point, SV40 was known to cause cancer in hamsters and other animals, but had not yet been proven to cause cancer in *humans*. So, for a while, the vaccine promoters were able to use this lame excuse to continue infecting us. But in 1961, SV40 was proven to cause cancer in human cells as well.[65] What did they do *then*? Pretty much the same thing—nothing. Well, they did *something*; they covered it up.

You might think these cover-ups were all part of the pharmaceutical companies' efforts to protect their investment here, but Merck actually told the Surgeon General, Dr. Leroy Burney, that they thought it unwise to continue making either type of polio vaccine until the SV40 issue was adequately handled. Burney begged them to continue making the vaccine, citing the above excuse—that it hadn't been proven to cause *human* cancers yet. In May of 1961, Merck finally came to the conclusion that they *couldn't* make the vaccine safe, so they simply stopped making polio vaccines altogether. In June, Maurice Hilleman (of Merck) told the government's Safety Technical Committee that it should withdraw use of the Salk vaccine as the contamination with SV40 was a "fearful thing," but the committee refused. At that point, the government found another pharmaceutical company, Lederle, who was willing to look the other way regarding SV40 and produce the unclean vaccine for them. The FDA then instructed Lederle scientists to only test their vaccine for SV40 contamination for 14 days, as the virus wouldn't show up in the tests for at least 21–28 days. This allowed them to say that they had tested the lots for SV40 and found them to be clean, even though they most certainly were not. This is how it is still being done today.

Ironically, and luckily for Sabin, the process of digestion inactivated or killed the SV40 in his sugar cube vaccine. Patients who received *this* form of vaccine do not have detectable SV40 antibodies. However, as of January 2000, the Sabin vaccine is no longer being used in the United States (except in rare instances) because of the nasty side effect of it sometimes *causing* polio. (It is, however, still used in many underprivileged countries.) So now, in the U.S., we're back to using the Salk vaccine. People who have received this type of polio vaccine *do* have SV40 antibodies in their blood, indicating they've been infected by the virus.[66] If you, or your parents, or perhaps any of your sexual partners received the Salk vaccine, you may have SV40 in your genes along with possibly dozens of other monkey viruses that are simply not tested for.

Was AIDS Caused by the Polio Vaccine?

There are many interesting theories on where AIDS came from (some of which we'll be covering in Chapter 12), but several of them point to monkey viruses somehow mutating and getting mixed up with humans. Edward Hooper, author of *The River: A Journey to the Source of HIV and AIDS* suggests that Hilary Koprowski's oral polio vaccine, administered to 325,000 Africans over three years beginning in 1957, may have been contaminated with a monkey virus called SIV (Simian Immunodeficiency Virus). This virus is similar to HIV (though it does not cause immune deficiency in monkeys or humans and thus is misnamed) and some think it could have evolved or mutated into HIV.[67] The attenuation process, described above, could certainly account for this mutation if SIV was present in the kidney tissues used to grow the virus.

In an article, which appeared in a 1959 issue of the *British Medical Journal*, Albert Sabin reported that he had discovered an "unidentified cell-killing virus" in the vaccine being used in the Belgian Congo area of Africa. Interestingly, according to some sources, the first known case of "AIDS" appeared in the Belgian Congo in 1959. Within the next few years, several more cases were reported in the same area. The area where this vaccination effort was most concentrated, Burundi, the Congo, and Rwanda, are now considered to be the center of the AIDS epidemic.[68] Coincidence?

This hypothesis was reported in *The Lancet* in 1992 in an article titled: "Simian Retroviruses, Polio Vaccine, and the Origin of AIDS." [69] On March 19, 1992, *Rolling Stone* picked this up and ran a story called: "The Origin of AIDS; A Startling New Theory Attempts to Answer the Question 'Was It an Act of God or an Act of Man?'" [70]

But why was AIDS so concentrated in the gay community here? Here's one theory. In the U.S. in the late 1970s homosexual men were given a stronger version of the oral polio vaccine as a treatment for genital herpes.[71] (*"But polio and herpes are two completely different viruses,"* you say. *"How could giving one possibly help with the other?"* Good question! Remember that thing about giving cowpox shots to prevent smallpox? This is kind of like that. It's all very scientific. Hey, don't look behind that curtain!) Since oral polio is a live vaccine and the poliovirus is found in the stools, this provides a logical way for the dissemination of the disease among gay men.

SV40, which we've already discussed, is also a powerful immunosuppressor, and quite possibly a trigger for HIV. In fact, it has been reported to cause a condition similar to AIDS.[72]

Biologist Richard de Long wrote:

During the last twenty years a number of new and very serious diseases has arisen. Some of these are Reye's syndrome, Kawasaki disease, Lassa fever, Marburg disease, non-A non-B hepatitis [now called hepatitis C], Ebola hemorrhagic fever, and acquired immune deficiency syndrome... Since 1961 we have been immunizing the human population with attenuated viral vaccines en masse. Such unparalleled use of live viral vaccines may be the reason for the appearance of new diseases... Since most humans in the world are now harboring live vaccine viruses of different kinds within their cells, the probability of genetic recombination between these viruses and other viruses as they infect cells becomes quite high... All the new diseases listed above appeared after the mass administration of the live poliomyelitis vaccine and followed by mass immunization with other live viral vaccines.[73]

Though there is certainly some fairly strong circumstantial evidence for this theory, as you'll read in Chapter 12, there are better explanations for what caused the AIDS crisis. Also, after publication of *The River*, they supposedly checked the original vaccine lots used in those areas of Africa and found no SIV or HIV contamination.

Did The Polio Vaccine Really Wipe Out Polio?

The Salk and Sabin vaccines are generally given credit for wiping out polio. In fact, when people defend vaccination as being an effective public health measure, they usually point to how well it worked for polio. But the reality of the situation is actually very similar to what we've just seen with the smallpox vaccine. Whether polio is truly caused by the poliovirus, by heavy metals in pesticides, by some other toxin, or some combination, by all accounts, its incidence had waned tremendously long before the government launched its mass administration of the Salk polio vaccine on April 12, 1955. In fact, it was all but gone by then. Once the vaccine was introduced, however, the disease seemed to make a comeback.

> When epidemics strike, people begin a natural quarantine process. When there's an outbreak at school or your child is sick, you simply keep your kids at home. My father told me how his parents wouldn't let him go into town or swim in the public pool when he was young because of their fear of polio. Also, as mentioned in the section on smallpox, sanitation, hygiene, and living conditions were continuing to improve throughout this time with the advent of indoor plumbing, etc.

Only 13 days after the vaccine's launch, where it had been described as one of the greatest medical discoveries of the century, the Salk Vaccine hit its first major snag, known as The Cutter Incident. The problem: Cutter Laboratories' vaccines had not been fully inactivated, causing live, unattenuated poliovirus to be injected into some 400,000 children.[74] Eighty of these children were immediately infected with polio. Within two weeks, the number was up to 200. Seventy-five percent of the victims were paralyzed. Eleven children died.[75]

President Eisenhower was up in arms, as he had endorsed the vaccine. He asked the Surgeon General to call a temporary halt to vaccine production. Other countries immediately suspended their nascent programs as well. Salk and the vaccine manufacturer discovered that there were lumps in the vaccine, apparently preventing some of the viruses from being killed by the formaldehyde. It was suggested that the lab mix the vaccine more thoroughly. After a five-day halt, the public was told the problem was solved and that there was no longer anything to worry about. But more problems were yet to come.

In the next four months, Boston reported more than 2,000 cases of polio in vaccinated individuals. The entire previous year, they had only had 273 cases. New York and Connecticut saw their number of polio cases double; Vermont's cases tripled; and both Rhode Island and Wisconsin saw five-fold increases in polio, all among the vaccinated, and often the symptoms were in the vaccinated arm. In July, Canada suspended its vaccine program. By November, all of Europe had done likewise.[76]

In May 1956, after one year of vaccinating, the *New York Times* reported that there had been a 12 percent *increase* in paralysis over the previous year.[77] By January 1957, 17 U.S. states had stopped distributing the vaccine. By 1959, in the five cities/ states that had made the vaccine compulsory, each saw a 300–400 percent increase in polio cases.[78] Dr. Bernard Greenberg, the head of the Department of Biostatistics at the University of North Carolina testified at a Congressional hearing in 1962 that since beginning the vaccination efforts, infantile paralysis had increased by 50 percent from 1957 to 1958 and by 80 percent from 1958 to 1959.[79] Not only were there more cases of polio, but the cases were more serious.

Clearly, the vaccine was making the epidemic worse rather than better. Someone was going to have to do something; otherwise, the public would start to refuse the shots.

Far from being the slam-dunk victory they were hoping for, the February 1961 issue of the *Journal of the American Medical Association* stated,

"It is now generally recognized that much of the Salk vaccine used in the U.S. has been worthless." [80] That was putting it rather *mildly*.

At that point, the United States switched from the Salk to the oral Sabin vaccine, which we continued to use until 2000 when we switched back to the Salk vaccine. Why did we switch back? Because the Sabin vaccine caused polio, too.

Now, of course, the responsible thing to do would have been to stop the vaccinations, throw out all the dangerous lots, and admit the attempt had failed, at least until they were sure they had a safe and effective shot. But what did they do instead? Just as the vaccine advocates had done for smallpox, they decided to simply change the criteria for diagnosing polio.

One of the ways they did this was to exclude from the statistics all cases of polio that occurred within 30 days of vaccination under the pretext that such cases were "pre-existing" and therefore the shot could not have protected them anyway.[81, 82] This insulated them from most, if not all, of the cases they actually *caused* with the shots.

So, here's one of the tactics the vaccine pushers use to help their statistics: When a vaccinated child gets the disease s/he was being vaccinated against, they do not say the vaccine failed or worse yet *caused* the disease. They simply call it "pre-existing" or a "non-preventable case" or they say that the child was still susceptible to the disease because s/he had not yet been fully immunized.

Another change was to increase the amount of time required before a polio diagnosis could be made. Before the vaccines came out, the term "paralytic poliomyelitis" included all children who had been paralyzed for at least 24 hours. But in 1956, they upped the requirement to at least *60 days* of paralysis.[83, 84, 85] Since most cases lasted fewer than 60 days, this requirement meant *far* fewer cases of polio being reported.

Another tactic was to simply change the name, just as they did with smallpox. Before the vaccines were introduced, thousands of cases of non-paralytic polio were diagnosed in children who actually had aseptic meningitis. In other words, prior to the vaccine, these two similar diseases were lumped together under the heading of polio. Doctors were cavalier about using the diagnosis because polio was "going around." However, once the vaccination was in place, doctors were asked to distinguish between the two and report them separately. According to the *Los Angeles County Health Index: Morbidity and Mortality, Reportable Diseases*, "Most cases reported prior to July 1, 1958 as non-paralytic poliomyelitis are now reported as viral or aseptic meningitis." [86, 87, 88] This caused the number of meningitis cases to go from practically zero to many thousands, while the number of polio cases did the exact opposite. Amazingly, *even if the poliovirus was present*, it was still to be considered meningitis.

Other cases were called Guillain-Barré syndrome, cerebral palsy, muscular dystrophy, or hand, foot, and mouth disease—basically, anything but polio.

Even after doing all of this, there were still too many cases of paralytic polio to suit the authorities, so they renamed *these* "acute flaccid paralysis." [89] It was decreed that two stool samples would be taken from these paralyzed patients to see if they contained the poliovirus, in which case the polio diagnosis would theoretically be made. Interestingly, the poliovirus is rarely found in the stools of these paralyzed children and so the diagnosis is almost never used anymore—at least in this country.[90] *This* is how the fight against polio was truly won, and yet, the vaccine manufacturers take full credit for ending polio in the West.

> The World Health Organization (WHO) reports that acute flaccid paralysis is now rampant and on the rise in many parts of the world, especially in areas like Southeast and East Asia where pesticide use is high and where they (WHO) are trying to stamp out polio with repeated injections and oral polio vaccines.[91] Hmm.

I suppose we could rid the world of AIDS in a similar manner. First, we'll raise the public's awareness of the problem and get them sufficiently scared. Then we'll declare all out war on the disease with the goal of total, worldwide eradication. Perhaps we can sell some red ribbons to get the start-up money together. Then we'll formulate our vaccine. I suggest using pure sugar water. We'll test our vaccine on a few rats to make sure they don't die right away, then go to the FDA for approval. If we have any trouble with the FDA, we'll give some of the Advisory Board members some stock options in our new venture. It's perfectly legal, so why not? Then, once we're approved, we'll simply start giving everyone in the population injections of our sugar water vaccine. We'll need a catchy slogan. Something like: *AIDS? No. Sugar H_2O!* No need for double blind, placebo-controlled tests. We don't have time for that. Can't you see there's an epidemic out there? If we have to, we can grease a few palms in Washington to have the vaccine mandated so that all schoolchildren will need the shot before entering school, but if we get people scared enough, I don't think that will be necessary.

Now, here's the important part: Anyone who's *had* the injection who comes down with AIDS symptoms is given the diagnosis of Kaposi's sarcoma, Pneumocystis carinii, oral thrush, candidiasis or whatever. Feel free to be creative here. Those who *haven't* had their sugar water injections will get the diagnosis of AIDS. And we'll make sure those few cases are well publicized! We don't want people becoming complacent about this or we could have a full-blown pandemic on our hands.

Once people see how effective our vaccine is, they'll line up in the streets for their injections. And most of them will pay whatever we ask. Once everyone in the population has had their shots, we will have wiped out AIDS and we can pat ourselves on the back for a job well done. Of course, everyone will need booster shots for life because, well, you gotta make a living somehow.

This is essentially what they have done with both polio and smallpox with one exception: Our sugar water injections won't have any side effects nor will they cause any new cases of the disease.

- In spite of all of this creative diagnosis, which makes polio statistics practically impossible to decipher and therefore meaningless, polio still occurs in Africa, Southeast Asia, and the eastern Mediterranean—presumably because they haven't completed Operation Vaccinate Everyone/Change the Name yet. There have been no cases of "natural polio" (I assume this means paralysis of more than 60 days with a positive stool sample, not occurring immediately after a vaccine) reported in the entire Western hemisphere since 1991 and no cases in the U.S. since at least 1979.[92] There *have* been more recent cases of polio in the U.S., but they have all been caused by the vaccine. Even the Centers for Disease Control admits that all cases of polio in the U.S. since 1979 have been caused by the vaccine.[93] (Yet we still vaccinate for this disease four times before a child enters school.)[94] In fact, in 1977, Jonas Salk, the inventor of the first polio vaccine said, *the current live virus polio vaccine developed by Dr. Albert Sabin is "the principal if not the sole cause of the 140 polio cases reported in the U.S. since 1961. At the present time the risk of acquiring polio from the live virus vaccine is greater than from naturally occurring viruses."* [95] Between 1980–1985, there were 51 documented cases of polio in the U.S. that were all caused by the live "Sabin" vaccine.[96] As mentioned, we no longer use the oral vaccine in the U.S. for this reason; instead, we ship it to *less fortunate* countries.

Some Final Thoughts on the Polio Vaccine

Besides the three polioviruses (hopefully inactivated) and the ever-present, cancer-causing wild monkey viruses, there are some other things in the current polio vaccine that you may not necessarily want injected into your body or that of your child, namely: formaldehyde, phenoxyethanol, and the antibiotics neomycin, streptomycin, and polymyxin B.[97] Of course, these are just the things the manufacturers know about and admit to.

As mentioned previously, formaldehyde can cause paralysis, the very thing we're trying to avoid here. It's the main ingredient in embalming fluid and is a known carcinogen (i.e., causes cancer.) Phenoxyethanol is an alcohol and is used as a preservative. Antibiotics, as you've just recently read, can lead to problems as well.

So, do polio vaccines work, and if so, are they worth the risks? I guess that depends on who you believe. I, for one, do not trust what the pharmaceutical companies, who stand to gain so much from the sale of those vaccines, have to say. Until we have true, long-term, double blind, placebo-controlled, independent studies proving the safety and efficacy of vaccines, I think the best we can say is, the jury is still out. However, here is a quote from one of the most credible people on earth on the topic of vaccination.

"Official data has shown that the large scale vaccinations under-taken in the U.S. have failed to obtain any significant improvement of the diseases for which they were supposed to provide immuniza-tion. In essence it was and is a failure." [98]

—Dr. Albert Sabin, 1985

DIPHTHERIA, PERTUSSIS, TETANUS (DPT)

Diphtheria is caused by the bacteria *Corynebacterium diphtheriae.* These bacteria produce a poison that can enter cells and kill them. In the throat, this can cause a thick, gray membrane to grow, which can sometimes choke a patient to death. The poison can also travel to other parts of the body, damaging different organs or the nervous system. The heart is a common target. In the nineteenth century and early part of the twentieth century, diphtheria killed thousands of children every year. Today, the disease is very rare. In 1992, there were four cases, including one death, which were attributed to diphtheria in the United States. The first vaccine for diphtheria came along in the 1920s. It was combined with vaccines for pertussis and tetanus in 1946.

In 1969, there was an "epidemic" of diphtheria in Chicago, which led to 16 deaths. Nine of the 16 had been vaccinated. You'll find statistics like this for many of the vaccines we'll discuss in this chapter. Statistics like this, go a long way toward proving the *in*effectiveness of vaccines. But whether this vaccine works or not, it's no longer necessary. Erythromycin, a common antibiotic, will kill these bacteria should someone happen to catch this incredibly rare disease. Still, every child in America is vaccinated for this dreaded disease four times by the time they are 18 months of age, and six times by the time they are 16 years old, the first being within the first six to eight weeks of life.

Tetanus is also bacterial and very rare. It is caused by the bacterium *Clostridium tetani*, which lives in soil, manure, and the digestive systems of animals and people. These bacteria are anaerobic, which means they cannot live in the presence of oxygen. This is why they thrive in deep puncture wounds. Stepping on a rusty nail is a common way to contract this disease.

Once in the body, the bacteria produce a poison that blocks the nerve signals that allow muscles to relax. The result is strong, painful, sustained muscle spasms that have the ability to break bones. The disease is commonly called "lockjaw" because of the commonality of severe jaw muscle spasms, which prevent the person from opening his/her mouth. In 1992, there were 45 cases of tetanus in the United States. Nine of them were fatal.

Because this vaccine seems to be relatively innocuous, and because the death rate of tetanus is fairly high in those who get it, and because it is a horrible disease to have or die from, this is one vaccine I would consider at least marginally useful. I still wouldn't give it to an eight-week-old infant though. It does not give permanent immunity, so booster shots are recommended every 10 years or so. It *can* be given by itself, though your pediatrician may balk at the request.

There *are* certain risks with this vaccine though. In 1992, *The Lancet* reported finding optic neuritis and myelitis associated with the tetanus toxoid, which is found in the shot. There is also evidence, reported by the Institute of Medicine in 1994, that the diphtheria and tetanus vaccine (called Td or DT) can cause brachial neuritis and Guillain-Barré syndrome, a condition very similar to polio, characterized by progressive deterioration of the muscles, nerve inflammation, shock, paralysis, and death.

There's also no evidence that I'm aware of that shows getting a tetanus shot *after* a puncture wound will help prevent lockjaw. This seems a little like locking the barn door after the horse is gone. Following a puncture wound that *might* have contained tetanus with a puncture wound that *definitely* contains tetanus defies logic, and yet, it's common practice. Injecting an antibiotic into the surrounding tissue would make more sense.

Pertussis is the fancy doctor's name for whooping cough. It, too, is a bacterial infection—this time caused by the bacterium *Bordetella pertussis*. Whooping cough gets its name because of the characteristic sound infected children make when struggling to breathe through mucus-blocked airways. Although it can affect any age, infants and small children have the highest risk of dying because they have smaller airways to begin with.

The disease starts out as a mild cough that becomes progressively worse. By the third or fourth week, the coughing can be so severe that the child may gag, vomit, or even stop breathing. Antibiotics can help stop the spread to others, but they do little to help the suffering patient. Many children need to be hospitalized for weeks in order to suction the mucus from their airways. The entire course of the disease may last two to four months. Thankfully, most people who recover from the disease are conferred with lifetime immunity. Whooping cough appears to be cyclical, coming back around every three or four years.

Though pertussis killed up to 10,000 people per year in its heyday, most of whom were children, today, it is very rare. The vaccine became available in 1906. In 1970, pertussis reached its all time low of 1,010 cases, but since then it has been increasing steadily. In 1993, there were 6,335 cases—the highest number reported in 26 years. A study in the July 1994 issue of the *New England Journal of Medicine* found that over *80 percent of the children under five years old who contracted whooping cough that year had been fully vaccinated.*[99] This indicated to the authors that the vaccine may be becoming less effective. Similar findings have been found in countries like Norway, Denmark, and the Netherlands. Scientists are also finding more and more mutated strains of pertussis.

So, what's in this chemical concoction that we inject into all of our healthy children at two months, four months, six months, 15–18 months, and four to six years of age (plus a DT shot at 11–16 years)? Well, from its inception until 2004 (or 2005, depending on which company the shots came from), DPT was stabilized with thimerosal, which is 49.5 percent organic mercury—a known neurotoxin with an affinity for brain tissue (see box below). It has always and still does contain formaldehyde, the main ingredient in embalming fluid, which as we've mentioned is a known carcinogen. It also contains aluminum, another toxic heavy metal, which has been implicated as a major cause of Alzheimer's disease.[100]

Mercury is one of the most potent neurotoxins on the planet. It is the third most toxic metal on earth, and *the most* toxic non-radioactive element. It attacks the brain, kidneys, and bone marrow. It has been implicated in many of today's most crippling diseases such as MS, ALS (Lou Gehrig's disease), autism, and Alzheimer's disease. The phrase, "mad as a hatter" and the character in Lewis Carroll's *Alice's Adventures in Wonderland*, the Mad Hatter, came from the fact that people who made hats used to work with mercury and it consequently destroyed their brains. *Inorganic* mercury is so toxic that if you break a thermometer in a school, you have to call in a Hazardous Materials team to clean it up. This is also the type of mercury we get from silver dental fillings. *Organic* mercury, which is what is in thimerosal, is about a thousand times *more* toxic than inorganic mercury. And *this* is what we're injecting into our children. Thimerosal has also been widely used in over-the-counter products such as eye drops, nasal sprays, and topical antiseptics.

Adults have what is known as a blood brain barrier, which among other things helps protect our brains from many neurotoxins by only allowing certain things to enter. But we are not born with this protection intact. It takes many months or years for this barrier to be built up, and even then it's not impenetrable. Certain drugs like anesthetics can pass through this barrier. Certain chelating agents used in chelation therapy like DMSA and DMPS can also penetrate this barrier. Chelation therapy is frequently used to help remove heavy metals like mercury, lead, and aluminum from cells and nerve tissue.

With all of these toxic materials (known neurotoxins, carcinogens, etc.,) being injected into a brand new baby with a barely formed and as yet untested immune system, and a not-yet-functioning blood brain barrier, surely they must have tested to make sure this was all safe, right? Well, kind of, but not really. You see, they *did test* thimerosal, (once) but they *didn't* find it was safe. In fact, all the test subjects died. (As far as I can tell, they've *never* tested the safety of using aluminum or formaldehyde in these injections.)

"You mean to tell me since 1929 we've been using thimerosal and the only test that you know of is one that was done in 1929, and every one of those people got meningitis and they all died?"

—Congressman Dan Burton, June 19, 2002

How can this be, you ask? It's quite simple really. The FDA has never required testing of thimerosal's safety or a determination of safe levels of exposure in newborns or children. In fact, you'll find that the FDA has been quite lax when it comes to the testing of *any* vaccine for safety or for efficacy.

The only safety testing that's ever been done on the DPT vaccine, which, by the way, was the first instance of three vaccines being combined together, was an unproven method called the Mouse Weight Gain Test. Here's how this "scientific" study works: The vaccine is injected into the stomachs of baby mice. If the mice don't die right away and continue to gain weight, the vaccine is assumed to be safe for humans. That's it! This bogus test was done once back in the 1940s and that was enough for the FDA to approve it for administration to every human being on earth. With FDA approval, we began immediately injecting this unproven vaccine into our eight-week-old children en masse.[101]

Now do you think that just because something is good for mice or bad for mice, that it's necessarily good or bad for us? What about other animals? Are humans just really smart monkeys? You've heard me mention in this book that we humans need to have a certain amount of vitamin C in our diets or we'll get scurvy and die. But did you know that human beings and guinea pigs are the only animals on earth that need to *consume* vitamin C? Every other animal on earth, monkeys, rats, dogs, cockroaches, you name it, all make their own vitamin C. Does that mean we should be using guinea pigs as our—well—guinea pigs? Not necessarily. It turns out that guinea pigs can eat strychnine (one of the deadliest poisons to humans), and penicillin *kills* them. What about other animals?

Belladonna, another poison to humans, is harmless to rabbits and goats. Digitalis *lowers* blood pressure in humans, but *raises* it in dogs. Sheep can swallow enormous amounts of arsenic and suffer no consequences. So now, do you feel that a Mouse Weight Gain Test is sufficient to begin a campaign of injecting all the children on earth with an otherwise untested vaccine?

By the way, the mixing of these three bacterial vaccines was done simply to make the doctor's job easier. The same was done later with the viral vaccines for measles, mumps, and rubella (MMR). But no one has ever studied what happens when we mix vaccines together. The result is that nobody knows, to this day, if or how the three vaccines in DPT or in MMR interact with one another. The problem is, sometimes when viruses are mixed together they make each other more potent. Other times they inactivate one another or weaken the effect.

For nine years, beginning back in 1959, Parke-Davis tried adding the polio vaccine to DPT to save the doctors even more time. Unfortunately for the doctors, "Quadrigen" killed so many kids and Parke-Davis was getting sued so frequently, that they were eventually forced to quit making it.

But that didn't stop the vaccine makers from trying again. In 2002, GlaxoSmithKline introduced "Pediarix," an experimental mixture of DTaP, hepatitis B, and polio vaccines. In the trials assessing the vaccine's safety, five children were killed.[102] Apparently that was an acceptable number for the FDA though, as they approved the shot for use on our newest generation. The CDC also says it's fine to give this five-vaccine mixture along with Hib and Prevnar (for a total of seven vaccines at a time). Yet in the same sentence, they admit that they have no safety information on doing this. Like I said, it's all very scientific. Kind of like playing Russian roulette. In fact, when you do a little research into the *real* story behind vaccines, you find that *we (or our children)* are the real guinea pigs in the grand vaccine experiment. Pediarix is currently recommended at six weeks (because waiting until eight weeks was just too risky), 10 weeks, and six months.

So, what *do* we know about the safety of DPT? A 1981 study in the journal *Pediatrics* stated that convulsions or collapse and shock resulted in one out of every 875 DPT shots.[103] It has been estimated that at least two children are killed or severely injured by the DPT vaccine every day. In 1991, the Institute of Medicine found compelling evidence that DPT causes acute inflammation of the brain (encephalopathy, encephalitis, encephalomyelitis), shock, collapse, and prolonged, continuous crying.[104] A study published in a 1992 issue of *The American Journal of Epidemiology* showed that children die at a rate of eight times greater than normal within three days of getting a DPT shot.[105] I know personally one person who had a grand mal seizure right after receiving his DPT vaccine. Had his parents not been EMTs, he would have died in his crib that day. Nevertheless, he came away from the experience with permanent brain damage. DPT is also suspected of causing bacterial meningitis and Sudden Infant Death Syndrome (SIDS), previously known as crib death, where babies just stop breathing for no apparent cause.

The *Physicians' Desk Reference* (*PDR*), which is the drug bible, lists the following as adverse reactions to the DPT vaccine: anaphylactic shock, death, convulsions, hives, joint pain, difficulty breathing, encephalopathy, brachial neuritis, Guillain-Barré syndrome, SIDS, seizures, intussusception, vomiting, central nervous system demyelinating diseases, rash, low blood pressure, respiratory tract infections, lack of muscle tone, ear pain, and cellulitis.[107] Remember, these are the adverse reactions that the drug makers *admit* are due to the vaccine. Not coincidentally, many of these are also the symptoms of mercury poisoning.

Pertussis, by far, is the most problematic of the three vaccines included in the DPT shot. A 1994 study in the *Journal of the American Medical Association* found that children who had received the pertussis vaccine were five times more likely to have asthma.[108]

In the 1970s, Japan became frustrated with the "whole-cell" pertussis vaccine, which was being used in the DPT shot, because of numerous infant deaths. They refined the vaccine, leaving only a few components of the bacteria, producing a somewhat safer "acellular" pertussis vaccine. This became available in Japan in 1981. But here in the United States, we stoically, bravely, and stubbornly continued using the older, more dangerous, whole-cell pertussis until 1996. By the mid 1980s, around 300 lawsuits had been filed against the makers of DPT. One of them was filed by Barbara Loe Fisher, whose son had had convulsions following his fourth DPT shot and was left with multiple, severe learning disabilities and attention deficit disorder. She, along with another mother, formed the National Vaccine Information Center (NVIC). Barbara also co-authored a groundbreaking book with Harris Coulter, Ph.D., called *A Shot In the Dark*. This book brought the risks vaccines pose into the light of day. That book, along with the NVIC, was instrumental in finally getting acellular pertussis (DTaP) approved and released in the United States.

The NVIC continues to lead the fight for safer vaccines, true informed consent, better research, and making shots optional instead of mandatory.

Japan also blazed the trail in another way pertaining to the DPT shot. When they began compulsory vaccination with DPT at four months old, they noticed a sharp increase in SIDS. (Remember, we vaccinate for DPT at *two* months.) When they decided to hold off on vaccinating their children until they were at least two years old and their immune systems had developed a little, SIDS disappeared. Later, when they started vaccinating earlier again, like we do in the West, SIDS reappeared. This finding correlates nicely with a study that was done in 1991, which monitored infants' breathing before and after receiving a DPT injection. The researchers found the vaccination caused a significant increase in episodes where breathing either stopped completely or nearly did so. This continued for several months after the vaccination. Recall that polio deaths also resulted from breathing cessation. (Could this be the cause of sleep apnea in adults as well?)

Many feel that SIDS is not some mysterious disease, but merely a deceptive label to cover up the fact that yet another child has become a victim of an adverse vaccine reaction. There are countless incidents of healthy children being vaccinated for DPT one day and their mothers finding them dead in their cribs the next morning. SIDS has been on the rise ever since mass vaccination programs began. Are *these* deaths being attributed to iatrogenic causes? I seriously doubt it.

Most of Europe now vaccinates for DPT at six months to two years of age, if they do it at all. But here in the U.S., we still vaccinate for DPT at six to eight weeks. We also see 6,000 to 8,000 cases of SIDS every year. The truth is, very few countries in the world still mandate this shot. In Japan, when the government had to start paying for vaccine-related injuries and deaths, they stopped compulsory vaccination altogether. Sweden discontinued compulsory pertussis vaccination in 1979. In fact, the vaccine is *banned* in Sweden because of the inherent dangers associated with it. By the way, Japan and Sweden have the two lowest infant mortality rates in the world.

In 1950, the U.S. had the third lowest infant mortality rate in the world. By 1986, we had dropped to 17th place. In 1995, we had fallen to 24th. We are one of the richest countries on earth. We have plenty of food and clean water, good sanitation, etc. And we spend far more money on healthcare than any other country (about two times more per capita as our nearest competitor). We also vaccinate far more than any other country. These are our pitiful results. Our government's answer to the problem: More vaccines are needed!

"Vaccination is the single most prevalent and most preventable cause of infant deaths."

—Australian researcher Dr. Vierra Scheibner, author of
Vaccination: The Medical Assault on the Immune System

MEASLES, MUMPS, RUBELLA (MMR)

MMR was added to the mandated schedule of shots in 1978. It was approved after a study lasting only 28 days. To this day, no medium or long-term studies have been done on this vaccine.

Measles is usually a mild, self-limiting, viral disease of childhood, which commonly resolves in about a week. Once you've had the disease, you have lifetime immunity. The symptoms are a red bumpy rash on the skin, fever, a cough, runny nose, redness and inflammation of the inner eyelids, and fatigue. The danger, and the reason we vaccinate, is that measles can be complicated with encephalitis, which can be deadly.

Back in 1901, measles killed almost 12,000 people in the U.S., but those numbers declined on their own until 1966 when only 44 people died of the disease.[109] The measles shot was licensed in 1968, long after the major threat was gone. Once again we have a disease that had once been a threat and had been nearly wiped out—before the vaccine ever made it to market.

Is the vaccine effective? In 1978, after 10 years of vaccinating for the disease, half the cases of measles were found in vaccinated children.[110] In 1989, the CDC reported that in schools that had 98 percent (or higher) vaccination rates, 89 percent of the children who got measles that year had been vaccinated against the disease.

Reports like this led the Mayo Vaccine Research Group to say that, "the apparent paradox is that as measles immunization rates rise to high levels in a population, measles becomes a disease of immunized persons." **Worse, the World Health Organization (WHO) reported that those vaccinated have a 15 times greater chance of catching measles than those not vaccinated.**[111]

Between the years 1983 and 1989, the occurrence of measles in the U.S. increased tenfold. In 1990, the incidence increased another 50 percent and we saw 27,000 cases of measles, including 100 deaths.[112] *The Arizona Republic* reported that in the 1990s, the death rate for measles was 20 times higher than it was before the vaccine was in widespread use.[113] Another report by the CDC, which appeared in *Clinical Immunology and Pathology*, in May 1996, stated that the measles vaccine "produces immune suppression which contributes to an increased susceptibility to other infections." [114]

Great vaccine, right?

Mumps is another self-limiting disease of childhood, usually lasting about a week with no complications. Symptoms include swollen salivary glands, fever, and headache. Once you've had it, you have immunity for life. The only danger with mumps is for males. If they don't get the disease as children and catch it as adults, it may cause a painful swelling in the testicles. Even if this happens, which is rare, the risk of sterility is very low because it usually only affects one testicle. And while no man would wish a painful, swollen testicle on his worst enemy, why do we vaccinate girls? Answer: To protect the males. But if the boys (or men) are vaccinated, and the vaccination actually works, aren't they already protected? Hmm. Add to this that several studies show an *increase* in the number of mumps cases after beginning the vaccination program, almost all of which occurred in people who had been vaccinated.

The mumps vaccine should be reserved only for adult males who never got the disease as children and who want the added peace of mind. But seeing as how the vaccine may be weakening our collective immune system as a race, even this should be discouraged. Also, it doesn't seem to be very effective. The Minnesota Department of Health reported 769 cases of mumps in school children, 632 (82 percent) of which occurred in children who had been "immunized" for mumps.

Rubella, also known as German measles or three-day measles, is basically just a milder form of measles. Fever, rash, and sore throat are the usual symptoms. Once you've had the disease, you are imparted with lifetime immunity. Like mumps, there is only one part of the population who is really at any risk with this disease. That group is the unborn fetus whose mother happens to catch rubella during the first four months of pregnancy. That's a pretty small group to risk injecting poisons into the entire population.

If we're committed to protecting these early fetuses, the people we want to prevent from getting this disease are women of childbearing age who never had the disease during childhood. Why, then, do we vaccinate children, especially male children? Answer: To protect pregnant women from catching rubella from those children. The problem is, when those children grow up, they are no longer protected, because whereas the *disease* confers *lifetime* immunity, the vaccination wears off by the time adulthood rolls around. Thus, women of childbearing age—those we most want to protect—are unprotected. In other words, by the time having immunity to the disease is really important, the vaccine's effectiveness has completely worn off. Don't try to make sense of the logic here. You'll only frustrate yourself.

Before 1969, when the rubella vaccine became available, 75 percent of the cases of rubella occurred during childhood (i.e., only 25 percent occurred in adults). By 1977, people aged 15 and up made up 62 percent of the cases of rubella. Because we are only giving people temporary immunity, we have artificially turned this childhood disease into an adult disease and, thereby, put those early fetuses more at risk than ever.

Ironically, if a woman had the disease as a child, she would still have antibodies to rubella as an adult, which she could then pass on naturally to her offspring through her milk. This transference would quite possibly make the baby immune to the disease for life as well. This type of immunity strengthens the species as a whole. This is one way evolution works. When we as a species learn how to combat a virus by building antibodies to it and then pass those antibodies on to our offspring, the gene pool is strengthened. Vaccinations prevent this from happening. So, we've substituted temporary immunity for lifetime immunity and we're vaccinating the wrong population. Like many things in medicine, it's completely backwards.

A study in the February 20, 1981 issue of the *Journal of the American Medical Association* found that 90 percent of obstetricians and 75 percent of pediatricians refused to take the rubella vaccine.[115] What was that bit about protecting the pregnant moms?

The rubella vaccine should be limited to females over 18 years old who have never had the disease and want the added protection for their future offspring. In all other cases, it should be banned as it prevents the strengthening of our species' immune system. It would be much better, of course, to simply make sure your immune system is working well. Why would anyone want to have foreign chemicals injected into her body, especially before going into pregnancy?

Two of the adverse reactions associated with the MMR vaccine include immune thrombocytopenic purpura (a bleeding disorder caused by a lack of platelets in the blood) and diabetes. In the next chapter we will discuss one more very big problem with the MMR vaccine.

HEMOPHILUS INFLUENZA TYPE B MENINGITIS (HIB)

This shot has nothing to do with the flu or influenza. Hemophilus influenzae bacteria are found in the mucus membranes of normal people and can cause a mild, self-limiting infection of the nose and throat. But a certain strain (Type B) can, on rare occasions, cause meningitis, usually in children under five years old. Antibiotics have helped prevent the death of many cases of bacterial meningitis, but many children are still left with mental retardation or epilepsy. Thus, the need for a vaccine arises.

Early research on the first Hib vaccine showed no efficacy at all in children under 18 months of age.[116] (The current schedule recommends four doses of Hib by that age.) In fact, according to a preliminary study by the CDC, *children who were vaccinated were found to be five times more likely to contract the disease than children who had not received the vaccine.* The research was also "uncertain" as to whether the vaccine did any good in children under 24 months. *The New England Journal of Medicine* published a study of 55 cases of Hib in 1988. All of the children in the study had received the vaccine. Thirty-nine of those children got meningitis, three died, and six were left deaf.[117]

More recent versions of Hib have proven more effective. It still gives only limited and temporary immunity, but at least it's directed at the population most at risk for the disease. However, it also carries risks. Adverse reactions include high fever, crying, seizures, serious allergic reactions, hives, wheezing, rapid heart rate, dizziness, thrombocytopenia (decrease in the number of blood platelets), and Guillain-Barré syndrome. Of course, many of these adverse reactions may be because the Hib vaccine also contains aluminum and mercury—or rather, it did until 2004 or 2005, depending on the manufacturer. The Hib vaccine has also been implicated as a possible cause of insulin-dependent diabetes. Furthermore, Hib is only one of many forms of meningitis and the vaccine is only protective against this one form.

CHICKENPOX

Chickenpox is caused by the varicella zoster virus, a relative of the herpes virus. It is usually a mild, self-limiting disease of childhood. Once you've had the disease, most people have lifetime immunity. The shot was originally developed to protect patients who were at high risk for developing complications from chickenpox—in particular, children with leukemia, kidney disease, or immune suppression. Unbelievably, in 1995, the chickenpox vaccine was added to the list of mandated shots and is now given to all children 12–15 months of age and individuals over 13 years old who have not yet had the disease.

Merck, the vaccine's manufacturer, claims the shot only gives immunity for five years. Oddly, the American Association of Pediatrics originally recommended the shot at one year and then not again until 11 years. Hmm. Perhaps a simple adding error. Then, for no apparent reason, in 2002, they dropped their recommendation down to only one shot at 12–18 months. In 2007, they raised the recommended dose back to two shots. (Again, don't strain your brain trying to figure out the logic here—there is none.)

As with measles, the adult version of chickenpox is much more serious. Therefore, unless your child gets booster shots every five years for the rest of his/her life, you are putting them at much greater risk by giving them the shot than they would be if they just got the disease.

Ever hear of chickenpox parties? Wise parents throw these when one of their children comes down with chickenpox. Rather than *quarantine* the sick child, all of the child's playmates and neighborhood kids get invited over for a party with the goal of having all the children go through this rite of childhood at once. This way they all get the disease out of the way when they're young, when it's least dangerous. And of course, as opposed to the vaccine, the children are all left with *lifetime* immunity.

Don't forget in all of this that these childhood diseases are like exercise for the immune system. Like other systems in the body, (especially the muscular, skeletal, and cardiovascular systems) the immune system thrives on a challenge and it gets stronger with each hurdle it overcomes. The phrase "use it or lose it" is an apt one here. Vaccinations *appear* to work within this premise, but because they are injected rather than entering the body through the usual routes, and because they use killed or weakened germs, they do not activate the whole immune system and they only give partial, temporary immunity at best. When we use antibiotics and vaccinations, we are weakening, not only our individual immune systems, but our collective immune system (the human genome) as well, *and* we're creating stronger bugs at the same time. Whenever we try to use science and medicine to replace our inborn intelligence, we lose ground in the battle for survival.

Of course, if you'd *rather* just give your child partial, temporary immunity, that's your choice, but shouldn't it be just that—*your choice*? Why are we allowing the government, our doctors, and especially our school systems to dictate what sort of medical care our children get?

So what is the justification for mandating *this* shot to all children? A CDC study estimated that $439 million per year is spent by parents in time lost from work caring for children with chickenpox. So, this time it's not even about protecting the kids; it's to keep mom and dad from having to take time off from work. But isn't it worth a few days off of work to give your child lifetime immunity to a disease that is much more dangerous for adults?

We learned earlier that the polio vaccine is cultured on monkey kidneys. "What is the chickenpox vaccine cultured on?" you ask. No, it's not *chicken* parts. The chickenpox vaccine is cultured on human embryonic lung cell cultures—in other words, aborted human fetuses. I had a hard time believing this when I first heard it, so I looked it up in the drug bible, the *Physicians' Desk Reference (PDR)*.[118] It's true.

Like all the other vaccines we've studied, there have been no long-term studies done on the safety or efficacy of the chickenpox vaccine to date. In fact the 2002 *PDR* states, "...no placebo-controlled trial was carried out with Varivax using the current vaccine." [119] Once again, your children are the guinea pigs in this massive, uncontrolled experiment. My prediction: More adults getting chickenpox in the near future, more people dying from chickenpox, and lots more cases of herpes zoster (shingles).

ROTAVIRUS

Rotavirus is the leading cause of severe diarrhea in infants. Almost all children will suffer from a case of diarrhea caused by rotavirus by the time they reach five years; however, most cases are mild and self-limiting and many infections cause no symptoms at all. When symptoms *are* present, the only recommended treatment is re-hydration (i.e., water or IV fluids) and staying close to the toilet.[120] Worldwide, some 500,000 children die from rotavirus per year, but here in the U.S., the CDC estimates the death rate at only 20–40 people per year.[121] Deaths from the infection occur most often in the Third World where poor sanitation, overcrowding, and starvation are rampant.[122]

In 1998, Wyeth-Ayerst unveiled RotaShield, its answer to this horrible scourge on society. Six months before it was approved by the FDA, the CDC was already recommending this oral vaccine for universal use. (Although rotavirus is mainly a problem in the Third World, in order to make the vaccine's distribution to the poorer countries possible, it would need to be sold at $80/dose, or $240 for the series of three, to the richer countries as well.)

The vaccine was actually created by the NIH (your tax dollars at work) by mixing Rhesus monkey rotavirus with human rotavirus strains to create a genetic hybrid human/monkey rotavirus strain that is not found anywhere in nature. This genetic aberration was then tested on monkeys, but not humans. Once licensed, the vaccine was immediately added to the mandated schedule. The three doses were to be given at two months, four months, and six months of age.

As is typical in these cases, one of the CDC's Board of Advisors members, Paul Offit, M.D., had a slight conflict of interest pertaining to the vaccine. He was a co-owner of the patent! And while he admitted in a Congressional hearing that he would make money if the vaccine were to become routinely recommended, he claimed that he was "absolutely not" biased.[123] I'll bet.

But there was a problem. Almost immediately after its release, parents started reporting that after receiving the shot, their infants would suffer from a painful condition called intussusception, where the bowel folds in on itself causing an obstruction. This almost always requires surgery and without treatment, it can be fatal. The CDC investigated and found that RotaShield caused intussusception in about one in every 5,000–10,000 children vaccinated. At least one infant died from the vaccine. There were also many cases of severe vomiting and diarrhea reported. The problems with this vaccine were so widespread that after only 11 months, the manufacturer voluntarily pulled the RotaShield from the market.[124]

However, the vaccine makers were not about to give up on their quest to rid the world of rotavirus, so in 2007, Merck launched a new vaccine called RotaTeq, which was quietly slipped into the mandated schedule. And wouldn't you know it. The new vaccine causes the same exact problem as the old vaccine—intussusception.[125] Maybe that's because it's almost the exact same vaccine. The only differences are the addition of one more strain of the virus, and instead of being a genetic hybrid of human and *monkey* viruses, it's a hybrid of human and *cow* viruses. Yeah, that's obviously much better.

The study that was done prior to the vaccine's release (funded by the manufacturer and co-authored by the co-owner of the patent) showed its efficacy was similar to a placebo. In other words, it didn't work. (At least they used human subjects this time though.) It also reported that of the 34,035 vaccine recipients, 803 of them reported some sort of serious adverse event. *Twenty-four of them died*, seven from sudden infant death syndrome.[126] (Remember, only 20–40 people in the U.S. die from the *disease* each year.) Still, the FDA approved this wonder drug with amazing speed. As might have been expected, within less than a month of its being added to the mandated schedule, the FDA had already cited 28 new cases of intussusception in children who had received the vaccine.[127] The manufacturer also warns that their mutant human/cow rotavirus could be spread to non-vaccinated individuals.

As of this writing, RotaTeq is still on the mandated schedule at two, four, and six months of age.

PNEUMOCOCCAL CONJUGATE VACCINE (PCV) "PREVNAR"

Prevnar is a vaccine that's marketed to protect against otitis media (middle ear infection), bacterial meningitis (inflammation of the meninges—the protective covering around the brain and spinal cord), and blood infections. Pneumococcal bacteria, of which there are more than 90 different strains, are found in the nose and throat of most healthy children. The bacteria only cause problems in those with weakened immune function. When kids *do* get sick, antibiotics are prescribed. However, the overuse of antibiotics (as detailed in Chapter 7) has caused at least seven strains of pneumococcus to become antibiotic-resistant. Prevnar was medicine's answer to that. It contains just those seven antibiotic-resistant strains. Oh, it also contains aluminum, but you probably could have guessed *that*. It was approved by the FDA in 2000 and added to the recommended schedule in 2002. Since its release, the vaccine has been marked by controversy.

The first controversy is that otitis media is generally a mild, self-limiting condition easily handled with pain medication, simple home remedies like garlic oil drops, and time. Chiropractic adjustments also seem to help many children recover quickly, and whole food nutritional supplements can help as well. (Dr. Freddie Ulan has noticed a strong correlation between otitis media and a weak heart, and found that the Standard Process supplement "Cardio Plus" often helps children with chronic ear infections.) The medical treatments for otitis media, such as antibiotics and tympanostomy tubes, have been discussed in Chapter 7 and should be reserved as methods of last resort. As was previously mentioned, antibiotics are what created the "need" for the vaccine in the first place. Another controversy: The FDA has never licensed Prevnar for use against otitis media. Perhaps that's because the studies show it only works about seven percent of the time.[128]

Bacterial meningitis can be a very serious condition, but according to the *New England Journal of Medicine*, it occurs in less than one in 100,000 people.[129] The CDC claims about 700 cases of pneumococcal meningitis per year in the United States. About 35 of those patients die from it.

The next controversy surrounding this vaccine is all the side effects it causes. In one safety study performed on the vaccine, paid for by the manufacturer, of course, rather than comparing the vaccine with a placebo, they decided to compare it with another experimental vaccine. Now, when you compare two unknowns with each other, the only results you can get are "unknown." But the really strange thing is, Prevnar proved to be less safe than the other vaccine, and yet still got approved![130] The manufacturer lists fever, vomiting, diarrhea, rash or hives, edema, pain and tenderness, hypersensitivity reaction, difficulty breathing, bronchial spasm, and anaphylactic reaction, as potential side effects.[131]

Between its release and it being added to the recommended schedule in 2002, the Vaccine Adverse Events Reporting System received 3,243 reports of reactions to this shot. Four hundred-and-seventy-six of these were considered serious; 79 resulted in death. And finally, like all the other vaccines we've discussed, Prevnar has not been evaluated for whether or not it causes cancer, birth defects, or infertility.

This shot is now recommended to children at two, four, six, and twelve months of age. According to the product insert, Prevnar may also decrease the efficacy of Hib, pertussis, and polio if given together with these other vaccines, which it is.

By the way, Prevnar made its manufacturer, Wyeth Lederle, $461 million in its first year on the market before it was even mandated. Now that's good marketing!

HEPATITIS A

Hepatitis A is primarily a disease found in Third World countries. In the U.S., it's very rare and getting even rarer (even before we started vaccinating for it). It's caused by ingestion of infected fecal matter. (In school, we used the pneumonic hepatitis

A=anal; hepatitis B=blood.) Therefore, it's found wherever there is poor sanitation, poor hygiene, poverty, and overcrowding. Symptoms, when present (most hepatitis A infections are subclinical, meaning the patient never even knows s/he is sick), include loss of appetite, nausea, vomiting, diarrhea, hives, joint pain, dark urine, and occasionally jaundice. These are all self-limiting (meaning they go away on their own in a few weeks). Once the infection passes, the patient has permanent immunity—and hepatitis A does *not* cause long-term liver damage.[132]

But this horrible disease of the Third World apparently needed to be prevented here in the U.S., so in January 2002, we added two shots of "Havrix" to the mandated schedule of vaccines. These are given between 12 and 23 months of age. One of the side effects of this amazing vaccine is...try and guess...hepatitis! Others include convulsions, encephalopathy, neuropathy, Guillain-Barré syndrome, multiple sclerosis, and anaphylactic shock.[133] The vaccine is made from infected lung tissue cells taken from an aborted 14-week-old male fetus. The infected cells are then filtered and attenuated with aluminum, formaldehyde, and 2-phenoxyethanol, and injected into healthy one-year-olds.[134] Amazingly, even though hepatitis A is much more prevalent *outside* the United States, we are the only country on earth that vaccinates against it.

Dr. Tim O'Shea summed up this insanity nicely when he said:

"[W]as it really necessary to introduce an infectious vector into the entire population of children in order to theoretically prevent a disease which is virtually nonexistent in the United States, and getting rarer? And is self-limiting, does not contribute to chronic liver disease, and confers lifetime immunity to the few who do get it?" [135]

HEPATITIS B

Hepatitis B is the most controversial of all the vaccines. Hepatitis B is an inflammatory liver disease that is spread through contact with infected blood and semen. At least 90–95 percent of victims recover on their own after four to eight weeks (or occasionally a few months) with no chronic liver disease.[136] The fatality rate is very low—approximately 0.2 percent.[137] Symptoms include nausea, fatigue, fever, headache, cough, lack of appetite, joint pain, jaundice, and tender liver.[138] (Sounds a lot like a bad flu to me.) Those who recover are left with permanent immunity. Hepatitis B is most prevalent in the Far East and Africa, with the lowest incidence in the world being in the U.S. and Western Europe (approximately 0.1 to 0.5 percent, almost all of which fall within the high-risk group). In the U.S. in 1995, there were fewer than 300 cases of hepatitis B in children under 14 years old.[139]

The hepatitis B vaccine was invented for those in the high-risk group: intravenous drug users, prostitutes, prisoners, and sexually promiscuous men and women. Healthcare workers who work with blood are also at some risk for contracting the disease, therefore, many are required to get the vaccine prior to employment. If a mother is infected with hepatitis B, she can also pass it to her infant during the birth process. Even though this is not a deadly disease and only around 0.001 percent of infants are actually at risk,[140] and those who *are* at risk can be easily screened by simply testing the mother for hepatitis B, in 1991, the CDC and the American Academy of Pediatrics (AAP) began recommending the vaccine for *all* newborns. It is usually given within the first 12–24 hours of life.

Assuming the mother does not have hepatitis B, why then would we subject infants to this shot on their very first day of life? The official answer is, "to protect the child when s/he becomes sexually active." Okay. So, apparently they're concerned that certain extremely precocious children may be having sex with prisoners or IV drug users before they even get out of the hospital. As ridiculous as this sounds, it *must* be the case if we are expected to believe their official explanation. Otherwise, why not wait a few years? But wait, it gets even more confusing.

According to the manufacturer of the vaccine, "...the duration of the protective effect of Recombivax HB in healthy vaccinees is unknown at present, and the need for booster doses is not yet defined." [141] The CDC states that, "Between 30 to 50 percent of persons who develop adequate antibody after three doses of vaccine will lose detectable antibody within 7 years." [142] They also state that "...up to 60 percent of vaccinated people lose detectable antibody 9 to 15 years after vaccination." [143] Wait. The immunity wears off in seven to 15 years?! But those three doses are all given within the first year-and-a-half of life and there are no boosters recommended unless you take a job in the healthcare field.

So, not only are they expecting these extremely precocious children to become sexually promiscuous by the age of eight, but they also seem to think that they will then suddenly find themselves in a monogamous relationship by the time they reach nine.

Clearly, the official answer of protecting the child once s/he becomes sexually active doesn't make *any* sense. If the above facts are true and protecting the child is truly the goal, then why not wait until the child is at least in high school when sexual activity is more likely to be starting? According to the AAP schedule, children are supposed to get a final dose of tetanus and diphtheria at the age of 11–16 years. Why not hit them with hepatitis B *then* if you feel you must? At least then it would make more sense.

When the official story doesn't add up with the facts, there must be another reason they're not telling us. Hmm. What could it be? Well, it certainly couldn't be the $1 billion a year in hepatitis B vaccine sales for the three and a half million babies born into this country every year. That would just be unethical. Okay, then the only answer

I can think of is the following scenario: A careless nurse walks out of the room of a patient who has hepatitis B, carrying an uncapped, infected needle. On her way to the lab, she passes another nurse who is carrying a baby. Unexpectedly, the rubber toe of her white nurse's shoe catches and grabs on the tile floor causing her to trip. As she lunges forward, falling out of control, she jabs the infected needle into the unprotected infant infecting her with hepatitis B. Honestly, this is the most realistic possibility I can come up with. Of course even if this impossible scenario were to happen, the baby has better than a 95 percent chance of surviving with no permanent liver damage and will have permanent immunity from hepatitis B for the rest of her life. Hmm. Maybe it's just the money thing then.

Well, if they're giving it to babies not even one day old for no apparent reason, surely the vaccine must at least be safe, right? Surely there must be some long-term studies showing its safety and effectiveness, right? Surely the hospitals, the CDC, the FDA, and the pediatricians wouldn't force something on not-even-one-day-old infants without double blind, placebo-controlled, scientific studies up the wazoo, right? Uhh...well...no. But then you could probably guess as much by now.

The insert label for the vaccine itself says that the test subjects (children up to 10 years old) were only monitored for five days.[144] (By the way, there are many reports of adults in Canada who have suffered from central nervous system and immune system dysfunction or who have died following hepatitis B vaccination.) For any other class of drugs, this would be completely unheard of. At the very most, the drug would be considered in the very early stages of "experimental" classification. But in the case of vaccines, this is typical. A five-day study or a Mouse Weight Gain Study and the next thing you know, the vaccine is being not offered, but *forced* upon everyone. Once again, we are the guinea pigs in this grand experiment; there's no control group; and nobody's monitoring the results.

The first hepatitis B vaccine was developed in the early 1980s. It carried the live virus and it was feared that it may actually *cause* hepatitis B. So, in 1986, they developed the very first genetically engineered vaccine containing recombinant (or altered) DNA. It also contained mercury, aluminum, and formaldehyde.[145]

Why do we warn pregnant mothers not to smoke, drink, or take drugs while they're pregnant, encourage them to take prenatal vitamins, get plenty of rest, etc.; and then let the mother put herself through the agony of "natural childbirth" (i.e., no drugs); and then as soon as the baby is born, rush to inject them with as many poisons as their little bodies can handle for no apparent reason? Doesn't this seem like a huge paradox to you?

The EPA has stated that the "safe" level of mercury for *adults* (it's never been established what a safe level for an infant with no blood brain barrier or other protective mechanisms is) is 0.1 microgram per kilogram per day.[146] Up until 2004/5, that first hepatitis B shot contained about 30 times that amount. Injecting 30 times the safe amount of a known neurotoxin with an affinity for the brain into the system of an unprotected baby, not yet one day old, with no blood brain barrier, for a disease he or she is not even at risk for seems rife with controversy and not very scientific to me. And yet this is what the medical profession pats itself on the back for, claiming they're practicing "preventive healthcare."

In 2000, amid rising pressure from angry parents, vaccine makers finally succumbed and produced a hepatitis B shot with no thimerosal, though it took several years to fully phase the preservative out. The 2009 *PDR* lists four different hepatitis B vaccines. Twinrix is hepatitis A and B together. It no longer contains thimerosal. However, it does contain aluminum hydroxide, aluminum phosphate, phenoxyethanol, and neomycin (an antibiotic). Another, Engerix B, contains no thimerosal but contains aluminum hydroxide. Comvax contains both Hib and hepatitis B. It does not list thimerosal as an ingredient, but it does list formaldehyde and aluminum hydroxide. Since it contains Hib, it is not approved for children under six weeks of age. The last one is called Recombivax HB and is produced by Merck. It apparently has two forms, one *with* thimerosal (50 mcg/mL of mercury) and one without. Both versions, however, contain formaldehyde and aluminum hydroxide.[147] So, now you have the real story. Which poisons would you like injected into your infant?

Apparently, my concerns about the safety of this vaccine are not unfounded. As of 2001, the Vaccine Adverse Events Reporting System (VAERS) had received over 60,000 reports of adverse reactions associated with the hepatitis B vaccine. *Between 1990 and 1998, there were at least 439 deaths and 9,673 serious reactions allegedly linked to the vaccine*[148] (all to prevent, *at most*, 300 cases per year of what basically amounts to a bad flu you can only get once in your life).

But thousands of adverse events are never reported to VAERS because the parents don't make the connection between something their pediatricians did, which they assumed was a safe practice, and their child's symptoms. Thousands more are falsely dismissed by officials as not being due to the vaccine. One parent of a child who died as a result of the vaccine, claimed that the coroner called VAERS and never received a call back. In fact, the FDA admits that VAERS reports represent *only about 10 percent* of the actual cases that have occurred. If this is true, the actual number of adverse reactions could be well over 600,000. According to another survey, conducted by the National Vaccine Information Center (NVIC), only about 2.5 percent of adverse events are actually reported by doctors. This would put the numbers even higher.

In 1986, Ronald Reagan signed the National Childhood Vaccine Injury Act. This law, which basically admits that vaccines *do* injure and kill a certain number of children every year also states, *"...no vaccine manufacturer shall be liable in a civil action for damages arising from a vaccine-related injury or death."* The federal government actually protects vaccine makers from being sued if they kill our children— even if it's obviously their fault! So, here's the politics of vaccines in a nutshell: Vaccines are mandated by our government, insisted on by our schools, and pushed on us by our trusted doctors, hospitals, and pediatricians. (Parents have actually been accused of "neglect" for not vaccinating their children. One couple was even held back by armed guards while doctors forcibly vaccinated their child against their will.) The vaccines themselves are not adequately tested (except perhaps on us, in which case, they're still not monitoring the results). And the vaccine makers aren't even liable should they make a bad batch and kill thousands of children. And when they *do* make a bad batch (which they call a "Hot Lot") they literally do *nothing* about it. They don't rush to their shelves and remove all the bad vaccines, nor do they have a massive recall on the doses they've sold to hospitals and doctors' offices. They simply take note of it and keep right on selling the dangerous vaccines. Why? Because the government shields them from all liability. They literally have *no* motivation to make the vaccines safer. Why do they continue to put mercury, formaldehyde, and aluminum into vaccines even though we know it isn't safe? Because they have no reason *not* to. It's just easier for them not to change. No testing, no liability, patents to protect against competition, and a government-enforced program to ensure universal participation. Pretty sweet deal. Vaccines truly are the Holy Grail to them.

The VAERS was formed in 1991 by the FDA and the CDC as an offshoot of the National Childhood Vaccine Injury Act. Before that there was no central reporting agency for vaccine injuries. Thus, we have no records of what was going on between 1902, when mass vaccination began in the U.S., and 1991. As I've said before, we are involved in a massive "experiment" with no controls and nobody's even keeping track of the results.

A number of studies have documented adverse reactions to the hepatitis B vaccine. Here are a few of the more serious reactions, followed by the journals the studies appeared in: myasthenia gravis (*Archives of Internal Medicine*)[149]; Reiter's syndrome and reactive arthritis (*British Medical Journal*)[150, 151]; systemic lupus erythematosus (*Nephron*)[152]; central nervous system demyelinating diseases such as multiple sclerosis (*The Lancet*)[153]. In 1994, the Institute of Medicine reported that, *"The evidence establishes a causal relation between hepatitis B vaccine and fatal anaphylaxis."* [154]

On July 8, 1999, Jane Orient, M.D., the Executive Director of The Association of American Physicians and Surgeons, called on Congress to issue an immediate moratorium on mandatory hepatitis B vaccinations for school children because of the dangerous side effects. She said that the *deaths and adverse reactions to hepatitis B vaccines are "...vastly underreported, as formal long-term studies of vaccine safety have not been completed." And that "...for most children the risk of a serious vaccine reaction may be 100 times greater than the risk of hepatitis B."* [155]

According to the September 2000, *Townsend Letter*, as of 1999, the number of reported severe adverse reactions to the hepatitis B vaccine surpassed the number of cases of hepatitis B. [156]

In October 1998, the French government suspended hepatitis B vaccines for schoolchildren. The reason was that 15,000 citizens filed a class action lawsuit against the government citing hundreds of neurological and autoimmune disorders including multiple sclerosis following hepatitis B vaccination.

HUMAN PAPILLOMA VIRUS (HPV) "GARDASIL"

The Human Papilloma Virus, of which there are more than 100 strains, causes genital warts in both men and women. HPV is the most common sexually transmitted disease in the U.S., affecting more than six million women per year. Ninety percent of these infections clear up on their own. But genital warts have long been *associated* with cancer of the cervix. (So have other things, of course, such as the artificial hormone DES, which was given to pregnant women in the 1960s to prevent miscarriage and caused cervical cancer in the daughters of these women. But let's not talk about drugs or other toxins causing cancer. That could hurt vaccine sales.)

Cervical cancer is relatively rare. According to the American Cancer Society, about 3,870 women die in America from cervical cancer each year. It's also one of the most easily treated cancers, provided it's caught within a reasonable time via a pap smear. Also, keep in mind that if HPV *does* cause cervical cancer, it could be almost totally prevented simply by using condoms.

We will be discussing cancer in depth in a future book, but for now let me just say that medicine has been searching for years to find a virus that causes cancer, and HPV may just be a case of wishful thinking. (Before HPV was implicated in cervical cancer they were trying to blame herpes.) As you learned a few chapters back, it's just as likely that cancerous cells create HPV, as it is that HPV causes cancer. In any case, "association" does not equal "cause," and they've never proven that HPV *causes* cancer; they've merely observed that they often occur together.

In order to prove a virus causes cancer, you'd have to satisfy certain requirements called Koch's Postulates. In brief, Koch's Postulates say you would have to first, find the virus in every case of that type of cancer. Then, you'd have to grow a culture of the virus in a lab. When you took that culture and infected someone or something else with the virus, it would have to get that type of cancer, too. This has never been done with HPV or any other virus. But this hasn't stopped the drug makers from making the claim that HPV *causes* cervical cancer. In fact, Merck, the maker of the HPV vaccine, falsely makes this claim in the *PDR*.[157]

Gardasil, the HPV vaccine, contains just four of the 100 plus strains of human papilloma virus, though it is claimed that two of those strains (type 16 and 18) are the "cause" of over 70 percent of cervical cancer cases.[158] The vaccine also doesn't contain the actual virus, but genetically engineered "virus-like particles." Now remember, the human immune system is very precise. You can have antibodies to last year's flu but still "catch" the flu this year. So, with the immune system, being a close match doesn't really cut it. It has to be exact.

As mentioned, HPV is sexually transmitted. The more partners one has had, the higher the chances one has been exposed. Gardasil is currently recommended for 12-year-old girls, and yet Merck only claims the immunity from their shot lasts for five years—because that's as long as they studied it. Any claims to efficacy beyond this are mere speculation. There are currently no booster shots recommended (though three shots are recommended in order to confer this supposed immunity). This means by the time a girl reaches 17, her immunity (if there ever was any) may be already wearing off or gone completely. (The average age for cervical cancer is 50, by the way.)[159] And in case you're thinking about waiting until later in life to get your shots, the vaccine's safety and efficacy has not been evaluated in women over 26 years of age. Clearly, the decision to vaccinate 12-year-olds was made by Merck's marketing department rather than by anyone with a scientific background or even rudimentary math skills.

As if HPV were the Plague, all female immigrants between 11 and 26 years of age entering the U.S. must now submit to the HPV vaccine prior to receiving a green card.

The three shots cost between $420 and $825, depending on where you live. Conservative estimates predict annual sales for this shot of more than $4 billion by 2012.[160] But those estimates are based on vaccinating just *half* the population, which would only give Merck half the potential profit on this life-saving vaccine. Surely, selling their concoction to *all* of the population is the ultimate goal, just as we've seen with the other vaccines we've discussed. The problem is, how do you sell the "cervical cancer vaccine" to boys? Well, lest you worry about Merck's bottom-line too much, they've found a way of at least attempting to sell it to boys.

Oddly, their marketing department didn't just go with the easier, though less scary, preventing of unsightly penile warts or even penile cancer (which is incredibly rare and *not* associated with HPV). No, they're actually trying to convince the public that boys should be vaccinated for HPV because if they have oral sex with someone who has genital warts, they could potentially get *throat cancer*! If I wasn't so afraid people and our government would actually buy this outlandish line of fecal matter, I'd think this obvious ploy for dollars was funny. But the truth is, within a couple of years, this vaccine will probably be put into the mandated schedule for *everyone,* boys and girls alike, and nobody will bat an eye. Although it's reprehensible, I'm almost glad they're trying this tactic because it may just show people (at least those who are paying a modicum of attention) how the huge vaccine push is purely about profit and how little science is actually behind any of it. In this case, there is absolutely no science backing up this throat cancer claim. It is pure speculation, pure conjecture, and anyone who actually *does* vaccinate their male child with the intention of preventing throat cancer has fallen prey to snake oil salesmen of the worst kind.

So, does the vaccine actually work? Who knows? The massive experiment is just beginning. And once again, there's no control group; or at least there won't be once the vaccine becomes mandated, which it will. (No vaccine has ever been FDA approved that didn't eventually become part of the mandated schedule.) In fact, Texas' Governor, Rick Perry, who has financial ties to Merck, has already made Gardasil mandatory for all 12-year-olds in his state,[161] and at least 17 other states have shown their intentions to do likewise.[162]

Is Gardasil safe? Well, that depends on whom you ask. Merck will tell you it's completely safe, but they also report that it hasn't been evaluated for carcinogenicity or for causing fertility issues. *And* they say it shouldn't be given while pregnant. They also list a wide array of side effects in the *PDR* including fever, sore throat, dizziness, upper respiratory tract infection, gastroenteritis, appendicitis, pelvic inflammatory disease, nausea, and bronchial spasms.[163] The vaccine has also been associated with loss of consciousness, loss of vision, and seizures.[164] But that's just what the manufacturer says. According to the National Vaccine Information Center and CBS news, as of November, 2008, there had been 10,151 reports of adverse reactions to Gardasil, 152 of which were life-threatening or causing permanent disability. Included in that 10,151 are 16 strokes, 544 seizures, 23 blood clots, 9 heart attacks, and 29 deaths![165] Yes, you read that right. In less than two years of vaccinating, already 29 girls have died. All told in 2008, 20 percent of the reports received by VAERS have been related to the HPV vaccine. And remember, the vaccine's not even mandatory yet and it was only approved in 2006! Surely because of all this, Gardasil sales are now falling and many states have resisted putting it on their mandated schedules.

The cause for many of these injuries and deaths appears to be that two of the ingredients in the shot (L-histadine and Polysorbate-80) combine to increase blood clot formation by five-fold.

Stop the Bus; I Want to Get Off

The topic of vaccination has become a hot one lately and it's constantly changing as new vaccines are being added to the schedule at a furious rate. Just to give you some idea of how fast things are changing, when I started writing this book, the total number of vaccines given by age 18 was 40. Now it's 68, and there will surely be more added in the near future. There are experimental vaccines in the pipeline that they've been working on for quite some time like the "birth control vaccine" that makes women sterile—just the thing for all that overpopulation in the Third World. Then, of course there's an AIDS vaccine in the works (and it's not just sugar water in *their* vaccine). Whew! After reading all of this, can you imagine being the first one in line for your shot of (hopefully) inactivated HIV? Roll up your sleeve and pull the trigger.

Pretty scary stuff, huh? But this chapter was just the tip of the iceberg. The next chapter is where we *really* sink the vaccine ship. All aboard!

CDC'S 2010 RECOMMENDED VACCINE SCHEDULE		
Birth	Hepatitis B	1 Vaccine
1–2 Months	Hepatitis B	1 Vaccine
2 Months	Diphtheria-Pertussis-Tetanus, Polio, Hib, PCV, Rotavirus	7 Vaccines
4 Months	Diphtheria-Pertussis-Tetanus, Polio, Hib, PCV, Rotavirus	7 Vaccines
6 Months	Diphtheria-Pertussis-Tetanus, Hib, PCV, Rotavirus	6 Vaccines
6–18 Months	Hepatitis B, Polio	2 Vaccines
12–15 Months	Measles-Mumps-Rubella, Hib, PCV, Varicella	6 Vaccines
12–23 Months	Hepatitis A (Twice)	2 Vaccines
15–18 Months	Diphtheria-Pertussis-Tetanus	3 Vaccines
4–6 Years	Diphtheria-Pertussis-Tetanus, Measles-Mumps-Rubella, Polio, Varicella	8 Vaccines
11–12 Years	Tetanus/Diphtheria, HPV (3 Doses), Meningitis	6 Vaccines
15 Years	Meningitis	1 Vaccine
6 Months–18 Years	Influenza (yearly)	18 Vaccines
36 VACCINES BY 18 MONTHS OF AGE; 68 VACCINES BY 18 YEARS		

USA DEATHS

Year	Polio	Diphtheria	Pertussis	Tetanus	Measles	Influenza
1901		48,839	33,094	28,065	11,956	15,496
1906		28,225	26,436	16,318	10,837	10,109
1911		20,350	20,285	11,503	7,615	7,086
1916		15,623	21,382	8,596	7,926	54,283
1921	7,229	12,267	14,724	7,818	4,919	13,673
1926	6,038	7,074	13,047	6,040	3,994	17,602
1931	4,545	4,388	9,850	4,709	2,957	11,191
1936	3,666	2,189	6,809	3,275	1,238	8,449
1941	3,539	1,135	4,399	2,384	1,013	4,366
1946	3,799	<u>467</u>	<u>1,460</u>	<u>1,697</u>	469	1,736
1951	3,826	125	558	1093	268	1,178
1956	<u>1,604</u>	45	206	788	203	938
1961	1,076	22	82	550	162	553
1966	928	15	32	282	44	633
1971–75	0	12	122	122	<u>17</u>	491

*Underlined numbers represent the advent of the Polio vaccine,
the combined DPT shot and the combined MMR shot.

With Permission of Tim O'Shea, D.C.

10

Autism: How Incompetence, Greed & the Fear of Germs Led to The Biggest Healthcare Cover-Up in History

"...the biological case against thimerosal is so dramatically overwhelming that only a very foolish or a very dishonest person with the credentials to understand their research would say that thimerosal wasn't the most likely cause of autism. You couldn't even construct a study that shows that thimerosal is safe. It's just too toxic... If you inject thimerosal into an animal, its brain will sicken. If you apply it to living tissue, the cells die. If you put it in a Petri dish, the culture dies. Knowing these things, it would be shocking if one could inject it into an infant without causing damage."

—Boyd Haley, Ph.D., Chairman of the University of Kentucky Chemistry Department

Autism was first described by Leo Kanner, M.D. in 1943, a few years after thimerosal was introduced and used in the pertussis vaccine. He described autistic children as totally self-absorbed and alienated. (The word autism comes from the Greek "auto" meaning self.) They are in their own world, detached, unresponsive, unable to relate to others, hyperactive, and can be violently aggressive. A prominent feature is an inability to relate to or communicate with other humans in ways that are natural or meaningful. About 75 percent have some degree of mental retardation. Another 10 percent are known as autistic savants. Many also suffer with epilepsy, cerebral palsy, and other neurological disorders.

Autism has become a hot topic lately. The reason—autism has reached epidemic proportions. Once virtually unheard of, there are now some 500,000 autistic children living in the United States and pediatricians are diagnosing more than 40,000 new cases a year. In 1983, approximately one child in every 10,000 was autistic. In the early 1990s, studies indicated that the number of children affected by autism spectrum disorders (ASD), which includes milder forms of autism such as Asperger's syndrome, was at one in 1,500.[1] In 2002, the National Institutes of Health (NIH) and the Centers for Disease Control and Prevention (CDC) both estimated that one in 150 children was affected by ASD.[2] In 2006, the CDC put the number at one in 100.[3] In 2007, they increased their estimate again to one in 90.[4] Some experts now put the number as high as one in 10.[5] One out of every eight school children is now in special education for some sort of learning disability. The Autism Society of America projects that autism disorders are increasing by 10 percent per year.

Some have claimed this massive rise in numbers is due simply to increased awareness, but a recent study in California indicated that only 24 percent of the increase is likely due to increased awareness or a change in diagnostic criteria.[6] And as Dr. Boyd Haley, one of the world's foremost authorities on mercury toxicity says, "If the epidemic is truly an artifact of poor diagnosis, then where are all the 20-year-old autistics?" [7]

Lifetime care costs for each autistic child falls between $5–10 million.

The official stance, according to our all-knowing government, is that the cause of the autism is unknown. However, there is a plethora of scientific evidence indicating that autism is caused by two main factors: mercury and the MMR vaccine.

Mercury as a Cause of Autism

From the 1930s until 2005, thimerosal was included in many childhood vaccinations including DPT, DTaP, Hib, hepatitis B, and the flu shot. It was also used in shots given to mothers (both during and after pregnancy) whose blood type was Rh-negative. Thimerosal is *still* in most flu shots, which are now recommended to pregnant women and kids every year from the age of six months on. It's also used in adolescent and adult "booster" shots for DT, Td (Diphtheria and Tetanus), as well as in anti-venom shots for pit vipers, coral snakes, and black widows.

As you know by now, thimerosal is 49.5 percent mercury by weight. And, as stated previously, mercury is the third most toxic substance and *the most* toxic non-radioactive metal on earth. There is virtually a one-to-one correlation between the symptoms of autism and those of mercury poisoning. And yet, there is virtually no published research (in the United States) on using thimerosal in vaccines! The research that *has* been done all indicates that thimerosal is extremely toxic, especially to the nervous system, and ineffective at killing bacteria, which is its intended mission.

In its early history, autism was only seen among children born to affluent families. (See box below.) Perhaps that's because in those days, the upper class were the ones most likely to vaccinate their children as vaccines were not yet covered by health insurance. But by the 1970s, many more Americans were vaccinating their children. Vaccinations had become a large part of "well baby visits" to the pediatrician. The government was even willing to pay for those who could not afford the vaccinations. The result: Now we see that autism is evenly distributed over all socioeconomic classes.

Dr. Kanner believed at first that these affluent mothers were somehow colder to their children and that this coldness caused their children to become mentally unstable. This was his early explanation for the cause of autism. He later recanted this theory.

For many years, the pertussis vaccine (later combined with tetanus and diphtheria into the trivalent DPT) was the only shot that contained thimerosal. Autism was a rare disorder in those days and babies only received a handful of vaccinations in all. But in 1989, Hib was added to the recommended schedule of vaccines. In 1991, hepatitis B was added. Both of these vaccines contained thimerosal. Their addition to the schedule *tripled* infants' exposure to mercury! Hepatitis B, as we've stated, is given the day the child is born and followed by two more doses, one at two months and another at six to 18 months of age. Hib is given at two months, four months, six months, and 12 to 15 months of age. Babies were already being given four doses of mercury-containing DPT at two, four, six, and 12 to 18 months of age. As you can see from the graph below, the addition of Hib and hepatitis B corresponds *exactly* with the sharp increase in the number of autism cases we've seen since the early 1990s. The more thimerosal-containing vaccinations we add, the more autism we have. Do you really think this is a coincidence?

Thimerosal in Vaccines Implicated in Autism

Autism Prevalence and the Spread of Thimerosal Vaccines

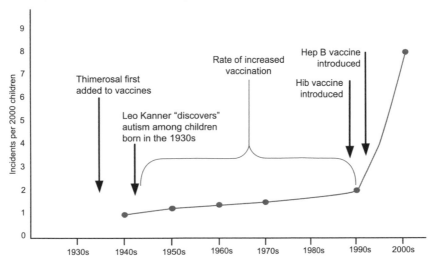

Reprinted with permission from the Coalition for SafeMinds

Ninety-three percent of all autism cases begin shortly after a child is vaccinated.

Re-assembling the Smoking Gun

The truth is, the government *knows* vaccines are the main cause of the autism epidemic, as well as other brain disorders like ADD/ADHD, and despite what you hear on the news, there's *tons* of information indicating that this is true. The reason they're lying about it is a matter of liability ("lie ability"?). Our government has not only *encouraged* vaccination, they've made it practically mandatory for everyone, implying that they're safe, effective, and necessary. How would it look for them if this "public health measure" caused the biggest, most tragic epidemic in the history of healthcare? As an ad put out by Generation Rescue said, "If you caused a 6,000 percent increase in autism, wouldn't you try to cover it up too?"

ARE WE POISONING OUR KIDS

IN THE NAME OF PROTECTING THEIR HEALTH?

COMPARISON OF CDC MANDATORY SCHEDULE
Children birth to six years (recommended month)

USA 1983 AUTISM RATE: *1 in 10,000*	USA 2008 AUTISM RATE: *1 in 150*

Influenza (prenatal)
Hep B (birth)
Hep B (1)
DTaP (2)
Hib (2)
IPV (2)
PCV (2)
Rotavirus (2)
Hep B (4)
DTaP (4)
Hib (4)
IPV (4)
PCV (4)
Rotavirus (4)
Hep B (6)
DTaP (6)
Hib (6)
IPV (6)
PCV (6)
Influenza (6)
Rotavirus (6)
Hib (12)
MMR (12)
Varicella (12)
PCV (12)
Hep A (12)
DTaP (15)
Hep A (18)
Influenza (18)
Influenza (30)
Influenza (42)
MMR (48)
DTaP (48)
IPV (48)
Influenza (54)
Influenza (66)

DTP (2)
OPV (2)
DTP (4)
OPV(4)
DTP (6)
MMR (15)
DTP (18)
OPV (18)
DTP (48)
OPV (48)

10   36

Green our vaccines. And administer them with greater care.

Mercury. Aluminum. Formaldehyde. Ether. Antifreeze. Not exactly what you'd expect-or want-to find in your child's vaccinations. Vaccines that are supposed to safeguard their health yet, according to our studies, can also do harm to some children.

The statistics speak for themselves. Since 1983, the number of vaccines the CDC recommends we give to our kids has gone from 10 to 36, a whopping increase of 260%. And, with it, the prevalence of neurological disorders like autism and ADHD has grown exponentially as well.

Just a coincidence? We don't think so. Thousands of parents believe their child's regression into autism was triggered, if not caused, by over-immunization with toxic ingredients and live viruses found in vaccines. The Centers for Disease Control and the American Academy of pediatrics dispute this but independent research and the first-hand accounts of parents tell a different story.

Why are we giving our children so many more vaccines so early in life?
Why do we only test vaccines individually and never consider the combination risk of vaccines administered together? Given the dramatic rise of autism to epidemic levels, isn't it time for the scientific community to seriously consider the anecdotal evidence of so many parents? We urge the CDC and the AAP to help us find the answers to these questions and learn why the increase in the number and composition of so many vaccinations has led to a surge in neurodevelopmental disorders. Our children deserve no less.

GENERATION RESCUE
www.generationrescue.org

We want to thank Jim Carrey and Jenny McCarthy for their generous support of Generation Rescue and their never-ending commitment to solving the growing challenges of autism.

Liability is also why lawmakers like former Senate Majority Leader Bill Frist have been working so hard to protect the vaccine makers like Eli Lilly from lawsuits for the past decade or so. And it's why the drug makers finally decided (after just 70 years) to *voluntarily* stop using thimerosal in most children's vaccines. They finally realized that people were on to them and that they weren't going to shut up about this issue until something was done about it.

To give you some idea of the amount of evidence there is on this topic and how it all fits together, I'd like to give you a historical timeline on mercury, autism, and vaccinations. Keep in mind as you're reading it, that this is just a taste of what's out there.

As mentioned in the opening chapters of this book, quack salvers or "quacks" (the forefathers of today's allopathic medical doctors) used quicksilver (mercury) to treat syphilis and other diseases. It "worked" because mercury kills virtually anything it touches. In 1929, a decade and a half before the penicillin era, ethyl mercury (thimerosal) was the best germicide medicine had. And back then, most people didn't realize how toxic mercury was. I've actually heard many stories of kids being given a bit of the slippery, silvery substance to play with. But how long have we known thimerosal isn't safe?

The drug companies have essentially known it from the beginning. The one and only "safety study" performed on thimerosal was done by a Dr. K. C. Smithburn in 1929. Dr. Smithburn had 22 patients who were dying from meningitis and, having nothing else to offer them, he decided to try a brand new drug called thimerosal. He injected each of his patients with varying amounts of the drug, then waited to see what would happen. Seven of the patients died within one day of receiving the injections. Every one of the patients died within a couple of weeks. This was not *particularly* surprising since they had been considered "terminal" even before the drug was introduced, but they also suffered from all sorts of nasty side effects that are not part of a typical meningitis case, like watching their skin slough off.

Eli Lilly, the original manufacturer of thimerosal, used the above experiment as their "safety study" on the drug when they applied to the FDA for licensure. They strategically left off the part about all of the patients dying and wouldn't let the FDA see the actual study, but apparently, this was good enough for the FDA. In 1931, Eli Lilly began using thimerosal in the pertussis vaccine as a "preservative." It was also used in many topical creams, eye drops, and other over-the-counter (OTC) drugs.

By 1935, veterinary vaccine maker, Pittman-Moore, began warning the folks at Eli Lilly that they had injected dogs with thimerosal-containing vaccines and half of them had become sick. They seemed concerned that the drug's manufacturer had made a mistake in using the highly toxic drug on humans and declared thimerosal "unsatisfactory as a serum intended for use *on dogs* [emphasis added]." [8]

During World War II, the Department of Defense required Eli Lilly to label vaccines containing thimerosal as "poison." With their asses now firmly covered, they then went ahead and injected the poison into our troops.

In 1967, a study performed by the Michigan Department of Public Health and published in the journal *Applied Microbiology* found that when mice were injected with pertussis vaccines containing thimerosal (a.k.a. Merthiolate), they died at a higher rate than when they received vaccines *not* containing thimerosal. [9]

In 1971, Eli Lilly discovered that thimerosal was toxic to cells in concentrations as low as one part per million. Typical thimerosal-containing vaccines contain 100 times that amount.

By 1972, the U.S. government recognized that mercury was a cumulative toxin that damaged brain cells.

On February 14, 1973, the FDA asked Eli Lilly for more information on the safety of thimerosal. Ely Lilly responded by saying:

...due to the length of time this product has been on the market, its efficacy and safety have been proven by over forty years of use throughout the world. Because of this long period of use, it would be difficult to get recognized researchers to conduct new studies for safety or efficacy. They believe that over forty years of wide usage has proven efficacy and safety beyond that which could be done in special studies.[10]

In August of that same year, an internal memo at Eli Lilly entitled "Merthiolate Toxicity" stated, "The effects of long term, intravenous use in man is not known, no long-term toxicity tests have been performed." [11]

In Toronto in 1977, 10 babies died after an antiseptic containing thimerosal was applied to their umbilical cords in the hospital. Also in 1977, a Russian doctor conducted experiments on adults using ethyl mercury (thimerosal). He found that even at doses much lower than what we give our children in America, these adults still suffered from brain damage years later. [12] This study helped lead to Russia's banning of thimerosal from children's vaccines in 1985. Denmark, Australia, Japan, Great Britain, and all the Scandinavian countries have since banned it as well.

In 1980, the FDA started to catch on that thimerosal might not be such a great thing and proposed banning it in all over-the-counter (OTC) products. An advisory committee studied 18 products containing thimerosal and found all of them either ineffective at killing bacteria or unsafe. They cited a study performed in 1935 that showed thimerosal was 35 times more toxic to a baby chick's heart tissue, which it was intended to *protect*, than it was to the staph bacteria it was meant to *kill*. They cited a Swedish study that showed 10 percent of children, 16 percent of military recruits, 18 percent of twins, and 26 percent of medical students had allergic reactions to thimerosal. And they cited a study from 1950 that showed, "Thimerosal was no better than water in protecting mice from potential fatal streptococcal infections." Their report stated, "The panel concludes that thimerosal is not safe for OTC topical use because of its potential for cell damage if applied to broken skin, and its allergy potential." [13]

At that point, the FDA began the lengthy process of removing ethyl mercury from OTC products including topical ointments, contact lens solutions, diaper rash creams, and contraceptives. Though there was no opposition from anyone, *including the makers of thimerosal*, the FDA didn't issue an actual ban on the germicidal preservative in OTC products for another 18 years!

In 1984, the 5th edition of *Clinical Toxicology of Commercial Products*, a textbook found in most hospital emergency departments and poison control centers, contained the statements, *"...ethyl mercury derivatives are virulent neurotoxins on either acute or chronic exposure... They are especially hazardous because of their volatility, their ability to penetrate epithelial and blood-brain barriers, and their persistence in vivo."* [14] In other words, just putting thimerosal on your skin could cause it to go to your brain and stay there, where it will just continue to kill brain cells in a powerful fashion forever.

In 1988, another Russian study concluded that, *"...merthiolate [thimerosal] is toxic in a dose of 0.8 micrograms/ml."* [15] At that time in the U.S., both the DPT and Hib vaccines contained 25 micrograms of mercury and kids were getting *four doses* of each before they were even a year-and-a-half old. In 1991, we added the hepatitis B shot to the schedule, which included 12.5 micrograms of mercury per dose. Given on the day they are born, this single dose represented about 30 times more than the weight-adjusted amount of *methyl* mercury that the EPA says is toxic for an adult! Remember, children are *much* more susceptible to mercury than adults are, and according to many studies, ethyl mercury (thimerosal) is even more toxic to brain tissue than methyl mercury.

Hepatitis B is given three times by the time children are a year-and-a-half old. Adding all this up, we see that by the time a child was six-months-old s/he had already received 187.5 mcg of mercury. By the time the child was a year-and-a-half old, his/her exposure would be as high as 237.5 mcg of mercury, not counting any flu shots (at 25 micrograms each), RhoGAM (10.5 micrograms) or BayRho (35 micrograms) injections, *or* any other fetal exposure, such as mom's "silver" fillings (which are about 50 percent mercury), or fish (methyl mercury) in her diet. And there are still more booster shots to come!

RhoGAM and BayRho are injections given to mothers whose blood is Rh-negative when their fetus is or may be Rh-positive. This is done to prevent the mother's immune system from attacking the fetus' blood. Many women receive multiple injections of these thimerosal-containing vaccines, both during and after their pregnancies. Mercury has been shown to pass through the placenta and is present in breast milk. About 50 percent of mothers of autistic children received RhoGAM shots during pregnancy.

In 1990, the Vaccine Adverse Event Reporting System (VAERS) was established by the CDC. In 1991, the Institute of Medicine performed a study looking into the risks of the pertussis and rubella vaccines. It concluded that the pertussis vaccine is linked to encephalopathy, or brain damage.[16]

In March 1991, an internal memo at Merck Pharmaceuticals stated that babies given the new recommended schedule of vaccines would be given 89 times the legally acceptable limit of mercury.

They stated, "It is reasonable to conclude that thimerosal should be removed from vaccines, especially where use on infants and young children is anticipated." [17] They did *not* remove thimerosal from any of their vaccines for another eight years, however, and continued *selling* thimerosal-containing childhood vaccines for another *ten* years.

Also in 1991, Eli Lilly ceased all manufacturing and selling of thimerosal. Other companies, however, continued to make and sell the drug.

In 1992, the FDA removed thimerosal from all small animal vaccines, but did nothing of the sort for children's vaccines.

In September 1994, the FDA issued an advisory on methyl mercury, the type of mercury found in fish. They stated:

> ...there is no doubt that when humans are exposed to high levels of methyl mercury that poisoning and problems of the nervous system can occur...the types of symptoms reflect the degree of exposure... During prenatal life, humans are susceptible to the toxic effects of high methyl mercury exposure because of the sensitivity of the developing nervous system... Methyl mercury easily crosses the placenta, and the mercury concentration rises to 30 percent higher in fetal red blood cells than in those of the mother... none of the studies of methyl mercury poisoning victims have clearly shown the level at which newborns can tolerate exposure... Pregnant women and women of child bearing age, who may become pregnant, however, are advised by FDA experts to limit their consumption of shark and swordfish to no more than twice a month.[18]

In 1997, the CDC received reports that Brick Township, New Jersey was seeing higher numbers of autistic children than ever before. The people of New Jersey asked the CDC to look into the possibility that the increase was being caused by vaccines. The CDC conducted two extensive investigations—one in New Jersey and another in Atlanta. In 1998, they released a report stating that the number of autistic children throughout the country had increased 10 times compared to what had been seen in the 1980s and early 1990s, but they refused to look into the vaccine connection.

In November 1997, Congress passed the Food and Drug Administration Modernization Act. Among other things, this act required the FDA to study mercury in FDA-approved products.

On April 22, 1998, the FDA finally banned thimerosal in all OTC products. In the 18 years since they had first proposed the idea, there was never any opposition to their doing so. In August of the same year, an internal "point paper" at the FDA declared:

> For investigational vaccines indicated for maternal immunization, the use of single dose vials should be required to avoid the need of preservative [thimerosal] in multi-dose vials... Of concern here is the potential neurotoxic effect of mercury especially when considering cumulative doses of this component in early infancy.[19]

In 1999, the FDA announced the results of its review of mercury in FDA-approved drugs. They discovered that if children were vaccinated according to the CDC's recommended schedule, by six months of age they would receive 187.5 micrograms of mercury, a level that exceeded the EPA's safety guidelines by more than 80-fold. It also exceeded the FDA's more relaxed guidelines, as well as the World Health Organization's guidelines on mercury.

Also in 1999, a Swedish study stated:

> In contrast to the toxic effects of metals, the concentration of the metal in a sensitized individual [those with an allergy] is of minor importance... Minute concentrations

of an allergen [mercury] can induce systemic reactions in sensitized individuals... In such a situation, metal induced inflammatory reactions in the brain or elsewhere could be triggered despite low concentrations detected in body fluids or locally.[20]

On June 20th and 21st, 1999, the CDC's Advisory Committee on Immunization Practices (ACIP) held a secret meeting in Atlanta to discuss the possibility of recommending thimerosal-free vaccines, which some companies had already moved toward producing. However, on learning that most vaccine manufacturers still had large inventories of thimerosal-containing vaccines and that they would incur huge financial losses if such a decision were made, they decided unanimously not to state any opinion on the matter. (This remains their stance to this very day.)

That same month, an FDA document stated that the Public Health Service had also agreed against publicizing any opinion on the matter because stating a preference could, "...result in unwarranted loss of confidence in immunization programs in the U.S. and internationally, shortages of childhood vaccines might ensue, and other potential far-reaching ramifications are envisioned." [21]

In June of 1999, Dr. Neal Halsey, Director of the Institute of Vaccine Safety at Johns Hopkins, drafted a letter to the members of the American Academy of Pediatrics (AAP) Committee on Infectious Diseases, of which he was the chairman. He wrote:

"In the past few days, I have become aware that the amount of thimerosal in most hepatitis B, DTaP, and Hib vaccines that we administer to infants results in a total dose of mercury that exceeds the maximum exposure recommended by the EPA, the FDA, CDC, and WHO..." [22]

Also in June of that year, Dr. Peter Patriarca, a former FDA official, wrote an e-mail to the CDC's Acting Director of the

National Vaccine Program Office. In discussing the pros and cons of removing thimerosal from vaccines, he said removal would:

> ...raise questions about FDA being "asleep at the switch" for decades by allowing a potentially hazardous compound to remain in many childhood vaccines, and not forcing manufacturers to exclude it from new products. It will also raise questions about various advisory bodies [like the CDC] regarding aggressive recommendations for use. (We must keep in mind that the dose of ethyl mercury was not generated by "rocket science." Conversion of the percentage thimerosal to actual micrograms of mercury involves ninth grade algebra. What took the FDA so long to do the calculations? Why didn't the CDC and the advisory bodies do these calculations when they rapidly expanded the childhood immunization schedule?)[23]

In July, 1999, the American Academy of Pediatrics and the U.S. Public Health Service issued a joint statement that recommended the removal of thimerosal from childhood vaccines, but also recommended to parents and pediatricians that children continue to be immunized according to the schedule, even if the pediatrician only had vaccines that contained thimerosal. Further, they admitted that "some children" had been exposed to levels of mercury that exceeded federal guidelines and yet asserted that there was no evidence that showed thimerosal causes any harm.

In August 1999, Merck Pharmaceuticals began manufacturing a single-dose thimerosal-free hepatitis B vaccine. However, they continued selling off their stockpile of the older thimerosal-containing vaccines until October 2001. Most doctors believed that all of Merck's hepatitis B shots were mercury-free during the transition period.

In the fall of 1999, epidemiologist Thomas Verstraeten began studying the CDC's Vaccine Safety Database in an effort to determine whether or not there was evidence of a link between thimerosal and neuro-developmental disorders. The analysis compared children who had never received thimerosal to those who had. It also took into account how much each child had received.

In November, he began analyzing the data he had amassed and discovered that several diseases/disorders were what he considered "high risks." Each of these disorders occurred well above the level needed to be considered "caused by the drug": autism, ADD, ADHD, coordination disorder, sleep disorders, tic disorders, speech and language disorders, convulsive epilepsy, and kidney disorders.

In one analysis of the data, Dr. Verstraeten eliminated children who received the hepatitis B shot at birth and found that in doing so, one-third of the autism cases disappeared and one-fourth of the other disorders went away. He also found that five of these disorders (autism, ADD, speech and language disorders, sleep disorders, and coordination disorders) were, "very much related." If a child had any one of these, s/he also had a 20 to 100 percent chance of having *at least* one other on the list.

In 2000, The National Academy of Sciences published *Toxicological Effects of Methylmercury*. (Again, this is the kind of mercury found in seafood.) In the report, they state that methyl mercury is highly toxic and can cause damage to the nervous system and kidneys, that the cardiovascular system becomes toxic at very low levels of exposure, that it can affect the reproductive system and cause damage to the immune system leading to increased susceptibility to infectious diseases as well as autoimmune diseases.[24]

Also in 2000, Dr. William Slikker, Jr. of the National Center for Toxicological Research at the FDA stated in the journal *Neurotoxicology* that, "Thimerosal crosses the blood-brain and placental barriers and results in appreciable mercury content in tissues including brain." [25]

On April 6, 2000, Representative Dan Burton of Indiana, whose grandson became autistic after receiving several of his "routine" childhood vaccinations in one day, began a three-year investigation into the link between thimerosal and autism. C-SPAN covered this story for six hours. The film shows one family after another getting up to testify how their happy, healthy children, who had been developing normally, became autistic soon after receiving an MMR or DPT shot. The families were followed by experts on the subject whose testimony concurred with theirs.

During the hearings, Congresswoman Helen Chenweth-Hage (R-ID) addressed the various government agencies who were still stubbornly denying the fact that thimerosal was toxic and could cause harm. She summed up the views and frustrations of many members of Congress when she said:

> You listened to the testimony just as I did, and you are willing to, with a straight face, tell us that you are eventually going to phase this out after we know that a small baby's body is slammed with 62 times the amount of mercury that it is supposed to have... It doesn't make sense. No wonder people are losing faith in their government. And to have one of the witnesses tell us it is because mothers eat too much fish? Come on. We expect you to get real. We heard devastating testimony in this hearing today, and we heard it last April. And this is the kind of response we get from our government agencies? I am sorry. When I was a little girl, my daddy talked to me about something about a duck test. I would ask each one of you to read this very excellent work by Sallie Bernard and Albert Enayati [discussed below], who testified here today. My daddy used to say if it walks like a duck and talks like a duck and sounds like a duck, for Pete's sake it is a duck. I recommend that you read this, side-by-side, page after page of analysis of the symptoms of

people who are affected with mercury poisoning compared to autism. This is the duck test, and you folks are trying to tell us that you can't take this off the market when 8,000 children are going to be injected tomorrow; 80 children may be coming down, beginning tomorrow, with autism? What if there was an *E. coli* scare? What if there was a problem with an automobile? The recall would be like that... Mr. Egan, [of the FDA] I will address this to you. You know, it was shown in the last panel that autistic symptoms emerge after vaccination. It was shown that vaccines contain toxic doses of mercury. It was shown that autism and mercury poisoning, the physiological comparison is striking. There is altered neurotransmitter activity, abnormal brain neuronal organization, immune system disturbance, EEG abnormalities. It goes on and on and on, the comparisons. That is why I say, I back up what the Chairman and the ranking members are all asking you, that we cannot wait until 2001 to have this pulled off. You know, if a jury were to look at this, the circumstantial evidence would be overwhelming. Let's do something before we see it in the courts.[26]

In June of 2000, just two months after C-SPAN's coverage of the House's hearings, another secret meeting was called by the CDC. It was held at the Simpsonwood Conference Center in Norcross, Georgia. There was no public announcement made and only 52 top government and corporate scientists were invited to attend, including officials from the CDC, the FDA, the World Health Organization, and representatives from all the major vaccine manufacturers.

The transcripts for this meeting were obtained by SafeMinds.org. They are available at: http://www.safeminds.org/government-affairs/foia/Simpsonwood_Transcript.pdf.

These scientists were repeatedly reminded that they were not to record, make photocopies, or take anything from the meeting with them. Once that was clear, they were told of the huge study that had been done by CDC epidemiologist Tom Verstraeten (mentioned above). Verstraeten had analyzed the CDC's massive database on childhood vaccines, including the medical records of 100,000 children and concluded that thimerosal appeared to be responsible for the autism epidemic as well as other neurological disorders in children. He told the audience, "I was actually stunned by what I saw." He then cited a staggering number of studies that linked thimerosal to speech delays, attention deficit disorder, hyperactivity, and autism. He also noted that since 1991, when the CDC and the FDA began recommending *three* vaccines laced with mercury—one (hepatitis B) being given within hours of birth—that the estimated number of autism cases had increased 15-fold from one in every 2,500 children to one in every 166 children.

Verstraeten said, "This analysis suggests that in our study population, the risk of tics, ADD, language and speech delays, and developmental delays in general may be increased by exposures to mercury through thimerosal-containing vaccines during the first 6 months of life." [27]

What did these esteemed scientists do with this data? They spent the next two days wishing the study had never been done and trying to find ways of covering it up. According to Robert F. Kennedy, Jr., in an article entitled *Deadly Immunity*, "The CDC paid the Institute of Medicine (IOM) to conduct a new study to whitewash the risks of thimerosal, ordering researchers to 'rule out' the chemical's link to autism." [28]

After receiving their marching orders, Dr. Marie McCormick, chairperson of the IOM's Immunization Safety Review Committee told her fellow researchers in January 2001, "We are not ever going to come down that [autism] is a true side effect" of thimerosal exposure. In fact, according to the official transcripts of the meeting, one of the committee's chief members, Kathleen Stratton, "predicted" that the IOM would conclude the evidence was, "inadequate to accept or reject a causal relation" between thimerosal and autism. She then added that this was what "Walt wants." [29] This was a reference to Dr. Walter Orenstein, director of the National Immunization Program at the CDC.

U.S. Representative David Weldon, a physician from Florida, told Robert Kennedy, Jr., that CDC officials are not interested in an honest search for the truth on this issue because "an association between vaccines and autism would force them to admit that their policies irreparably damaged thousands of children. Who would want to make that conclusion about themselves?" [30]

To help cover their tracks, the CDC told anyone who asked that Dr. Verstraeten's findings and his data had been lost and could not be replicated. They also gave their giant database on vaccines to a private company (America's Health Insurance Plans), declaring it off-limits to researchers and thus preventing it from being acquired through the Freedom of Information Act. Verstraeten then went to work for GlaxoSmithKline (a major vaccine manufacturer), reworked his data, which was published in the journal *Pediatrics*, and buried the link between thimerosal and autism.

In 2001, Kathleen Stratton and Marie McCormick, of the IOM, released a report stating, "The committee concludes that although the hypothesis that exposure to thimerosal-containing vaccines could be associated with neuro-developmental disorders is not established and rests on indirect and incomplete information...*the hypothesis is biologically plausible* [emphasis added]." [31] In other words, common sense tells us that this is possible and perhaps even likely, but because nobody's studied the issue (i.e., there's been no double-blind, placebo-controlled tests, which would require one group of children to *not* receive their shots), there's not enough evidence to say one way or the other. This study was apparently completed before the Simpsonwood meeting because, as you'll see below, these same authors came to an entirely different conclusion on the topic in 2004.

In April, 2001, an article by Sallie Bernard and Albert Enayati (mentioned above) entitled "Autism: A Novel Form of Mercury Poisoning" appeared in the journal *Medical Hypotheses*. The abstract states:

A review of medical literature and U.S. government data suggests that: (i) many cases of idiopathic autism are induced by early mercury exposure from thimerosal; (ii) this type of autism represents an unrecognized mercurial syndrome; and (iii) genetic and non-genetic factors establish a predisposition whereby thimerosal's adverse effects occur only in some children.[32]

On April 25, 2001, Dr. Boyd Haley, Chairman of the Chemistry Department at the University of Kentucky and expert on mercury toxicity testified before Congress. Besides stating that he believed thimerosal was the most likely cause for the autism epidemic, he also described one possible genetic risk factor regarding autism, which would help to explain why all children don't get autism from their vaccines. He described a brain protein called APO-E that removes toxins from the brain. Some people have the type of APO-E that is very efficient at removing mercury and some people have the kind that is very *inefficient* at removing mercury. He said:

If you look at the chemistry of the APO-E proteins, this can be reflected in the fact that it is a housekeeping protein that clears the brain of waste materials. If you have APO-E2, you can carry out two atoms of mercury for every atom of APO-E that goes out. If you have APO-E4, you can carry out none. He [Dr. Mike Godfrey of New Zealand] took this and looked at autistic children. When he did the screen of autistic children, there was a huge preponderance of them that had APO-E4, indicating that there is a genetic risk factor, which deserves further study. And it does imply that the inability to detoxify the cerebral spinal fluid may be at least part of the neurological aspect of this disease.[33]

Research has also indicated that patients with Alzheimer's disease have a similar genetic inability to detoxify mercury and other heavy metals out of their brain cells. It's likely the same story for patients with MS, Parkinson's, and ALS (Lou Gehrig's disease).

Hormones also play a part in autism. Autism affects boys about five times more often than girls.[34] This is because estrogen is protective against the effects of thimerosal, whereas testosterone actually enhances the toxicity of thimerosal a hundredfold.

In October 2001, Merck sent out its last batch of thimerosal-containing hepatitis B vaccines. With their statement in 1999 that all of their hepatitis B vaccines were being made without thimerosal, they had led doctors and the public to believe that all of the vaccines being *shipped* were also free of thimerosal. Those last thimerosal-containing vaccines did not actually *expire* until 2002. Other vaccines that contained thimerosal did not expire until 2003 and continued to be used by doctors despite all the evidence mounting against using them.

In 2002, the National Institutes of Health described autism as the fastest growing disability in the United States, affecting 1 in every 250 children. And yet, they invested just $56 million toward autism research. As a comparison, they spent $688 million on diabetes research and more than $2.2 billion on AIDS research. Similarly, the CDC spent $11.3 million on autism research, $62 million on diabetes research, and $932 million on AIDS research.

In spite of the massive amount of evidence against mercury that, by this point, was common knowledge, and despite the fact that most vaccine manufacturers were now voluntarily producing childhood vaccines (including RhoGAM and BayRho) without thimerosal, the CDC still refused to state a preference for thimerosal-free vaccines over those that contained the drug. They also, for the first time ever, recommended that pregnant women and infants between six months and 24 months get a flu shot. The flu shot was also recommended for kids every year from then on, even though virtually all flu shots contained 25 micrograms of mercury.

In November 2002, as a part of the Homeland Security Act, Senate Majority Leader Bill Frist, M.D. (R-TN) slipped in what is known as a "stealth amendment." This amendment, known as the "Eli Lilly Protection Act," was designed specifically to keep children who had been injured by thimerosal from receiving compensation from Eli Lilly, the former manufacturer of thimerosal. Adding insult to injury, it also prevented thimerosal-injured children from collecting from the federal Vaccine Injury Compensation Trust Fund, which is not even funded by the drug companies, but by surcharges on the vaccines. As you know, the Homeland Security Act did pass, but within three months, the uproar from angry parents and Senator Debbie Stabenow (D-MI) led to this amendment being repealed.

Dr. Frist has received over $873,000 in campaign contributions from pharmaceutical companies. In fact, Eli Lilly contributed $10,000 and purchased 5,000 copies of his new book on bioterrorism the day after he introduced the amendment.

In 2003, the *Physicians' Desk Reference* showed that there were still three childhood vaccines that contained the full dose of thimerosal: the DTaP shot by Aventis Pasteur, Hib by Wyeth, and hepatitis B by Merck.[36]

A key point to remember here is that the nervous system of a child is not completely formed when s/he is born. Neither is the child's blood brain barrier, or immune system. While the blood-brain barrier is still forming, nerve tissue is extremely sensitive to toxicity or any changes in its biological environment. According to a University of Calgary video shown during the Congressional hearings in December 2002, the artificial presence of mercury in the blood can prevent normal nerve formation.[35] Of course, the earlier the nerves are affected, the more severe the consequences. As was suggested by Japan's "experiment" with SIDS (discussed in the previous chapter), something that may be relatively harmless to a child at two-years-old can cause devastating, permanent problems at birth or at two months of age.

At birth, the fatty, myelin coating that surrounds and protects the nerves, like the insulation on a wire, is not yet completely formed making nerves even more susceptible to damage. The result of damaging nerves, especially at this early stage, is the potential for virtually any neurological disorder. Once attached to the nerves, or lodged in the brain, mercury (or other heavy metals like aluminum) can stay there indefinitely. This means that not only sudden or acute neurological disorders such as autism can occur, but also conditions like ADD/ADHD, learning disorders, Asperger's Syndrome, MS, ALS (Lou Gehrig's disease), Alzheimer's, and Parkinson's disease. Every one of these diseases is on the rise and there is mounting evidence that all are caused by heavy metal poisoning, with mercury being at the top of the list.

Another factor is that babies don't develop the ability to produce bile until they are four to six months of age. Bile is one route our bodies use to bind and rid ourselves of toxins. When the body can't get rid of a toxin, it stores it somewhere. Mercury has an affinity for brain tissue. In fact, it has an affinity for the very parts of the brain that are involved in autism: the cerebellum, the amygdala, and the hippocampus.

In May 2003, Congressman Burton's Congressional Subcommittee on Human Rights and Wellness completed their final report called "Mercury in Medicine—Taking Unnecessary Risks." The report criticized the FDA and the CDC and stated that mercury should be removed from vaccines and other drugs. Here's a sample of what was said:

Through a Congressional mandate to review thimerosal content in medicines, the FDA learned that childhood vaccines, when given according to the CDC's recommendations exposed over 8,000 children a day in the United States to levels of mercury that exceeded Federal guidelines... Thimerosal used as a preservative in vaccines is likely related to the autism epidemic. This epidemic in all probability may have been prevented or curtailed had the FDA not been asleep at the switch regarding the lack of safety data regarding injected thimerosal and the sharp rise of infant exposure to this known neurotoxin. Our public health agencies' failure to act is indicative of institutional malfeasance for self-protection and misplaced protectionism of the pharmaceutical industry.[37]

The July/August 2003 issue of the *International Journal of Toxicology* reported on a study using hair analysis that indicated autistic infants are significantly less able to detoxify mercury from their bodies than their non-autistic peers. It also showed that autistic children were exposed to more maternal mercury through their mother's silver fillings and RhoGAM shots.[38]

According to a 2003 article in the *Journal of American Physicians and Surgeons*, having mercury injected directly into the system makes the exposure level several *logs* (powers of ten) higher in concentration as compared to oral ingestion.[39] On the next page is an interesting graph from that study.

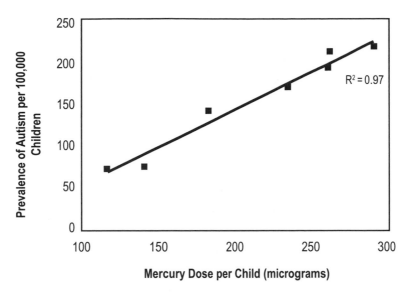

Reprinted with permission of the *Journal of American Physicians and Surgeons*

You don't have to be a scientist to be able to read this graph. The information is pretty simple: The more mercury, the higher the rate of autism.

In the fall of 2003, another study appearing in the *Journal of American Physicians and Surgeons* showed that when the chelating agent DMSA was used on children, those with autism excreted significantly more mercury (about three times as much) in their urine than those without autism, indicating that they had more mercury in their systems.[40] This, when combined with the studies above, indicates that autistic children have the unfortunate combination of more mercury and less ability to detoxify the metal on their own. (Note: DMSA is also being used successfully to *treat* autistic children.)

In February 2004, the California EPA Office of Environmental Health Hazard reported:

The scientific evidence that PMA (phenylmercuric acetate) and thimerosal cause reproductive toxicity is clear and voluminous... The evidence for its reproductive toxicity includes severe mental retardation or malformations in human offspring who were poisoned when their mothers were exposed to ethyl mercury or thimerosal while pregnant, studies in animals demonstrating developmental toxicity after exposure to either ethyl mercury or thimerosal, and data showing interconversion to other forms of mercury that also clearly cause reproductive toxicity.[41]

Another study in 2004, this one appearing in *Molecular Psychiatry,* showed how thimerosal and aluminum inhibit certain enzyme pathways which, "provides a potential molecular explanation for how increased use of vaccines could promote an increase in the incidence of autism." It also states, "The increased incidence of ADHD, which preceded the more recent rise in autism, could represent an alternative manifestation of vaccine-associated neuro-developmental toxicity..." [42]

Another study that year, appearing in *Toxicology and Applied Pharmacology* stated, "Our study clearly indicates that EtHg (ethyl mercury) is similar to MeHg (methyl mercury) with respect to the immunosuppressive effect on the immune system in vivo [living organisms]." They also stated that, "...thimerosal treatment subsequently leads to strong immunostimulation and autoimmunity..." [43] In other words, thimerosal causes the immune system to go haywire and can sometimes cause the body to attack itself. We'll come back to this point briefly when we discuss the MMR shot.

In May 2004, the Institute of Medicine released its updated report on the vaccine-autism issue. Their report in 2001 had stated the connection was inconclusive but "biologically plausible." The conclusion of the new report, however, was just as they had "predicted" during the CDC's secret Simpsonwood meeting back in June of 2000. The summary stated, "...the body of epidemiological evidence favors rejection of a causal relationship between thimerosal-containing vaccines and autism. The committee further finds that potential biological mechanisms for vaccine-induced autism that have been generated to date are theoretical only." [44] Interestingly, they also suggested that no further study be done on the topic.

Rather than listening to the scientists who were experts on this topic and who did not have ties to the vaccine industry, or study the CDC's giant database that Tom Verstraeten had had at his disposal, the IOM relied on four badly flawed European studies where the children receive much less thimerosal than kids in America do. They also cited Verstraeten's new, cleaned-up study from the journal *Pediatrics*.[45] Remember, Verstraeten now worked for GlaxoSmithKline, a major vaccine manufacturer.

However, this fabricated report fooled no one. Under pressure from angry parents, Congress, and even a few of its own members, the IOM reluctantly convened a second panel composed of different scientists to review the findings of the first. These scientists criticized the previous panel for its lack of transparency and urged the CDC to make its database available to the public. Thus far, only two people have managed to gain access to this information. Their names are Mark Geier, M.D., Ph.D., president of the Genetics Center of America and his son, David Geier. It took them a year of battling, along with the help of Congress, but they finally got the CDC to turn over their records.

As of this writing, the Geiers have completed six studies using the CDC's records that show a strong correlation between thimerosal and neurological damage in children. One study of educational performance showed that children who received higher doses of thimerosal had nearly three times the rate of autism and more than three times the number of speech disorders and mental retardation. Another study shows that since thimerosal has been eliminated from most vaccines, autism rates are beginning to decline. You can view much of their research online.[46] Dr. Geier, summarized the issue this way:

> This is about as proven an issue as you're going to see… what is occurring here is a cover-up under the guise of protecting the vaccine program. If we're not convinced thimerosal is causing autism, I recommend that we spend $10 or $20 billion to find out what is causing it. Nobody's doing that.[47]

In September 2004, the United Kingdom and California both banned thimerosal-containing vaccines. Also in September, a representative from Rhode Island introduced a bill to ban thimerosal-containing vaccines in his state.

In 2005, many other states followed suit, each filing bills with the goal of banning thimerosal in vaccines. In January, bills were filed in Florida, Maryland, Washington, New Hampshire, Illinois, Minnesota, and Nebraska. In February, bills were filed in Tennessee, Oregon, New York, and Ohio. In March, Vermont, Pennsylvania, and Nevada joined the fray. In May, bills were filed in Massachusetts and Missouri. Over the next several months, New York, Illinois, Iowa, Missouri, and Delaware passed their bills.

While all of this was going on, there had been several bills introduced into Congress that attempted to ban thimerosal from vaccines in the U.S. None of these bills even made it to the floor for a vote.

Meanwhile, Senator Frist and his Republican cohorts were still busy trying to protect their Big Pharma buddies from the mean old mommies of autistic kids. They had already introduced several bills that attempted to protect the vaccine industry from lawsuits. Like the Eli Lilly Protection Act, these were introduced as stealth amendments or "riders" that were tacked onto other bills that had little or nothing to do with healthcare. One such subversive scheme was the "Public Readiness and Emergency Preparedness (PREP) Act," which was tacked onto the 2006 Department of Defense Appropriations Bill. In the midst of the Iraq and Afghanistan wars, this bill was considered "must-pass" legislation. Knowing this, on December 19, 2005, in the middle of the night, after all negotiations on the bill had been concluded and Frist had actually assured representatives that the PREP act would *not* be attached, he slipped it into the bill.

This provision would give vaccine makers unprecedented immunity, even in the case of willful misconduct where they'd acted negligently or recklessly; it would allow thimerosal to be used in vaccines even in states where it had been banned; and it would give immunity for damages caused by *any* drug, provided the Department of Health and Human Services considered it a "countermeasure for an epidemic." [48]

On December 21, the senate approved the bill unanimously. Nobody was even aware that the provision had been attached when they voted on it. On December 30, President Bush signed the bill into law.

As of 2005, there were at least 4,200 parents of autistic children involved in a class action lawsuit against Eli Lilly, GlaxoSmithKline, and other companies that use thimerosal.

In February 2006, Senator Edward Kennedy and 20 other Democrats from the House and Senate sent a letter to Senator Frist protesting his underhanded tactics.

On January 1, 2006, the Illinois ban on thimerosal-containing vaccines took effect. Hospitals, physicians, and pharmacies were not informed of the change, but this point was moot because that same day the ban was suspended by the Illinois Department of Health for fear of vaccine shortages.

In July, California's ban on thimerosal-containing vaccines went into effect, but just three months later, in October, several organizations, including the California Medical Association, requested an exemption on the new law due to shortages of preservative-free flu shots, claiming this was an "emergency situation."

In April, The Institute for Vaccine Safety at Johns Hopkins School of Medicine made note of the fact that there were over 200 new vaccines in various stages of development and that their manufacturers have plans for most, if not all of them, to be added to the Recommended Childhood Vaccine Schedule.

Also in 2006, New Jersey, Hawaii, Kansas, and Kentucky filed bills to ban thimerosal in vaccines. Washington's governor signed the bill banning thimerosal-containing vaccines into law. Both houses in Hawaii approved the ban on thimerosal, but the governor vetoed the bill under pressure from the American Academy of Pediatrics.

In November 2006, PutChildrenFirst.org released the results of a survey of over 9,000 Americans. The results showed:

- 74 percent did not know the flu shot contained mercury.
- Upon learning that the flu shot contains mercury, 74 percent said they would be less likely to take it and 86 percent of parents said they would be less likely to allow their child to get a flu shot.
- 78 percent disagreed with the CDC's stance on vaccinating pregnant women and children with mercury-containing shots.
- 73 percent believed the government should warn pregnant women NOT to get a flu shot that contains mercury.

- Over 70 percent felt that Congress, doctors, and medical groups like the American Academy of Pediatrics should take responsibility for making sure no vaccines contain mercury.
- 82 percent of parents said they would be willing to pay the additional $2.50 for a mercury-free flu shot.

On December 19, 2006, The Combating Autism Act was signed into law by President Bush. It authorized nearly $1 billion over five years toward the screening, education, early intervention, prompt referrals for treatment and services, and research of autistic spectrum disorders. The act was not fully funded, however, and though earlier versions of the bill would have allotted $45 million to study the possibility of "environmental causes" of autism, these were stripped from the final bill.

In 2007, Vermont, Nebraska, and West Virginia introduced bills to ban thimerosal-containing vaccines, and Florida introduced its second bill on the matter.

In November 2007, the House and Senate both approved the 2008 Health and Human Services-Labor-Education Appropriations Bill, which included $37 million for autism services and treatment programs and fully funded the already passed Combating Autism Act. President Bush *vetoed* the bill, however, because of "objectionable provisions," such as the measure to ban the use of thimerosal-containing flu shots, *and* because he did not agree that the Combating Autism Act should be fully funded. The House of Representatives came within two votes of overriding President Bush's veto.

The Bushes have close ties to Eli Lilly and Big Pharma. The first President Bush sat on the Eli Lilly Board in the late 1970s. W's White

House Budget Director was a former Vice President at Eli Lilly. Sidney Taurel, who advised Bush II on domestic security, was Eli Lilly's CEO. W also received $891,208 in campaign contributions from Big Pharma.

That same month, the Department of Health and Human Services (HHS) conceded on a case alleging that a child had developed autism from her vaccinations. They stated:

> In sum, DVIC [Division of Vaccine Injury Compensation] has concluded that the facts of this case meet the statutory criteria for demonstrating that the vaccinations CHILD received on July 19, 2000, significantly aggravated an underlying mitochondrial disorder, which predisposed her to deficits in cellular energy metabolism, and manifested as a regressive encephalopathy with features of autism spectrum disorder.[49]

By conceding the case before it went to trial, they stopped any evidence and testimony from being presented, which would have been part of the public record. The HHS also barred the parents or their attorney from ever being able to speak about the details of the case. Despite conceding this test case, the HHS continued to deny that vaccinations can cause autism.

Also that month, more than 2,000 parents in Maryland were ordered to appear in court and allow their children to be vaccinated with the hepatitis B vaccine. If they refused, they would receive a $50 fine for every day that they did not comply or face 10 days in jail.

In March 2008, the parents of Hannah Poling (whose father, Jon, is an M.D. neurologist and whose mother, Terry, is a nurse and a lawyer) and their attorney held a press conference at the federal court in Atlanta, Georgia. Hannah was the child in the case that the HHS had conceded was injured by her vaccines and thus resulted in autism. They stated, live on CNN, that Hannah had been a perfectly normal little girl until she received nine vaccines in one day at the age of 19 months. Shortly after receiving those shots, she regressed into autism. It was discovered later that she had a mitochondrial disorder, which apparently predisposed her to the condition.

In an interview with the *Atlanta Journal-Constitution* regarding the case, the president-elect of the American Academy of Pediatrics stated:

> It raised a lot of questions for us... Our responsibility is to make sure the public is given good information and make sure the hype doesn't distract from public health. I still would not think that we're going to have evidence showing a role of vaccines actually causing autism.[50]

These words were echoed by Julie Gerberding, Director of the CDC, who said people should, "...set aside this very isolated, unusual situation." [51]

David Kirby, author of *Evidence of Harm*, who also writes for *The Huffington Post*, wrote a scathing article regarding the government's handling of the case. The article was entitled, "The Vaccine-Autism Story: Trust Your Government or Be a Patriot and Get on Google." [52] In the article, he sarcastically translated the "spin" the government was giving the public. For example:

> ...CDC Director Julie Gerberding told the media that the American people need to "set aside this very isolated, unusual situation," even though "the court apparently made the decision that it is fair to say that vaccinations may have been one of the precipitators."

TRANSLATION: (Middlebrow Bureaucratese) "I am either an exceedingly ignorant, untruthful or misleading Director, because there is no evidence at all that this situation is 'isolated and unusual' (indeed, the evidence points to the opposite), and because the court 'decision' was not made by the court at all, but rather by medical doctors who work for the U.S. Secretary of Health and Human Services," otherwise known as Dr. Gerberding's boss.

He also translated an email from a Dr. Paul Jarris, the Executive Director of the Association of State and Territorial Health Officials. The email said:

The case was settled because the vaccine worsened the child's underlying and previously undiagnosed disorder, causing impaired brain function. These symptoms of impaired brain function then led to an autism spectrum disorder. The federal government maintains that vaccines do not cause autism, and that this case does not indicate any change in their position on the issue.

TRANSLATION: (An Anti-Syllogism) "Vaccines cause brain impairment, and brain impairments cause autism. Therefore vaccines do not cause autism."

He also stated, "The next time someone tells you that this girl does not have autism, but only the 'symptoms' of autism, you tell them that the definition of autism is having the symptoms of autism." Well said.

On March 10, 2008, parents of autistic children began flooding the White House with phone calls demanding Julie Gerberding's resignation as Director of the CDC. This came at the request of actress, author, and activist Jenny McCarthy, whose son became autistic after receiving his routine vaccinations.

On June 4, 2008, the "Green Our Vaccines" rally took place in Washington, D.C. More than 8,500 people showed up to march. The event was hosted by Talk About Curing Autism (TACA) and led by Jenny McCarthy and her partner, Jim Carrey. Also speaking at the event were Robert F. Kennedy, Jr., Dr. Boyd Haley, Congressman Dan Burton, and Congresswoman Carolyn Maloney.

So, how do you feel now about the appeasing statements made by our government officials or doctors when they say that there's nothing to this whole vaccination/autism issue? Do you believe them? Do you still think this issue was created out of thin air by a bunch of hysterical parents looking for someone to blame or someone to pay for their children's shortcomings? Or, are you starting to see that this is part of the biggest cover-up (at least in healthcare) in history? This is bigger than tobacco; it's bigger than asbestos; it's bigger than thalidomide; it's bigger than DES... This is nothing short of our government knowingly sacrificing thousands of children's and their parents' lives in order to protect the profits of the multi-billion-dollar drug industry. It's utterly reprehensible.

But just in case our timeline didn't fully convince you, here are a few more fun facts regarding thimerosal and autism:

Wikipedia states, "Thimerosal is very toxic by inhalation, ingestion, and in contact with skin, with a danger of cumulative effects. When applied to human nerve cells, it changes cell membrane permeability and induces programmed cell death." And yet, in the preceding sentence, they paradoxically state that, "the World Health Organization has concluded that there is no *evidence* [emphasis added] of toxicity from thimerosal in vaccines and no reason on safety grounds to change to more-expensive [hmm, could this be a hint?] single-dose administration [which does not contain thimerosal]." Perhaps there's "no evidence" because, as they state a little further down, "Few studies of the toxicity of thimerosal in humans have been performed." [53]

Two points here deserve comment. First, there is overwhelming evidence indicating that the thimerosal in vaccines is toxic and dangerous. The problem is, the people in charge choose to ignore that research. It's just like Jim Carrey said recently, "There's no evidence of the Lincoln Memorial if you look the other way and refuse to turn around. But if you care to look, it's really quite impressive." [54]

Second, what the hell are they doing injecting even a "potential" toxin into kids for 70 years without studying it? As Dr. Tim O'Shea says:

> The key point here that no one seems to be pointing out is that research should be done <u>before</u> mandating a vaccine into the bloodstream of American children! You don't just start mass-injecting something into a population and then stand back and defy independent scientists to prove it isn't safe! That's exactly what we've done here. As a nation, as a government, and as parents, Americans should be very certain, beyond a reasonable doubt, that any substance being injected into an unformed little nervous system is absolutely safe and does no harm. That should be the minimum requirement.[55]

When Eli Lilly was making thimerosal, they were required to put out a Material Safety Data Sheet on it. I was able to find an actual scan of this document on the Internet. Here's the meat and potatoes of what it says: "Mercury poisoning can occur. Early signs of mercury poisoning are nervous system effects, including narrowing of the visual field and numbness in the extremities. *Exposure in utero and in children can cause mild to severe mental retardation and mild to severe motor coordination impairment* [emphasis added]." Hmm. Sounds a bit like autism to me. They also classify thimerosal as a "Poisonous solid." [56]

Oh, by the bye, with the massive explosion in autism cases, guess who's coming to the rescue? Eli Lilly has come out with a new slant on their ADHD drug "Strattera." They're now recommending it for the "off label" treatment of autism and autism spectrum disorders. Remember that discussion way back in Chapter 3 about how drug companies sometimes like to create new markets for themselves?

EMD Chemicals is another producer of thimerosal. Here's what *their* safety sheet says, *in all caps*: DANGER! POISON! MAY BE FATAL IF INHALED, ABSORBED THROUGH SKIN OR SWALLOWED. VERY TOXIC TO AQUATIC ORGANISMS. CAUSES EYE AND SKIN IRRITATION. CONTAINS MATERIAL WHICH MAY CAUSE DAMAGE TO THE FOLLOWING ORGANS: KIDNEYS, RESPIRATORY TRACT, SKIN, EYES, CENTRAL NERVOUS SYSTEM, EYE, [yes, they list the eyes twice in this sentence, as well as the] LENS OR CORNEA. MAY BE HARMFUL TO ENVIRONMENT IF RELEASED IN LARGE AMOUNTS. WARNING: This product contains a chemical known to the State of California to cause birth defects or other reproductive harm." [57] Now, keep in mind that these safety sheets are designed for occupational, i.e. primarily *topical* exposure. And we are to mutely accept that it's perfectly safe to *inject* this poison into not-even-one-day-old infants? Gee, what harm could possibly come from *that*?

Mark Geier, M.D., Ph.D. determined that "thimerosal contributed to about 75 percent of the neuro-developmental disorders he'd studied, while the MMR vaccine (discussed below) contributed to about 15 percent." The remaining 10 percent, he says, were related to mercury from RhoGAM shots, dental mercury, and other mercury sources.

Harris Coulter, Ph.D., author of *Vaccination, Social Violence and Criminality: The Medical Assault on the American Brain*, associates autism with what is known as post-vaccinal encephalitis. Encephalitis is brain inflammation and it can be caused by severe infection, trauma to the head, and severe burns. These causes are rare, however, when compared with what he says is the major cause of encephalitis—vaccination. Infectious encephalitis was epidemic back in the era of 1910–1930, and mental institutions were filled with patients suffering from post-encephalitic syndrome. These conditions were virtually identical to what we are now seeing in vaccine-damaged children.

Dr. Coulter also co-authored the book *A Shot in the Dark*, with Barbara Loe Fisher. In their book, they estimate that 12,000–15,000 children suffer from severe neurological damage every year. Dr. Coulter has said that he believes the prevalence could be much higher, and that, "one child in five or six is [neurologically] affected to some degree by the vaccination...about 20 percent of the population."[58] Many of these neurologically damaged children are autistic.

"Awareness of the relationship between these neurological disabilities and the post-encephalitic syndrome has been blocked... by reluctance to admit that the childhood vaccination program is the only possible cause of a mass epidemic of clinical and sub-clinical encephalitis."

—Harris Coulter, Ph.D.

The Amish: Our Top Secret Control Group

And finally, let's put one more nail in the thimerosal coffin, just to really seal the deal. We've discussed at various times in the past two chapters the idea that we are all part of this grand vaccine experiment and that there is no control group (people who have *not* received vaccinations) with which to compare ourselves. Well, that seemed to be the case, until an investigative journalist named Dan Olmsted realized that the Pennsylvania Amish don't vaccinate their kids and could serve as an outstanding control group in the issue of whether or not vaccines cause autism. Using national averages, he figured out that the Amish population *should* have about 130 autistic kids to care for. What he found, however, was that they only had four. Of those four, three of them, including one who had been adopted from China, *had* been vaccinated, and the fourth had had environmental exposure to mercury from a power plant.[59]

MMR as a Cause of Autism

The evidence showing a link between the MMR vaccine and autism isn't nearly as voluminous as the link with mercury, but there *is* some very interesting research being done by some very good scientists around the world on this topic. And, as you're about to read, it may be a combination of these two things (MMR and mercury) along with a genetic susceptibility that leads to autism in some children.

Before thimerosal was removed from the hepatitis B, Hib, and DTaP shots, children had already been exposed to at least 187.5 micrograms of mercury before they had their first MMR shot. As we've discussed, this amount of mercury can have many effects on the body, including compromising the immune system. The MMR shot does *not* contain mercury. It does, however, contain at least three live, mutated (a.k.a. "attenuated") viruses. If this toxic amount of mercury has compromised an infant's immune system, some children may have a difficult time mounting an appropriate immune response to these viruses being injected directly into their bodies.

Autistic children frequently have gastrointestinal problems. In 1996, Andrew Wakefield, M.D., a London gastroenterologist, began studying this problem and discovered large bleeding masses called "lymphoid nodular hyperplasia" in the intestines of many autistic children. Apparently, the body thinks these masses are waste and tries to pass them, but since they're attached to the wall of the intestines, it sometimes causes the same folding up, or telescoping of the colon we discussed previously (under the category of rotavirus—another live virus vaccine) called intussusception. As mentioned, this can be fatal and in any case, it's very painful. Dr. Wakefield calls this new bowel condition "autistic enterocolitis."

In most of the cases he studied, the parents or the physician reported that the child's health problems began soon after receiving the MMR shot. Using a technique that can distinguish one virus from another, it was discovered that in almost every case of autistic enterocolitis (24 out of 25) they found a persistent measles infection in the inflamed intestines of these children. This technique is so accurate and precise, that it can distinguish between the virus from the *disease* and the virus from the *vaccine*. Guess which one it was. It was from the vaccine! And in case you're wondering, only one child in 15 without autism has this virus in his/her gut.

Dr. Wakefield also found this same chronic measles infection

Psychoneuroimmunologists are now reporting that over half of the immune system is in the gut and that the gut, the brain, and the immune system are all intimately linked.

present in 75 percent of children with Crohn's disease (another chronic intestinal disease), traditionally an adult disorder following years of dietary abuse. The inflammation that results from this infection can cause what is known as "leaky gut syndrome." This is where large proteins and other harmful substances can be absorbed into the blood and are then carried to the brain and other tissues. This can lead to major food allergies and autoimmune diseases. Many of these substances, such as casomorphin (from milk proteins) and gluteomorphin (from wheat and other gluten-containing foods) can cause abnormal behaviors. Both of these substances have mild opiate-like effects.

Dr. Wakefield and 12 other British scientists wrote up their

> Many parents of autistic children find that a diet free from casein and gluten helps their children to function more normally.

research and had it published in *Lancet* on February 28, 1998.[60] Of course, this report was met with harsh criticism from the pro-vaccine groups in America including the CDC and the AAP. In typical fashion, the CDC ignored the science and stated that children's health problems following vaccination were coincidental and not caused by vaccination. Funny, they never say the so-called benefits of vaccination are coincidental—only the adverse events.

Vijendra Singh, Ph.D., a neuroimmunologist and expert on autism, found that autistic children had experienced an autoimmune reaction in which their bodies, for some reason, attacked the lining of their nervous system. He calls it a "hyper-immune response to the measles virus." He found that 55 percent of the families he worked with reported the symptoms of autism appeared soon after receiving the MMR shot, and 33 percent said they appeared soon after the DPT shot.[61]

Mary Megson, M.D., assistant professor of pediatrics at the Medical College of Virginia, has found that autistic children have a major deficiency of vitamin A. She suspects it's the MMR vaccine that's causing this. She's also found that the pertussis vaccine disrupts a protein that is needed for retinal formation. Interestingly, many autistics have night-blindness and loss of 3D vision. She's had success treating autism, dyslexia and other learning disabilities using cod liver oil, which is high in natural vitamin A.[62]

The Politics of Vaccines

By now you must be thinking, is this crazy chiropractor right about all this vaccine business? And if he is, why would the system be set up this way? Well, I hate to use the old cliché again, but when something defies all logic and common sense, follow the money. But let's get more specific, shall we?

1. **Why would the FDA approve (virtually) untested vaccines for universal use on children?**

    If you remember, back in Chapter 4, we talked about the incestuous ties between the Advisory Board members of the FDA and the pharmaceutical companies. These people with the power to approve or disapprove drugs are often employees or stockholders of the drug companies. In some cases, they actually own the patent on the drug they're voting on. Well, vaccines are among those drugs. And since vaccines fall into that Holy Grail category of drugs that are forced upon virtually every person on earth, these board members are anxious to get the vaccines approved as soon as possible.

    Answer: Money.

2. **Why would the federal government protect vaccine manufacturers from liability when children are obviously being killed and permanently damaged by vaccinations?**

    Let me answer that question with another question:

Where do you think all those huge campaign finance contributions come from? The pharmaceutical corporations are among the richest companies in the world.

Answer: Money.

3. **Why would pediatricians, doctors sworn first to "do no harm" and to uphold their patients' health as the utmost, knowingly go along with the vaccine scam and become frontline enforcers of it?**

Well, first of all, strange as it may seem, most of them don't know as much as you now know about vaccinations. Medical doctors know the *rationale* behind vaccination and even I'll admit, the *theory* sounds good. But they're not taught, nor do they take the time to research the information I've presented in these last two chapters—or any of the rest of this book for that matter. (In fact, you might want to give your doctor a copy of this book.) Unless they take a special interest in the subject and are willing to investigate it on their own time *and* have the moral fortitude to shun what their own profession says, they are unlikely to know about the mercury and other toxic ingredients that go into these shots and how dangerous they really are. Vaccinations are also a big part of the "Well Baby Visits" to your pediatrician. They are the biggest reason they want to see children when they're not sick. Dentists get people in the door for bi-yearly cleanings and check-ups. Pediatricians get kids in for their shots. Vaccines are also considered the "standard of care" for pediatricians. Most medical doctors feel bound to abide by the standards for their specialty, and vaccines fall into that category.

Answer: They've been brainwashed to believe it's their job. In other words, money.

4. **Why would state supported schools be a part of upholding this scam against the very children they are supposed to be educating and protecting?**

   The states get $100 from the federal government for every fully vaccinated child. The schools are supported by the states. The schools therefore become one of the primary enforcers of these vaccine mandates. Schools get even more money if a disabled child attends their school, so if one becomes autistic as a result of his/her being fully vaccinated, they stand to gain doubly. I'm not suggesting that there is any maliciousness by the individuals running our schools; only that the system is set up to encourage more vaccinations and more disabled children.

   Answer: Money.

My wife is an elementary school teacher. When she learned about the dangers of vaccinating, she immediately wanted to warn all of the parents at the school where she works. But when she inquired about this, she was told she was not allowed to say anything, implying that it would be illegal for her to do so. She was told she couldn't even mention that there was a waiver to get around the mandate.

5. **Why would the federal government want to give money to the states for vaccinated children when they know that vaccines injure and kill many children every year, especially if the federal government is going to foot the bill for all those injuries?**

Oh, wait…is this about that campaign finance thing again? Yes. The drug companies don't give the money to the federal *government*, they give it to the people who *run* the government. The people who *run* the government don't pay the states nor do they pay for the vaccine-injured babies. *We* do. That's right. So, follow the bouncing "$". Pharmaceutical companies give money to the people who want to run things in Washington. They get elected and pass laws to support and protect their benefactors. Thousands of infants are injured and killed, and we pay for their compensation through our tax dollars and a special surcharge that's placed on every vaccine. Pharmaceutical companies and elected officials win. Taxpayers and one in 100 babies (and their parents) lose.

Answer: Money.

I don't think I can put things much more clearly than that, but here are some quotes by some who can:

"What if it's really true that the prime cause of autism turns out to be vaccines? Vaccines are the Sacred Cow of medicine. As the infrastructure for a lifetime of dependence upon medicines, vaccines are above reproach, above criticism. The best journals ask: how could vaccines—the crowning achievement of scientific medicine—be the cause of disease? It's the question that cannot be asked, the thought which cannot be entertained. American science is absolutely dominated by economics. In such a system, true scientific discovery is fatally handicapped."

—Tim O'Shea, D.C., Author of *The Sanctity of Human Blood:*
Vaccination Is Not Immunization

"It is apparent that critical medical decisions for an entire generation of American children are being made by small committees whose members have incestuous ties with agencies that stand to gain power, or with manufacturers who stand to gain enormous profits from the policy that is made… We suspect financial ties between vaccine manufacturers and medical groups such as the AMA and the American Academy of Pediatrics… Public policy regarding vaccines is fundamentally flawed. It is permeated by conflicts of interest. It is based on poor scientific methodology (including studies that are too small, too short, and too limited in populations represented), which is, moreover, insulated from independent criticism. The evidence is far too poor to warrant overriding the independent judgments of patients, parents, and attending physicians, even if this were ethically or legally acceptable.

"Children younger than 14 are three times more likely to die or suffer adverse reactions [to the hepatitis B vaccine] than to catch the disease… It's one thing to bar a student from school if he is carrying an infectious disease posing a threat to other children. But to require a questionable medical treatment as a condition of attendance crosses over the line to practicing medicine… Vaccines use school children as research subjects without informed consent, in violation of the Nuremberg Codes. School administrators and government bureaucrats could be prosecuted as war criminals.

"AAPS [American Association of Physicians and Surgeons] believes that parents, with the advice of their doctors, should make decisions about their children's medical care—not government bureaucrats… Measles, mumps, rubella, hepatitis B, and the whole panoply of childhood diseases are a far less serious threat than having a large fraction (10 percent) of a generation afflicted with learning disability because of an impassioned crusade for universal vaccination… The AAPS calls for a moratorium on

vaccine mandates and for physicians to insist on truly informed consent for the use of vaccines."

—Jane Orient, M.D., Executive Medical Director of the American Association of
Physicians and Surgeons (Quotes taken from various speeches)

"A common myth is that thimerosal is added to vaccines in 'trace' amounts. The concentration of mercury in a multi-dose flu vaccine vial is 50,000 parts per billion. To put this in perspective, drinking water cannot exceed 2 parts per billion of mercury, and waste is considered hazardous if it has only 200 parts per billion. Is it really safe then to inject pregnant women, newborns, and infants with levels of mercury 250 times higher than what is legally classified as hazardous waste?"

—Mike Wagnitz, Senior Chemist at the University of Wisconsin who
has over 20 years of experience in evaluating materials for mercury

"There is a great deal of evidence to prove that immunization of children does more harm than good and that there is no rationale for enforcing immunizations."

—Anthony Morris, M.D., Head of Biological Standards for the U.S. Department of Health

By the way, he was fired the day after he said this.

"The greatest threat of childhood diseases lies in the dangerous and ineffectual efforts made to prevent them through mass immunization. Much of what you have been led to believe about immunization simply isn't true. If I were to follow my deeper convictions, I would urge you to reject all inoculations for your child... There is no convincing scientific evidence that mass inoculations can be credited with eliminating any childhood disease. If immunizations were responsible for the disappearance

of these diseases in the U.S., one must ask why they disappeared simultaneously in Europe, where mass immunizations did not take place."

—Robert Mendelsohn, M.D., Author of *How to Raise a Healthy Child In Spite of Your Doctor*

"Immunizations, including those practiced on babies, not only did not prevent any infectious diseases; they caused more suffering and more deaths than has any other human activity in the entire history of medical intervention. It will be decades before the mopping-up after the disasters caused by childhood vaccination will be completed. All vaccinations should cease forthwith and all victims of their side effects should be appropriately compensated.

"Any country which mandates an extremely invasive medical procedure (vaccinations), with a lack of scientific foundation, its many known dangers and documented ineffectiveness, is not a free country. It is a plutocracy of vested interests using the citizens as their guinea pigs and slaves to further their greedy designs."

—Vierra Scheibner, Ph.D., Author of *Vaccination: 100 Years of Orthodox Research*

It is time for a paradigm shift. As a bare minimum, vaccinations must become voluntary and parents should be truly educated and warned about the benefits and the risks of these procedures as well as the poisons contained in these toxic chemical cocktails we so blithely call "immunizations."

Why have we allowed our government and the pharmaceutical companies this much power over our health and the health of our children? We have allowed them to lull us into a deep, submissive sleep, trusting them to do the right thing. Well, they have *not* done the right thing. In fact, in far too many cases, they have done the exact *opposite* of the right thing. They no longer deserve our trust. We must wake up and take the responsibility for our health back.

More vaccines are on the way, not fewer. We *must not* allow this assault on our children to continue or it will surely and swiftly lead to the demise of our species. We must make a stand. There *are* times that call for civil disobedience and this is one of them.

Call your politicians. Educate them. There's a long list of references at the end of the next chapter. Buy some of the books and send them to your representatives. Read them yourself and then donate them to your local libraries. Hold a neighborhood meeting and show one of the videos. Push for true informed consent.

Parents who are truly educated on the benefits and informed of the risks and still choose to vaccinate their children should be allowed to do so if they wish, but parents who choose *not* to vaccinate should not be harassed by their doctors and other authorities, or forced to do so against their will.

Push for independent research on the safety and efficacy of vaccines. Support the NVIC and other organizations like it that are trying to get the truth out to parents. And finally, tell others what you've just read. Get this issue out in the open where it can be discussed and debated.

Let's start a revolution. Together, we can make a positive change in this world. Please do *something*, and do it right now while you're still fuming and frothing at the mouth from what you've just read.

Lastly, remember that leading scientists are now declaring that germs are not the cause of diseases, but are rather the product of sick cells. Those cells are sick most often because of toxic accumulation, stress, and malnutrition.

11

Vaccine "Schmaccine"!
How **<u>NOT</u>** to Vaccinate Your Kids

"The only wholly safe vaccine is a vaccine that is never used."

—Dr. James Shannon, National Institutes of Health

N ow that you know the other side of the vaccine issue, you may be wondering if there's any way to get around them. The good news is, in most cases, there is. Vaccines are *mandated*. This does not necessarily mean they are *mandatory*. There *is* a way out.

In every state, there are waivers, which will allow children to attend public schools without being vaccinated. These waivers are not usually made public; you have to know they exist and actually ask for them. In some cases, school officials may not even know they exist.

All states have a **medical exemption**. This requires a note from a doctor saying that your child could be in danger if s/he is vaccinated. A few reasons for medical exemption are reactions to previous vaccines, a weakened immune system (patients taking steroids or those with cancer, AIDS, etc.), if they've been a recipient of blood products or blood transfusions containing antibodies, or if you can prove your child is already immune to the disease. Also, if you believe your child may have a genetic predisposition to vaccine reactions—perhaps you or one of the child's siblings has had a severe reaction to a vaccine in the past.

All states except Mississippi and West Virginia allow a **religious exemption** for vaccinations. Some states require proof that you belong to a religion that specifically prohibits the use of vaccination such as the Church of Christ, Scientist or Jehovah's Witnesses. You may have to submit something from a pastor, priest, or rabbi and defend your position.

Several states, including California, Arizona, New Mexico, Utah, Colorado, Washington, Idaho, Louisiana, Maine, Michigan, Minnesota, North Dakota, Ohio, Oklahoma, Rhode Island, Vermont, and Wisconsin, also have a **philosophical exemption** for vaccination. This simply requires a written statement (or the signing of a waiver form) of your philosophical objection to vaccination. The waiver for California can be found on my website: www.HealthIsNatural.com.

Other options: Many private schools do not require proof of vaccination. Home schooling is also becoming more and more popular.

Religious and philosophical exemptions have been under attack lately by the pro-vaccine camp and some states have lost these options already. If your state allows them, be prepared to fight for the right to *not* vaccinate. Your state may be next on the chopping block. If your state *doesn't* allow these exemptions, this would be an *excellent* cause for you to fight for. The government has no right to force a risky, largely untested medical procedure that amounts to injecting poisons and foreign viruses into our next generation.

There are some laws which are immoral to *obey*. For example, German officers were prosecuted during the Nuremberg trials for following immoral orders—orders from their own commanders, that they had been trained (brainwashed) not to question, but merely to execute. Isn't killing and/or damaging the brains, intestines, and immune systems of babies for minimal benefit (other than their own finances) also immoral? Shouldn't America's pediatricians be held accountable for injecting known neurotoxins, carcinogenic chemicals, wild monkey viruses, etc., into generations of children, even though they were "following orders" (standards of care handed down from the Centers for Disease Control)? Shouldn't they be prosecuted or at least reprimanded for causing the autism epidemic, SIDS, ADHD, learning disorders, Alzheimer's, Lou Gehrig's, Parkinson's? Certainly the drug companies should be. So should the CDC and the FDA, as they are *all* responsible for these problems that vaccines have created. They've certainly all patted themselves on the back hard enough for the *good* supposedly done by vaccines. It's time they faced up to the *other* side, the *darker, scarier* side of vaccines—the side they've been trying so hard to pretend doesn't exist.

Some laws simply outlive their usefulness. If vaccinating everyone to achieve "herd immunity" was ever useful, it has definitely outlived its usefulness. The proof of this: Far more babies are now being seriously injured by the hepatitis B vaccine than are being protected from the disease. The only people in this country who've gotten polio since the 1970s are people who've gotten it from the vaccine. Mild childhood diseases like chickenpox are becoming more problematic adult diseases like shingles.

It is wrong for the government to force *any* medical procedure on *anyone* unless perhaps the whole population is truly at risk. This is often the excuse that is given for forcing vaccination on every child in the public school system—that the unvaccinated are putting everyone at risk. But if the vaccines work, then those who have chosen to take the shots should be protected, no matter what the rest of us do. So their story doesn't hold water. Therefore, vaccines should not be mandated. The Surgeon General can *recommend* them if s/he wants, but we don't have to listen. Just like you can choose to smoke, drink, and take prescription drugs during your pregnancy if you want.

When enough people start refusing the shots because they realize the dangers of the shots are worse than the dangers of the diseases, things will start to change. Imagine if every parent at your child's school (or even a good percentage of them) stood up to the system and said, "We will not vaccinate our kids, no matter what you say." Now, imagine if that started happening all over the country.

Imagine our next generation growing up free from autism, SIDS, and learning disabilities. Imagine them growing up and never having to worry about Parkinson's, MS, Lou Gehrig's, or Alzheimer's disease. Wouldn't that be worth the minuscule risks associated with them having to deal with diseases like chickenpox, measles, mumps, rubella, rotavirus, hepatitis A and B, which are almost always mild, self-limiting, and immune *strengthening*? If your answer is no, then by all means, feel free to vaccinate your kids. However, no one has the right to make that decision for everyone, no matter what his/her position or motivation.

The children I know who have not been vaccinated are among the healthiest, happiest, brightest children I have ever seen. Far from the neglect or abuse many of these parents are charged with, these parents cared enough about their children's lives to research what was going to be injected into that brand new life they had just created and they cared enough to say, "No. We will accept the hassle of finding a pediatrician who will respect our wishes and not brow beat us for bucking the system. We accept the responsibility of finding a school that will accept our unvaccinated child. We will seek out the waivers and do whatever it takes to protect the nervous system of this precious little child of ours. But we will *not* allow the government to make medical decisions for us, especially when those decisions are clearly based on money rather than science, or even common sense and logic."

Personally, I would not live in a state or a country where my child was forced to take a vaccine that I did not feel was safe. I would leave the country before allowing my child to be forcibly vaccinated.

I know I've been harping on this issue for many pages now, but it's because I feel it's a very important one. In fact, I feel vaccination is one of the biggest healthcare issues facing this country. Cancer, which we'll be covering in another book, is the other big issue. Not coincidentally, both of these issues are about lack of choice and loss of freedom. Virtually every other issue in healthcare is simply a matter of overcoming dogma and ignorance, and this can be dealt with through education of the masses. Nobody can *force* you to take Lipitor or Prozac. There are no government mandates on these drugs. If you wanted, you could choose to lower your cholesterol or deal with your depression using natural methods. Not so with vaccination and cancer. Freedom and choice have been all but removed in these cases. As long as we have freedom and choices available, there is hope. But these freedoms are being eroded away.

The things our government has done to us are far worse than what our forefathers rebelled against in the Revolutionary War. That's why I feel it's time for a new revolution in America—a Natural Healthcare Revolution. And while this will *not* be a war of violence, I *am* advocating a little civil disobedience. When a law is immoral, it is immoral to follow that law. Understanding the immorality of the law, it then becomes everyone's civic duty to disobey that law until that law is changed. All I'm asking of you is that you educate yourself, then stand up for what is right. It is our children and the future of our species that is at stake here.

If You **Do** Decide to Vaccinate, Here Are Some Tips

If you decide this is all too difficult and just want to get your child vaccinated anyway, you can always wait until they're just about ready for school to do so. The older the child is, the stronger his/her immune system will be, and the better s/he will be able to tolerate the insult. Remember, many countries wait until the child is at least two years old before vaccinating, and their rates of infant mortality are much lower than ours.

Make sure your child is healthy when s/he receives his/her shots. Especially make sure there is no fever.

Make sure that if the vaccine is offered in a mercury-free form, that your doctor is using that form. Ask to see the package insert that accompanies the vaccine.

Try to spread out the vaccinations as much as possible. Insist that your child not be given multiple vaccines on the same day.

Give your child cod liver oil, flax seed oil, or other essential fatty acids before and after the vaccination. Put them on a good natural vitamin C product (Cataplex C, for example, from Standard Process). Standard Process also makes a product called Parotid PMG that helps pull metals and toxins from the tissues and another product called Cholacol II, which is a clay substance that will bind to the heavy metals and escort them out of the body safely. There are also good homeopathic remedies to help remove mercury and aluminum from the tissues. All of these things will help eliminate the vaccine toxins from the body.

You can also seek out someone who does allergy elimination work (NAET, BioSET, TBM, etc.) and have your child treated for the allergy/sensitivity to the vaccines prior to getting his/her shots. This may help to prevent any adverse reactions to the vaccines.

What to Do If Your Child Is Injured By a Vaccine

Report the reaction to your pediatrician.

Report the reaction to the Vaccine Adverse Events Reporting System (VAERS). They can be reached by phone at 1-800-822-7967 or by fax at 1-877-721-0366 or at www.fda.gov/cbeer/vaers/vaers.htm.

Contact the National Vaccine Information Center (NVIC). This is a non-profit group that is sympathetic to the cause that I am writing about. They are pushing our government for informed consent and choice on the vaccine issue. You can reach them at: 1-800-909-SHOT or 703-938-0342 or www.909shot.com or email: info@909shot.com. They could also use your support if you'd like to make a tax-deductible donation to this cause.

File a claim with the National Childhood Vaccine Injury Compensation Program. You can contact them at 301-443-6593 or 1-800-338-2382 or http://www.hrsa.cov/bhpr/vicp.

Treating Autism

The following recommendations are also effective for treating ADD/ADHD and other learning disabilities, MS, ALS, Parkinson's, and Alzheimer's disease.

Chelation therapy (pronounced "*Key*-lation") is often used to help pull heavy metals like mercury and aluminum from the brain and other organs. Since mercury is the most likely cause of autism, this is thought to be the one of the best ways to help autistic children. *Intravenous* chelating substances, however, are a bit of a double-edged sword, as they can also carry these metals *to* the brain. For this reason, it is best to do a good, thorough course of *oral* chelation first. By doing oral chelation first, you'll be removing all of the "low hanging fruit" so to speak, so you'll have less likelihood of carrying excess metals to the brain if and when you *do* move on to IV chelation. In other words, let's say your child has mercury in his system. For simplicity's sake, let's just say it's in his liver and brain. You don't want to use IV chelation at first because it could potentially pick up the mercury in his liver and bring it to his brain. It's best to use oral chelation to clean out the liver first, then move on to IV chelation to clean out the brain.

I use two different methods of oral heavy metal chelation in my office. From Standard Process, I use Parotid PMG and Cholacol II. About 1 per day of each should suffice for a child. The other method uses various homeopathic and herbal remedies. There's also an EDTA suppository supplement called Detoxamin that is supposed to work well.

Andrew Cutler, Ph.D., has written an outstanding book entitled *Amalgam Illness, Diagnosis and Treatment*, which describes the oral chelation process in detail. Don't be fooled by the title. Many parents of autistic kids have used the Cutler method with great success. Epsom salt baths (part of the Cutler method) will also pull toxins from the system.

Autistic children also improve when put on a gluten-free, casein-free (GF/CF) diet. Casein is found in dairy products; gluten is found in many grains including wheat, rye, barley, oats, and spelt. Gluten is also often hidden in things like soups, soy sauce, candies, cold cuts, malt, starches, natural flavorings, hydrolyzed and texturized vegetable proteins, no-fat and low-fat products, some drugs, vinegars, and alcohol. This results in a fairly limited diet, but there are many substitutes that can be used in place of these common food items. For example, rice milk can be substituted for dairy. (Do *not* use soy milk! Soy is genetically modified, it's an estrogen, and it's a toxin. It is not fit for human consumption, especially by human *children*. This topic will be covered in a future *Why We're Sick*™ book.) Authentic Foods carries a large line of tasty gluten-free products. They can be found at www.authenticfoods. com. They also have an autism blog. The book *Nourishing Hope for Autism*, by Julie Matthews is another great resource.

Autistic children should also avoid trans fats, artificial colors and flavors, preservatives, nitrates, sugar, and aspartame (NutraSweet). And of course, you should remove any known food allergens from your child's diet. The most common food allergens are eggs, soy, and corn.

Adding cod liver oil (which is high in vitamin A and essential fatty acids) to their juice also helps. Nordic Naturals makes a high quality, orange flavored cod liver oil that mixes well with juice. The dose is one teaspoon per day for a small child and one teaspoon twice a day for a larger child.

Other supplements to consider are a good multivitamin. Standard Process makes a great one for kids called Chewable Catalyn. Catalyn is a perfectly balanced, whole food supplement that contains every nutrient known and likely all the nutrients we've yet to discover too. I recommend one to three per day for kids.

Probiotics are also important, as are digestive enzymes. For these, I recommend Lact Enz, Zymex, and Multizyme from Standard Process at a dose of about one each per day. Okra Pepsin E3 may also help. One other supplement from Standard Process that may help these children is called RNA. Other supplements that are recommended for autistic children are the methyl donors glutathione, SAM-e, and Methyl B12. Antioxidant teas can also be helpful.

Other things that can help include installing a HEPA (High Efficiency Particulate Air) filter in your child's bedroom and changing from conventional cleaners to natural/organic cleaners. Infrared and hyperbaric oxygen treatments are also highly recommended. Don't cook on aluminum or Teflon cookware as the toxins from these pots and pans can leach into the food. I recommend cast iron or glass. Also, don't use fluoridated toothpaste as fluoride is a poison! (This too will be covered later in the *Why We're Sick*™ series.)

Doing all of this is a very good start; however, I don't recommend you try doing this on your own. It's very important to have someone who knows what they're doing help your child, especially with regards to getting rid of heavy metals. Find a doctor that specializes in holistic healing who can help remove the toxins from your child's system and hopefully make some improvements in the way their nervous system functions. Defeat Autism Now! (DAN!) practitioners are specially trained in treating children with autism. You can find a DAN! doctor at www.autism.com. My best advice is to find someone with experience in treating autistic children, be cautious, and always go slowly.

And remember, this is just the beginning. If you have an autistic child, there is help available. Autism *is* treatable.

For more information on this very important topic, please see:

Websites:
Safe Minds: http://www.safeminds.org/index.html
Defeat Autism Now!: http://www.autism.com/
Generation Rescue: http://www.generationrescue.org/
Talk About Curing Autism: http://www.talkaboutcuringautism.org/
Schafer Autism Report: http://www.sarnet.org/
Autism Facts (excellent timeline):
    http://autismfacts.com/index.php
No Mercury: http://www.nomercury.org/
Autism Research Institute: http://www.autism.com/
Autism Society of America: http://www.autism-society.org/
Unlocking Autism: http://www.unlockingautism.org/
Autism One: http://www.autismone.com/
MINDD Foundation: http://mindd.org/
Dr. Joseph Mercola's website: http://www.Mercola.com/
The Autism Autoimmunity Project website:
    www.http://casiquest.org/research_studies.html

Books:
Immunization, Theory vs. Reality: Exposé on Vaccinations,
    by Neil Miller
Vaccines: Are They Really Safe and Effective? A Parent's Guide to
    Childhood Shots, by Neil Miller
The Sanctity of Human Blood: Vaccination Is Not Immunization,
    by Tim O'Shea, D.C.

A Shot in the Dark, by Harris Coulter, Ph.D., and Barbara Loe Fisher
Vaccination: The Medical Assault on the Immune System,
    by Viera Scheibner, Ph.D.
*Vaccination, Social Violence and Criminality: The Medical Assault
    on the American Brain,* by Harris Coulter, Ph.D.
Louder Than Words: A Mother's Journey in Healing Autism,
    by Jenny McCarthy
Healing and Preventing Autism: A Complete Guide,
    by Jenny McCarthy and Dr. Jerry Kartzinel
The Consumer's Guide to Childhood Vaccines, by Barbara Loe Fisher
What Your Doctor May Not Tell You About Children's Vaccinations,
    by Stephanie Cave, M.D., FAAFP
Fear of the Invisible, by Janine Roberts

Videos:

Autism: Made in America, by Gary Null
The Dangers and Ineffectiveness of Vaccinations, Viera Scheibner,
    Ph.D. (2 hours)
Vaccines: The Other Side of the Story, with Barbara Loe Fisher (30
    minutes)

12

AIDS: Should You Be Worried?

"There is no AIDS. It is something that has been invented.
There are no epidemiological grounds for it;
it doesn't exist for us."

—Philippe Krynen (AIDS charity worker)[1]

A IDS, which has been dubbed, "the plague of the century," doesn't kill nearly as many people as cancer, heart disease, or allopathic medicine, but it's always been shrouded in controversy, myths, and tales of conspiracy. As with most of the topics covered in this book, the stories put out by the establishment as to what causes AIDS and where it came from are highly suspect—at least once one dares to take an objective look at them.

The official story, as told by the CDC and all of its affiliated AIDS groups, is that AIDS is caused by a virus, namely HIV or the Human Immunodeficiency Virus, a.k.a., "the AIDS virus." Makes sense, right? AIDS is caused by the AIDS virus—everyone knows this by now. Furthermore, you catch AIDS by having sex with someone who's infected with HIV, or by sharing needles, or any other way of coming into contact with the blood of a person infected with the AIDS virus. To reduce the spread of this dreaded disease, sexually active people are urged to use condoms. Abstinence is preached as well, because sex is now seen as a potentially deadly act. On a related note, having sex with an

HIV-negative person, when you know *you're* HIV-*positive,* has been equated to assault with a deadly weapon. (Many people have actually been imprisoned for this offense.) Intravenous drug users are given free needles in the hopes that the sharing of needles will stop and thus help to prevent the spread of AIDS. We've also heard that the virus mutates quickly, so an effective vaccine is probably impossible, but if it *is* feasible, it's still many years away. We've heard that AIDS is basically one hundred percent deadly and therefore infection with HIV is seen as a death sentence. As for how long between infection and full-blown AIDS, the virus, which has been classified as a "slow virus," seems to have no set timetable in mind. Originally, we were told it could take up to 10 months for AIDS to appear once a person has been infected, but now we are seeing increasing numbers of people living perfectly healthy lives with HIV for well over 10 years—and still going strong.

Regarding the origin of the disease in humans, we've heard crazy stories about people in Africa having sex with monkeys (monkeys that are about the size of a chicken, mind you—about 14 inches tall and 6.5 pounds), thereby contracting a wild monkey virus, which then mutated and was spread to other humans. Others say it was from a monkey bite, though it's never been demonstrated that the virus can be spread through saliva. Furthermore, we know that viruses very rarely jump from one species to another, but in the rare cases that they do, they are not then transmissible among that species.

Finally, we've been told that in addition to controlling the opportunistic infections that eventually kill all AIDS patients, the drugs AZT, ddi, ddc, and similar types of poisonous chemotherapy medications are the best we can offer this poor hopeless bunch. In essence, this is the story that virtually everyone on earth knows to be true.

"If you tell a lie long enough, eventually it will be believed as truth... [And] the greater the lie, the more people will believe it."

—Adolf Hitler, *Mein Kampf*

But what if everything you "know" about AIDS were a lie? What if you found out the official story was nothing but a fairy tale designed and destined to glorify the jobs and the lives of a certain breed of research scientist (especially one particular scientist who happens to be a total fraud and was asked to leave the National Institutes of Health because of blatant scientific misconduct concerning the discovery of HIV)? And what if you found this out, knowing that the United States has spent billions of your tax dollars studying every facet of this fairy tale, and yet no one has ever actually proved that the central tenet of this theory (that HIV causes AIDS) is true? And after learning this, what if you found out that alternative theories on AIDS aren't even *discussed* by those in charge, let alone funded or studied, but instead are written off as ludicrous, completely without merit, or conspiracy theories to be disdained and ignored? If any of this would upset you, then hold on because it's gonna be a bumpy ride.

Have you ever wondered, what if AIDS isn't really caused by HIV? What if those in charge mistook or selectively overlooked certain facts, jumped to the wrong conclusion, reported this falsehood to the world, and never looked back?

When I first heard this theory I thought, "Ridiculous. There are thousands of Ph.D.s all over the world who have been studying AIDS nonstop since the early eighties. They *must've* proven time and time again that HIV is the cause of AIDS." But I had to admit that I didn't really know that for sure. I'd never really studied the issue in depth and I'd never seen any *proof* that it was the cause. I realized that, like most of the rest of you, I'd simply accepted what I'd heard from authorities like the CDC, and believed their story because I had no reason to doubt it. After having wrestled myself to the neutral zone where I could finally admit to myself that it was at least *possible,* I still had a million doubts that would need to be overcome before I would be convinced of such a contrary theory. In short, it would be a very hard sell to convince me after all these years, that HIV wasn't the cause of AIDS.

Now, if a story like "HIV doesn't cause AIDS" comes from ole' Jim down at the barbershop, you might just write it off as another crazy conspiracy theory with no merit whatsoever, but when it comes from 1.) A researcher who won the Nobel Prize for inventing the PCR test, the definitive test for detecting HIV viral loads in the blood, 2.) The man who first discovered HIV (although he is officially considered the "co-discoverer" of HIV), 3.) The man who mapped out the genetic sequences of the first retroviruses discovered (HIV is a type of virus known as a retrovirus), who's also the recipient of many research prizes and other awards, and is a professor at the University of California, Berkeley, and 4.) hundreds or perhaps thousands of other knowledgeable scientists in the fields of virology, biology, and related fields, you stop and give them a chance to tell their tale. Such was the case when I picked up a copy of *Inventing The AIDS Virus*, a 700-page tome by Dr. Peter Duesberg.

Duesberg is a member of the science "hall of fame," known as The National Academy of Sciences, and in the 1970s, he was one of the first to study retroviruses. He's credited with having initially mapped the genetic structure of retroviruses and at one point he claimed they could cause cancer in humans. After doing more research, however, he changed his mind and claimed that retroviruses were more or less harmless and lived harmoniously within human cells. This remains his stance today—even in the face of AIDS and HIV. In 1985, at a science conference in West Germany, Robert Gallo, the "father of human retroviruses" and the other co-discoverer of HIV (not the one mentioned above), introduced Peter Duesberg as a man of extraordinary energy, unusual honesty, an enormous sense of humor, and a rare critical sense "that often makes us look twice, then a third time, at a conclusion many of us believed to be foregone." [2] This is exactly what he did for me with his book.

One of the first things you need to understand is that AIDS is not a disease; it's a syndrome. A syndrome is a group of symptoms, or in this case a group of diseases, that are lumped together under one heading with the *assumption* that there is a single cause. In the case of AIDS, we now have over thirty different diseases that, in the presence of immune deficiency (low T-cell counts) and/or HIV, make up the syndrome. Not one of these is a new disease; each has been around and recognized for decades. Most only occur in the immune compromised patient. Having a compromised immune system is nothing new either, however, in the late seventies, new techniques were developed that allowed the measuring of a certain component of the immune system called T-cells. It was this new technology that led to the discovery of AIDS.

AIDS was "discovered" in 1980 by Dr. Michael Gottlieb, a researcher studying immune deficiency diseases at the UCLA medical center. There, he found a patient suffering from a yeast infection in the throat and a rare fungal pneumonia caused by yeast that inhabits the lungs of almost every person walking the earth called *Pneumocystis carinii*. It's a rare pneumonia because this fungus usually only affects cancer patients whose immune systems have been destroyed by chemotherapy drugs. But this was a young man in his early thirties who was not on chemo. When Gottlieb measured the patient's T-cells, he found they were almost non-existent.

He spent the next several months searching and was eventually able to find four more cases displaying yeast infections of the throat, *Pneumocystis carinii* pneumonia, and low T-cell counts. Interestingly, all five men were homosexuals.

With these five cases discovered, Gottlieb alerted the CDC, claiming he had discovered a new syndrome. Circumstantial evidence began mounting, leading many at the CDC to the conclusion that the "gay pneumonia" was acquired through sexual contact. However, Gottlieb had also noticed another common factor among all five men: They had all reported being heavy users of the recreational drug known as "poppers" or nitrite inhalants, which were used in the fast-track homosexual community for their ability to help maintain erections, prolong orgasm, and facilitate anal intercourse by relaxing sphincter muscles.

By 1982, many toxicologists, including some from the FDA, thought they knew what caused AIDS. They published a number of papers declaring the syndrome was caused by drugs, both prescription (steroids and antibiotics) and recreational (especially inhaled drugs like poppers and crack cocaine). Several doctors also claimed to have cured AIDS patients simply through detoxification methods. However, that same year, the CDC, which was, and is, dominated by virologists, declared that AIDS *must* be caused by a virus, just as they were so sure that polio was decades earlier. They also declared that the virus must be spread by sex. Therefore, the CDC ordered that all future government-sponsored research be directed at finding and combating this virus. But these declarations were only *assumptions* based on the fact that these men were having lots of sex, while ignoring the fact that they were also inhaling lots of drugs. Since they hadn't even found the virus yet, there was no real science backing these claims.

Once Gottlieb's paper was published, more cases of immune deficiency and low T-cell counts were reported—all of them in homosexuals who reported frequent use of poppers, antibiotics, and other recreational drugs. However, the search was now being widened beyond *Pneumocystis carinii* pneumonia to include a rare blood-vessel tumor known as Kaposi's sarcoma, the "gay cancer."

In those early days of AIDS (before it had even taken that name), the CDC offered just two hypotheses: Either it was sexually transmitted/contagious, or it was caused by a *bad batch* (or particular brand) of poppers. Amazingly, they never considered the possibility that it might actually be caused by the *long-term* use of poppers (which could be likened to long-term smoking causing lung cancer or long term drinking causing liver cirrhosis) even though they were known to be carcinogenic biochemical toxins. When no bad batch of poppers was found, and short-term studies on mice caused no serious ill effects, they were left with the only other option they had given themselves—that this new syndrome must be sexually transmitted and contagious.

To "prove" it was contagious, the CDC used what's called a cluster study, where they tried to trace the alleged infectious agent from one man to another. Since each man had had hundreds or thousands of sexual encounters (averaging 250 per year), they had their work cut out for them, but this huge pool of men also allowed researchers to connect one immune deficient patient to another in many instances. It also led to the identification of "Patient Zero," a Canadian airline steward who seemed to be at the center of the outbreak and had apparently spread the disease far and wide. This cluster study was the only "proof" offered by the CDC that this new syndrome was sexually transmitted and not caused by the use of poppers or some other agent.

Needing a name for the new syndrome, people had begun referring to it as GRID, which stood for Gay Related Immune Deficiency. But the CDC was having a hard time getting any support for a gay disease. That's when someone noticed that other groups (besides the homosexuals) were suffering from their own versions of immune deficiency problems. These new groups included IV drug users and hemophiliacs.

As you'll see shortly, each of these risk groups had their own risky behavior that could cause immune suppression, so, many researchers came to the logical and early conclusion that just as AIDS included many different diseases, it also had different causes, depending on which subgroup you were talking about. As Dr. Duesberg put it:

Hardly anybody can remember that [in 1984] AIDS was still considered by many scientists a collection of diseases acquired by the consumption of recreational drugs. Since nearly all early AIDS patients were either male homosexuals who have used nitrite and ethylchloride inhalants [poppers], cocaine, heroin, amphetamines, phenylcyclidine, LSD, and other drugs as sexual stimulants, or were heterosexuals injecting cocaine and heroin intravenously, early AIDS researchers named these drugs as the causes of AIDS. Drugs seemed to be the most plausible explanation for the near-perfect restriction of AIDS to these risk groups because drug consumption is their most specific common denominator.[3]

Before the discovery of HIV and the umbrella term of "AIDS," the only thing these different groups of people had in common was that their T-cell counts were depressed, leaving them susceptible to acquiring opportunistic infections. Now, as you may have learned by this point in the book, there are many things that can weaken or destroy a person's immune system. As Edward Hooper says in *The River: A Journey to the Source of HIV and AIDS:*

...since the dawn of *Homo sapiens*, there had been a low but fairly constant background level of cases in which humans died, not as a result of HIV infection, but because their immune systems had been destroyed by other factors. These included congenital immunodeficiency, exposure to ionizing radiation or radionuclides, exposure to toxic substances, undiagnosed cancer, and cancer treatments...[4]

So the fact that these well-circumscribed groups of people had depressed T-cell counts does not necessarily mean they had anything *else* in common. But once these diseases were all lumped together under the AIDS banner, the race to find a common cause was on—and lo and behold, they found one—sort of.

The Germ Hunters

In the 1870's Antoine Béchamp and Louis Pasteur told the world about bacteria. About 20 years later, an entirely new kind of germ was discovered. These new germs were so small that they could not be seen with the most powerful microscopes of the day.

Because they could not be seen, they were given the designation "virus," which means poison. In the 1940s, along came penicillin, which effectively put an end to the most deadly infectious diseases on the planet. But viruses were not so easy to kill. Even today, the only effective way to kill viruses is with a healthy immune system.

When the polio epidemic struck, many scientists were drawn into the burgeoning field of virology, which was soon flooded with young, eager scientists looking for a cure for the disease. Around that same time, the organization that later became known as the Centers for Disease Control was founded. Because the CDC's primary mission is dealing with infectious disease, it has always been run by men with a background in hunting germs. In fact, because modern medicine is basically founded on Pasteur's theory, by this point in our timeline germ hunters had secured many, if not most of the top jobs in medical politics, including leadership positions at the National Institutes of Health (NIH) and the National Cancer Institute (NCI).

When polio was "eradicated," suddenly, all these virus hunters were like soldiers without a war. Other than the common cold or the flu, there were very few infectious diseases left to conquer, at least here in the United States. And what does a virus hunter do when there are no more *important* diseases left to fight? He starts *inventing* diseases and blaming *other* diseases on viruses that show no signs of being infectious at all, like cancer. He creates mass hysteria with unfounded predictions of pandemic bird flu, SARS, West Nile Virus, swine flu, or seasonal flu, and busies himself with feeble attempts to combat these made up pandemics with poisonous cocktails of vaccinations mixed with heavy metals and other toxins. He makes himself out to be more important than he really is with advertised shortages of vaccines, which as anyone can tell you, only creates more demand for these worthless shots. If I were to sum it up, I'd have to say that the job of the virus hunter is largely to keep everyone on the planet deathly afraid of germs, in spite of the fact that today, only one percent of all deaths in the industrial world are actually caused by an infectious organism.[5]

We'll be discussing cancer in depth in a future book, but for now, you need to know that with the possible exception of a few rare cancers, most of which occur in other species, there is no evidence that cancer is caused by an infectious organism. But those few incidental cancers that *seemed* to have a viral origin in *some* cases (such as the theory that cervical cancer is sometimes caused by the Human Papilloma Virus) caught the imagination of the virus hunters, and so they went about trying desperately to prove that all cancer, or at least *other* cancers, were also caused by a virus.

When Nixon signed the National Cancer Act in 1971, suddenly, all these virus hunters were back in the game for a while. But after years of searching, the public finally started to figure out that the virus hunters were never going to find a virus that caused cancer. So, once again, many virologists were faced with no way to justify their salaries and no war to fight. And then AIDS came along.

If it could somehow be proven that AIDS was caused by a virus, these researchers would have something to occupy their time for many years to come. This would be difficult, however, since AIDS, much like lung cancer, did not act like an infectious disease (for example, it didn't spread outside of the risk groups— each of which participated in their own brand of immune destroying behavior). In order to prove that AIDS was caused by a virus, it would require the bending and breaking of some very well established rules in the field of infectious disease. In fact, it would require much more than that.

Koch's Postulates
"Medical teachings nowadays have become too hung up on a model of illness that looks for single microbes that cause disease. The bench scientists in their high-tech labs search the body for

viruses and then try to find diseases for them. It is the ultimate form of reductionism... This approach...moves science away from a study of environmental conditions and lifestyles, in other words, away from the complexities of the world." [6]

—Joseph Sonnabend, early discoverer of AIDS

We've seen in previous chapters the folly of over-utilizing an incomplete and inaccurate germ theory. However, once Pasteur's theory caught hold of the scientific community, researchers and doctors, anxious to leave their mark, rushed to be the first to discover the hidden germ that was causing a particular disease. Soon, anything and everything was being pinned on germs, and often, the germs receiving credit did not deserve it. Shoddy science, of the sort Pasteur was wont to use, became pervasive as a new branch of medical research struggled to find its feet. In those burgeoning years of microbiology, all one had to do to "prove" the cause of an illness was find a new germ somewhere in a sick body and point an accusatory finger at it. To stop this rampant blame game, Robert Koch, the microbiologist who discovered the germs responsible for anthrax and many other diseases, developed three postulates that germs must live up to if they are to be considered the cause of the disease rather than merely an innocent bystander.

These rules were put into place because the vast majority of germs, such as the bacteria we refer to as normal flora, are merely passengers, i.e., they don't cause any disease and are merely along for the ride. Because they cause no disease, they usually go on living in their host undetected and thus are harmless parasites at worst. Since they don't kill or harm their host, they are very successful parasites, which is why these "passenger germs" far outnumber pathogenic organisms.

Koch's postulates are based on scientific, logical thinking and have been the gold standard for determining the true cause of infectious diseases since 1884, just as the double-blind, placebo-controlled trial is the gold standard in pharmaceutical research.

Koch's postulates say:

1. The microbe must be found growing abundantly in every patient and every diseased tissue.
2. The microbe must be able to be isolated from the host and grown in a pure culture.
3. The isolated microbe must then reproduce the original disease when introduced into a susceptible host.

If an organism doesn't meet *all three* of these postulates, it's not the cause of that disease, plain and simple. There are no exceptions to these rules.

By contrast, here, taken directly from Peter Duesberg's book, is what scientists say about passenger viruses:

1. The time between infection by a passenger virus and the occurrence of any disease, if one occurs, is entirely unpredictable. It could be anywhere from a day to the lifetime of the patient. Since the passenger virus does not cause a disease, the time of infection is irrelevant to the onset of a disease.
2. A passenger virus can be active or passive, rare or abundant during any disease. Since the passenger does not cause disease, its activity is irrelevant to it.
3. The passenger virus can be present or absent during any disease. Since the virus is not pathogenic, disease can occur in the absence of the passenger virus.

Duesberg summarizes this by giving us an example: "In short, a virus that has been in its host for years before a disease occurs, that is typically inactive and rare during a disease, and that is not present in every case of that disease is not a credible suspect for viral disease. It is an innocent bystander or a passenger virus."[7] In fact, the virus he is describing here *is HIV*.

> *"I'm not afraid that HIV exists, because I think retroviruses are not much to be afraid of... HIV is just a latent, and perfectly harmless retrovirus."*
>
> —Peter Duesberg, Ph.D.

When one begins to look, s/he sees that HIV meets all the requirements for being a passenger virus and not one of Koch's postulates. This makes HIV innocent on all charges, no matter how many times you've heard the phrase, "HIV, the virus that causes AIDS." The truth of the matter is, most of the scientists studying AIDS are just as brainwashed as the rest of the public. They believe HIV causes AIDS for the same reasons you do. They've heard it over and over again from what they thought was a credible source, and they've been given no reason to doubt it. Most of them have never actually stood back from the situation and questioned it because they've had no reason to. Others, who *have* had some doubts, have seen the destruction of other scientists' careers who went against the tide and have chosen to simply toe the line as a means of survival.

Space does not permit a full discussion of the politics of research science, but one must understand that in this field, one is not rewarded for going against the tide. Research scientists must publish or perish. Without publishing new research, they receive no new funding. In order to get published, however, one's peers must approve the research, and research that contradicts one's peers does not often find its way into the mainstream peer reviewed journals. Nobel Prizes and other accolades also tend to go to those who toe the mainstream line, usually by being the first to discover something (like finding the virus that causes AIDS) or by taking known research to the next level, rather than those who break out of the mold altogether (like discovering HIV is *not* the cause of AIDS). In other words, one is rewarded for going with the tide and punished for going against it.

But getting back to Koch's postulates, let's examine each of them individually and see how HIV fails to meet each one.

The microbe must be found growing abundantly in every patient and every diseased tissue. Now this is a funny one. Do you remember back when we were discussing vaccines how the pro-vaccine camps for both smallpox and polio improved their statistics by changing the names of the diseases depending on whether the person was vaccinated or not? Well, with AIDS they've done something strikingly similar. This is how it works: When a person is diagnosed with any of the 30 plus diseases under the AIDS umbrella, *and* they're found to be positive for HIV, they are given the diagnosis AIDS. Anyone presenting with the exact same signs and symptoms, and, therefore, the same disease, who does *not* have the HIV antibodies in his or her blood, is either diagnosed with *that* disease (Kaposi's sarcoma, cervical cancer, etc.) or it's called ICL (Idiopathic CD4 Lymphocytopenia), which is basically AIDS without HIV.

Because this is such an important point, let me give you a little more detail on HIV-negative AIDS. The January 20, 1990 issue of *Lancet* contained a paper discussing six cases of Kaposi's sarcoma (KS) in HIV-negative homosexuals.[8] The authors of the study, not realizing the firestorm they were starting, came to the logical conclusion that HIV may not be the cause of Kaposi's sarcoma. But wait, outside the rare, usually mild case in older Italian or Jewish men, Kaposi's sarcoma has been practically synonymous with AIDS, especially in the homosexual population. It *is*, after all, the "gay cancer." This raises a serious question: If HIV doesn't cause Kaposi's sarcoma, does it still cause the other AIDS conditions?

> *"[W]e do not understand all the factors that contribute to KS development—HIV alone may or may not be the sole agent in epidemic KS, and if HIV is indeed a major factor, as I believe it to be, its role must be indirect..."*
>
> —Robert Gallo, Father of Human Retroviruses and co-discoverer of HIV
> (*Virus Hunting, AIDS, Cancer & the Human Retrovirus: A Story of Scientific Discovery*)

In 1992, just before the Eighth International AIDS Conference, *Newsweek* published a story about several more HIV-negative AIDS cases.[9] This story had the effect of pouring gasoline on the fire already started by the *Lancet* study and seemed to give researchers at the AIDS Conference the go ahead to unveil dozens more previously unpublished HIV-negative AIDS cases. Suddenly, after eight years of blind faith, the media started seriously questioning the HIV hypothesis and it became awkwardly apparent to those in charge that something would have to be done about the situation.

Top ranking AIDS officials from the NIH and the CDC promised to look into the matter. Three weeks later, they held a special meeting in Atlanta and announced that the HIV-negative AIDS cases reported by all these doctors were not really AIDS at all, but Idiopathic CD4 lymphocytopenia or ICL—a brand new disease they had just made up, which looked and acted exactly like AIDS, but occurred in people without HIV!

According to Edward Hooper, author of *The River*, this re-classification of HIV-free AIDS to ICL did not weaken the HIV=AIDS theory, but rather strengthened it by "making the description of true AIDS more specific."[10] Once again, we're being asked to follow the logic of a four-year-old: "Wait, they don't have HIV? Then that's not *real* AIDS. From now on, only call it AIDS if they have HIV."

Doing this, of course, meant that HIV would now be linked to AIDS 100 percent of the time, *by definition*. Furthermore, they dismissed ICL, calling it "insignificant" and stated that the number of diseases falling under this new syndrome, "was far too large and the diseases were too heterogeneous [dissimilar] to be caused by a single virus." [11] (Remember, the list of AIDS-defining diseases is now over thirty different diseases ranging from skin and cervical cancer to dementia to pneumonia and they are blaming all of this on HIV.)

Hooper also states in *The River* that besides being HIV-negative, the only other defining characteristic of ICL is that "the CD4+ lymphocyte [a type of T-cell] counts of ICL patients are often over 300 whereas those of AIDS patients are usually below 200." [12] Oh, I see, that's much more clear! But what about the facts that CD4+ lymphocyte counts are not constant in these syndromes, and though researchers find they are *not* good indicators of the severity of the disease, the assumption is that T-Cell counts will *decline* as the patient progresses toward his/her eventual demise? Can you see the impaired logic at work here?

The reality is, T-Cell counts can vary greatly—even in healthy people. Counts below 300 have even been found in healthy individuals with no indicators of AIDS. It's also been found that nitrite inhalants, crack cocaine, and even the stress of being told that you are HIV-positive can lower a person's T-Cell count significantly. In fact, the numbers are apparently so meaningless that as of 2002, the CDC no longer considers CD4 counts an important diagnostic criterion for AIDS.[13]

This AIDS conference and the immediate aftermath would have been the perfect opportunity for the people in charge of our public health to take another look at the "proof" they had on HIV, admit they may have made a huge mistake, and to come clean. Instead, they decided to cover things up by creating a new diagnosis in order to maintain their 100 percent correlation between HIV and AIDS. This is *not* what Robert Koch had in mind when he formulated his first postulate.

By 1993 there were thousands of patients on record (4,621 of them to be exact) with what appeared to be HIV-free AIDS—oops, I mean ICL.

In 1994 and 1995, several virologists confirmed that Kaposi's sarcoma, which for 12 years had been considered one of the two hallmark AIDS conditions, was *not* caused by HIV, but a herpes virus, which came to be known as HHV8 or KSHV.[14] Alas, once again, logic goes right out the window. Rather than reassess the HIV-causes-AIDS theory, those in charge fell back on their four-year-old logic again and decided that after 12 years of equating it with AIDS, Kaposi's sarcoma is really not a good indicator of AIDS after all! Staggering.

What makes this whole thing even stranger is that the "AIDS test" doesn't even test for *HIV*; it tests for HIV *antibodies*. (The accuracy of this test will be discussed in a later section.) Remember, antibodies are components of your immune system that are specific to a particular antigen (in this case, a *patho*gen, or germ). These are the elements that "learn" how to kill a virus and then stay present in your blood for life, ever vigilant in case that virus should ever decide to rear its ugly head again.

In every (other) viral disease, when we find antibodies to the virus in a patient's blood, we know that that patient has found a way of successfully killing that virus. The war may not be over, but soldiers are patrolling the area, guns at the ready. However, with AIDS, we are expected to believe that HIV antibodies are not neutralizing at all and their presence actually means you *have* the virus. In reality, all that can be deduced from this test is that you (or one of your ancestors) may have been exposed.

Antibodies are what we're hoping to build up when we vaccinate against a disease. This leads one to ask, if our own HIV antibodies aren't protective against HIV (as they are proposing), how can we ever expect an AIDS vaccine to work? Perhaps this is why we are no closer to having a vaccine for AIDS today than we were when they started looking more than 20 years ago.

There *are* viruses that can lie dormant in the body waiting for the opportunity to strike again when the immune system is in a weakened state. The herpes and varicella (chickenpox) viruses are like this. These viruses lay hidden inside a cell, protected from the person's antibodies, then suddenly shift into high gear and produce millions of new viral particles. This overwhelms the already weakened immune system and causes a flare up of herpes or the onset of shingles.

In order for a virus to cause *any* disease, but in particular one capable of permanently destroying the immune system, there would need to be millions and millions of virus particles circulating throughout the body. (The human body produces 100 million to one billion T-cells every day!) But this doesn't happen with AIDS. *Even in people who are HIV-positive with full-blown AIDS, it's rare to find a single active HIV particle anywhere in the person's body.* In fact, it is *so* difficult that it borders on the impossible, and so, virologists never even *attempt* to find the whole virus. Rather, they mistakenly assume that a positive test for HIV antibodies (which is a highly inaccurate test) is proof enough to issue a death sentence.

But even if they *were* to find a whole, active HIV particle in an AIDS patient (and any evidence that they've ever done this is *very* shaky), that's still not nearly enough to point the finger of doom at it and say, "that's the cause." This postulate says an *abundant* supply of the virus, in *every* case. In other words, numbers matter. In fact, Albert Sabin, the creator of the Sabin Polio Vaccine, and one of the most respected virologists in the world has said, with regard to HIV, "Presence of virus doesn't mean anything in and of itself, because virologists know that quantities count." [15]

This brings us to postulate number two.

The microbe must be able to be isolated from the host and grown in pure culture. Assuming one can actually find an HIV particle in an AIDS patient, the only way to get it to become active and grow in a culture is by using extreme measures, if it can be done at all. This is how it's done: Millions of white blood cells must be harvested from the patient and grown in culture dishes for weeks. During this time, the scientists use chemical stimulants to shock the cells into growing or mutating. This *sometimes* forces a dormant (see box below) HIV particle to wake up. With lots of TLC, on occasion, a single active virus can be obtained. At that point, it can be made to multiply and infect other cells in the dish.

The "proof" that they've managed to find an HIV particle and caused it to replicate itself is not visual (electron microscopy is rarely if ever used when studying HIV or any other viral disease); rather, if the cells die, they simply assume that HIV did the killing! Never mind that they just shocked the cells with enough chemicals to make them mutate. *That* couldn't have been the cause of such rampant cellular death. Everyone knows that drugs and toxic chemicals are harmless; only *viruses* kill cells. *And* never mind the fact that research published in 2006 in the *Journal of the American Medical Association* shows that **HIV only kills four to six percent of the T-cells that are lost in AIDS cases**.[16] Why wasn't *that* story on the evening news?

Let me explain a little about the dormant status of these HIV particles. First, you must know that retroviruses such as HIV incorporate themselves into the DNA of the cell they infect. At that point, they have essentially become a gene of that cell. When that gene is active, it can produce new viruses that can go on to infect other cells. When it's not active, it is harmless. Remember, barring infection and mutation, every cell in your body has exactly the same DNA. We have nose DNA in our livers and liver DNA in our noses. But as long as the liver DNA in our nose is inactive, our nose does not produce liver cells. The same is true of HIV. As long as it's not active, it's not producing new HIV particles and therefore it's harmless. And yet the virus hunters would have you believe that these dormant HIV particles, which, in a full-blown AIDS patient appear, at most, in about one in a thousand white blood cells, are causing the destruction of millions or billions of T-cells per day, and thus, killing these patients. Even they cannot explain how this is possible. We're just asked to believe them despite the common sense, physiological facts, and research that shows they're wrong.

Because the virus is virtually impossible to find once antibodies are present, i.e., once you have a positive HIV test, it's also very hard to pass on to someone else. It's been found that it takes an average of 1,000 unprotected sexual encounters to pass along even one virus to someone.[17] It *is* however passed from mother to fetus fairly readily—approximately 50 percent of the time, just like a gene is passed to an offspring.[18] These findings could account for the fact that the number of HIV-positive cases since testing began back in the mid-80s has remained perfectly stable at about one million people in the U.S., no matter how many cases of AIDS there are.[19]

Three fourths of the estimated 1 million Americans who are HIV-positive have not developed AIDS and eight percent of those who are HIV-positive have been symptom free for over a decade.

According to epidemiological standards, a virus that remains at about the same level in a population over a given period of time has been with that population for a long time. With flu outbreaks, the bubonic plague, and other infectious diseases, we see a rapid increase in the number of cases early on in the process, followed by a peak or a plateau, and then a steady decline. But HIV figures have remained constant now for the entire time that we've been testing for it. (See box below.) This indicates that HIV is probably not a new virus—even to humans. To put this more simply, just because we finally discovered HIV in the mid-80s, doesn't mean it hasn't been around for decades, centuries, or even *millennia*. In fact, the evidence suggests that it's been around for a very long time, much as distant planets, stars, and galaxies have been around for a very long time when astronomers finally discover *them*.

When one reads the news, s/he sees that the number of *AIDS* cases *does* appear to be climbing, but this is (at least partly) because of two deceptive practices. One is the ever-expanding definition of what constitutes AIDS. The other is that the numbers you hear are usually cumulative numbers rather than new cases per year, so, of course, the numbers are going up. If one uses cumulative numbers, the numbers can never go down, even if AIDS were eradicated today.

So technically, HIV can be grown in a culture, but it takes extreme measures and what Peter Duesberg calls, "exhumations of viral fossils," to do so.[20]

Postulate Three: *The microbe must reproduce the original disease when introduced into a susceptible host.* Monkeys that are injected with the viruses that cause hepatitis, polio (if it's injected into the *brain* that is), and the flu, get those diseases. Thus, these viruses pass Koch's third postulate. It would seem that all one would have to do to prove that HIV causes AIDS is to do the same thing with HIV. Incredibly, this experiment has been done, though you probably haven't heard about it because it disproves the HIV hypothesis. In 1983, the blood from AIDS patients was injected into several chimpanzees. Once the AIDS test was invented, they found that these animals *were* infected with HIV, but none of them ever developed AIDS or any other sickness for that matter.[21]

In 1984, 150 chimpanzees were injected with "purified HIV." Within a month, each monkey tested positive for HIV antibodies, but to this day, not one of them has become sick with AIDS or any other disease.[22]

These experiments indicate one of two things: Either monkeys don't get AIDS from HIV, or HIV doesn't cause AIDS period. When you put these findings in context with all the humans who have HIV but no AIDS, and all the people with AIDS/ICL but no HIV, one starts to get an accurate picture.

The one undeniable finding in AIDS (as well as ICL) is the destruction of millions of T-cells. Yet Duesberg claims that HIV doesn't kill T-cells even when it is purposely *grown* in T-cells! (And as mentioned above, *JAMA* reported that HIV only kills about five percent of the T-cells in AIDS patients.) Reports from labs and biotechnology companies all around the world say the same thing: HIV grows harmoniously with the cells it infects.[23] In fact, this is exactly how the virus is grown to produce the HIV antibody tests or the so-called AIDS test.

If this is true, there can be only one conclusion: HIV is a harmless passenger virus.

Robert Gallo and many other scientists working today say that Koch's postulates are outdated; that they just don't work for today's complex diseases including those "caused" by retroviruses. But Koch's postulates are based on simple logic and the germ theory that these scientists revere. If anything doesn't work, it's the germ theory. It's too broad and taken far too literally, and if anything, it has too *few* rules guiding these researchers—not too many. This blatant disregard for Koch's postulates has brought us back to the early days of the germ theory where anything and everything is being blamed on germs and, once again, nutrition, toxicity, and the other causes of ill health have taken a back seat.

What Gallo and his germ hunting colleagues refuse to see in diseases and syndromes where Koch's postulates cannot be fulfilled (AIDS, polio, etc.) is the possibility that these diseases may not be caused by infectious agents at all, or at the very least, not the ones they're trying to implicate. Rather than opening themselves to these possibilities, they continually try to plug holes in their pet theory, inventing new and magical characteristics and ascribing them to these mysterious things called viruses.

Robert Gallo & the Magic Virus Theory

Viruses truly are amazing things, and since we're defending a virus that's been convicted of mass murder without ever having received a fair trial, you, the jury, should understand a little bit about them. The story we've been told about viruses is basically this: A virus infects a cell, uses that cell's machinery (organelles) to produce more viruses, then, when the cell is overrun, the viruses explode out of the cell, thus destroying it. Each of these new viruses then goes on to infect another cell, where the process is started all over. Viruses cannot reproduce themselves without the use of a host cell. This is because most viruses are little more than a short strand of DNA surrounded by a crystalline protein shell called a capsid. Viruses are neither plant, nor animal. In fact, they're not even considered living organisms.

Retroviruses, such as HIV, are a little different. Rather than DNA, they're made of RNA. In most viruses, and in all plants and animals, DNA is that organism's blueprint—the instructions for how to make any protein the cell or body needs and, of course, to reproduce the entire cell or organism when necessary. When the cell is not actively dividing, DNA is kept locked inside the nucleus of the cell.

What's the difference between DNA and RNA? As a simple analogy, one could say that DNA is like an unabridged dictionary— it contains all the words in a particular language. Genes then are like the words in the dictionary. Some you use a lot; others are used infrequently or never. RNA is kind of like the alphabet, only in mirror image. A protein would be like a sentence in this analogy, and a cell like a page of text. A human body would be like *The Encyclopedia Britannica*.

When a cell needs a certain protein to be made, RNA moves into the nucleus, creates a template for that protein using the DNA blueprint, and then moves back out of the nucleus. (This template is called "messenger RNA," or "mRNA." The creation of mRNA is called *transcription*. Remember that word.) Amino acids, which are like the alphabet *not* in mirror image, are laid down on top of the RNA in the correct order to produce the protein. The messenger RNA is then broken apart into individual pieces to be re-used again at a later date. Retroviruses are *a lot* like mRNA (we'll come back to this point in Chapter 14).

Inside their capsid, retroviruses also contain a special enzyme called reverse *transcriptase*. This enzyme, as its name implies, reverses the process of transcription, as described above, and basically turns viral RNA into a tiny new segment of DNA. This new segment of DNA is then uploaded into the nucleus of the cell it's infecting. In this way, a retrovirus could be viewed as a genetic parasite. It becomes a gene of the cell, able to be reproduced (or not) just as any other protein. Nestled safely inside a cell's nucleus, it's also completely impervious to the body's circulating immune cells.

Because they become a permanent part of the cell they're infecting (rather than just occupying and using the cell's machinery, as other viruses do), retroviruses are not known for destroying millions of cells, as they supposedly do in AIDS victims. This would be suicide for them, which goes against all natural laws, even for viruses. In fact, if anything, retroviruses are known for causing rapid cell *growth*, which is why they were first implicated in causing cancers. As Peter Duesberg says, "In short, no retroviruses ever killed cells, and only very rare ones caused tumors in immunodeficient animals. Virtually all retroviruses proved to be benign passenger viruses in animals outside the laboratory." [24]

One of the viruses pointed to in the craze to blame viruses for cancer has been the Feline Leukemia Virus (FeLV), a retrovirus found in cats. In the 1960s, a scientist named Max Essex found that young, inbred lab cats that were exposed to this virus for months at a time would sometimes develop leukemia. Sounds slightly ominous. What you need to know, however, is that approximately two-thirds of *all* cats either have or will eventually get this virus, which in most cases is detected and destroyed by the cat's immune system. However, leukemia only occurs in four of every 10,000 cats. Also, one-third of all leukemic cats (as well as one third of all healthy cats) have never been infected by FeLV. This seems to indicate that FeLV may just be another benign passenger virus.

But finding a virus that supposedly caused cat leukemia caught the imagination of the virus hunters and inspired more research into human leukemia. When the War on Cancer had its big kickoff and a huge influx of cash was funneled into cancer-virus research, Robert Gallo, whose sister died of leukemia when he was a child, saw an opportunity to make his mark *and* some money. Working at the National Cancer Institute (NCI), he began searching for a retrovirus that caused *human* leukemia.

When Gallo discovered reverse transcriptase (indicating the possible presence of a retrovirus—see box below) in some leukemic patients, he was named head of NCI's Laboratory of Tumor Cell Biology. It was later discovered that Gallo's finding of reverse transcriptase in these patients was false, but rather than be dissuaded, the search for a cancer-causing virus was stepped up.

In the early days of retrovirus research, it was thought that reverse transcriptase (RT) was only found where there were retroviruses. It was further assumed that all retroviruses were bad. Now we know that every cell in the human body, not to mention bacteria, plants, and animals, produces reverse transcriptase. We also know now that most or perhaps all of the retroviruses in existence are harmless to humans. In effect, Gallo's supposed discovery of RT in leukemic patients actually meant nothing.

In 1975, Gallo presented new findings to the Virus-Cancer Program's yearly conference. This time he claimed to have isolated an actual retrovirus from human leukemic cells. He was humiliated once again, however, when it was proved that his findings were a result of laboratory contamination, and that the retroviruses were actually from woolly monkeys, gibbon apes, and baboons. Gallo tried to save his already tarnished reputation by speculating that one of those monkey viruses caused human leukemia, but this didn't fly with his colleagues either.

In 1980, the same year AIDS was discovered, Gallo finally met with success when he discovered the first known human retrovirus, which he isolated from a patient with a rare skin cancer previously thought to be caused by a fungus. He claimed the cancer was spread through the lymph system and could be passed to others through sexual contact, though he offered no proof for making either of these claims. But having already made up his mind about it, he named the virus *Human T-cell Lymphoma Virus* or HTLV. Now all he needed to do was to pin his virus to a disease.

When Gallo heard of a rare type of leukemia called Adult T-Cell Leukemia (ATL) that occurs mainly on the Japanese island of Kyushu, he sent a team to investigate, apparently ignoring the fact that his virus came from a patient with skin cancer, not leukemia. The other thing Gallo apparently ignored was that the capital of Kyushu is Nagasaki, and I think we all know what happened there. Finding a rare type of leukemia on the island where we dropped the bomb was really no big surprise, even though it *was* found in children born after the bomb exploded. Gallo's team was able to find reverse transcriptase in these patients (again, no big surprise since it's produced by every cell in the body), though they could *not* find HTLV itself. Regardless, based solely on finding RT, Gallo and his team made the huge leap that ATL was caused by his HTLV. He then renamed his virus Human T-Cell *Leukemia* Virus, despite the fact that it had never actually been found in a leukemic patient. You see the kind of solid scientific logic we're dealing with here? Though there isn't a single epidemiological study showing higher incidence of ATL in people with HTLV than without, and though not a single American infected with HTLV by blood transfusion has ever gotten leukemia because of it, Gallo managed to convince people that HTLV was the cause of ATL.

The story linking ATL with HTLV has many similarities to the story linking AIDS to HIV. For example, there are many people who have the virus who do not have the disease; and there are many people with the disease and not the virus. To circumvent this problem, Gallo used his influence at the NCI to redefine the disease so that only those patients with HTLV may be diagnosed with ATL. Other patients with the exact same disease who do not have HTLV are given a different diagnosis. Since there were so many patients walking around with the virus and no disease, scientists arbitrarily chose a latent period (the time between infection and disease) of five years. Since then, the latency period has crept up to anywhere between 40 and 55 years. Also, if and when a patient *does* develop leukemia, the virus remains sound asleep throughout the entire process forcing scientists to test for the antibodies instead of the actual virus. Any of this sound familiar? But despite all this nonsense, Gallo was awarded the prestigious Lasker Prize for discovering HTLV and became known as the "father of human retroviruses."

In 1982, Gallo found another retrovirus, this one in a patient with a very rare leukemia called Hairy T-Cell Leukemia. He quickly named the new virus HTLV-II, and renamed his first HTLV-I. Since then, however, only one other patient with a similar leukemia has been found to be infected with this virus. This patient moved back to his native Australia, changed his diet, and recovered completely. As Peter Duesberg says, "Gallo's second virus, much to his chagrin, remains a virus in search of a disease."

When AIDS was discovered, Gallo was still too consumed with cancer to pay any attention to a homosexual disease. It took another virus hunter by the name of Donald Francis of the CDC to suggest that AIDS might be caused by a retrovirus. Francis convinced Max Essex (discoverer of the feline leukemia virus) that AIDS was like a cross between FeLV and hepatitis B, that is, a sexually transmitted retrovirus. Essex then convinced his old friend Bob Gallo to jump on the AIDS bandwagon and search for a retrovirus as the cause. (Please see box below.) Having had such pitiful luck in finding a virus that caused cancer, a non-contagious disease, Gallo decided to try his luck at a new disease that, at least according to the CDC, *was* contagious.

With all due respect, none of this makes any sense. First of all, AIDS is *nothing* like FeLV *or* hepatitis B. Leukemia is a cancer that causes abnormal white blood cells to reproduce out of control. With AIDS, the white blood cells disappear. Hepatitis B is a virus that affects the liver. The only connections between these three diseases were that some people at the CDC were assuming AIDS was sexually transmitted and carried in the blood, like hepatitis B, and that, like leukemia, it led to a loss of immune function. These are *extremely* superficial connections. Second, when you go looking for a particular thing to be the cause of a disease, chances are pretty good that you'll find the evidence you're looking for. People, even some scientists, tend to see what they want to see.

Rather than search for a new virus, Gallo and Essex both decided it would be easier to just blame AIDS on HTLV-I, so in separate articles published in *Science* magazine in 1983, they did just that.[25, 26] They were asserting, therefore, quite paradoxically, that HTLV-I could both cause T-cells to grow out of control (as in leukemia) or to die in mass numbers (as in AIDS). They did not find much support for this hypothesis however.

Around this time, a French retrovirologist named Luc Montagnier, working at the Pasteur Institute, isolated a retrovirus from a homosexual with swollen lymph nodes. (Please note: This patient did *not* have AIDS.) Montagnier called his new virus LAV (Lymphadenopathy-Associated Virus) and asserted that it may be a contender as the cause of AIDS. Gallo was irate over the idea that Montagnier may have beat him to the punch, so he immediately began denouncing LAV to his fellow scientists and continued pushing his theory on HTLV-I. Forced to deal with the issue, however, he offered to write a summary for Montagnier's paper on LAV. In that summary, he claimed, falsely, that LAV was closely related to his HTLV-I and HTLV-II. In other words, in case LAV *did* turn out to be the cause of AIDS, he at least wanted credit for finding the family of viruses that included the AIDS virus.

Gallo convinced Montagnier to send him a sample of LAV and then spent the next several months (almost a year) claiming that he could not grow LAV in his lab. In reality, however, Gallo *was* able to grow Montagnier's virus, and was simply biding his time, trying to figure out how he could scoop the bloody French now that, in his mind, they had found the AIDS virus (in a patient that did not have AIDS, remember). He apparently spent much of this time developing a test that could detect LAV antibodies, and after testing some AIDS patients and finding positive results in *some* of them (see box below), became convinced that LAV was indeed the cause of AIDS.

Gallo was never able to find the purported AIDS virus (LAV/HTLV-III/HIV) in AIDS patients, however, just the antibodies. In fact, in 1994 he actually said, "We have never found HIV DNA in T-cells." [27] He explained this apparent paradox by saying, "If infection leads to a decline in the population of infected cells, you may not find the virus by the time you get frank disease." [28] Of course, using this sort of circular logic, one can also prove that unicorns disappear as soon as you look at them.

Suddenly, as if out of nowhere, in March 1984, Gallo had four separate papers prepared on a new retrovirus he called HTLV-III, which he claimed to have isolated from a number of AIDS patients. (These papers were published in the May 4, 1984 issue of *Science*.)[29] In early April, he began a series of lectures, including one at the Pasteur Institute, declaring his discovery and claiming the French LAV had proved to be a failure. He also leaked the story to the press far and wide, including the *Washington Post*, the *Wall Street Journal*, the BBC, and others.

On April 23, before the research papers had even come out, the Department of Health and Human Services held a press conference and Secretary of Health Margaret Heckler declared to the world that Dr. Gallo's HTLV-III was the "probable" cause of AIDS. The press understood, however, that the word "probable" was merely scientific false modesty, and what she *meant* to say was, "We *found* the cause." Heckler added that they hoped "to have a vaccine ready for testing in about two years." By the next day, the world media had dubbed HTLV-III the "AIDS virus." As Peter Duesberg says, this was science by press conference rather than by scientific validation. He goes on to say:

Thus, before any other scientists could review and comment on Gallo's claim, it had been set in stone. The press conference marked a point of no return. Career-minded scientists immediately dropped all other AIDS research, including work on the Epstein-Barr virus, cytomegalovirus, and HTLV-I, as well as all remaining experiments on poppers. From that date forward, every federal dollar spent on AIDS research funded only experiments in line with the new virus hypothesis.[30]

Normally, a discovery of this magnitude would be verified by several different independent laboratories before abandoning any and all other research forever, but not so in AIDS. Since the AIDS virus itself was so difficult to find in AIDS patients, Gallo held all the cards. As far as the world knew, he had the only viable viruses in his lab and he guarded them jealously. He insisted on approving any research done on his virus and he denied *many* requests. Most importantly, ***he specifically forbade anyone from trying to verify his claim that HTLV-III was truly the cause of AIDS!*** Why the scientific community allowed this behavior (especially knowing Gallo's history of bungling things) is a colossal mystery. Gallo's *motivation* in doing so, however, is obvious. Surely *he* remembered what had happened with his previous claims regarding leukemia, HTLV-I, and HTLV-II, and wished to prevent his becoming a laughing stock once again. But Gallo had learned from his previous failures. With HTLV-III and AIDS, he stacked the deck and played every card perfectly.

Luckily for him, the window on this verification process was very short. Sooner or later, everyone moved on to researching different aspects of the supposed AIDS virus (how to stop it from spreading, how to make an effective vaccine, etc.), and once that window closed, nobody wanted to spend the time, money, and effort trying to re-open it. Gallo's hypothesis was by then considered a foregone conclusion. Most now ignorantly assume that the original science on AIDS was sound, and to go back at this point would be a waste of resources, but nothing could be further from the truth. And so now we find ourselves in the predicament that, *to this day, no one has ever verified Gallo's claim that HTLV-III (later renamed HIV) causes AIDS.* It is simply presumed (based on very shaky scientific principals and circular logic) to be true!

Gallo's hypothesis was also embraced by the gay community who wanted desperately to believe that AIDS was not caused by their lifestyle, per se, but by a virus. With a vaccine just a couple years away and condoms in the meantime, the party could continue.

There's a lot to this story that's not included here because of space, most of it involving money, politics, and gigantic egos. Very briefly, it must be remembered that Gallo was a government scientist. The Reagan Administration had completely ignored AIDS until this point in the story, presumably because it was "a homosexual disease." But by 1984, with AIDS being found in hemophiliacs and even babies, pressure was mounting on them to do something. More importantly, Reagan was now campaigning for his second term. All of this, along with Gallo's pride, arrogance, and a burning desire for the Nobel Prize, led to the announcement that the virus had been found before it was ever confirmed.

But there were some, including writers for the *New York Times* who suspected Gallo had stolen his virus from the French. In January 1985, when Gallo and Montagnier both published the genetic sequences of their viruses, it became clear that Gallo's HTLV-III was *so* similar to Montagnier's LAV that researchers, including Don Francis, concluded it was not only the same *kind* of virus, but *the same virus from the same patient!* Suddenly, the scientific community knew that Bob Gallo had screwed up again.

When confronted with the fact that the two were in fact the same virus, Gallo claimed he had found the virus himself around the same time Montagnier had, but had failed to report it for almost a year. When asked how it could be so similar in genetic sequence, he proposed the far out (essentially impossible) theory that the viruses had been isolated from different patients who just happened to have been sexual partners, even though one was found in France and the other supposedly was American.

Gallo's claim to have isolated the virus from several AIDS patients also proved bogus. When asked to see these other viruses, he claimed that dozens of his samples had been destroyed through a series of lab accidents. In reality, none of Gallo's AIDS patients were found to actually have HTLV-III, just the antibodies to the virus, and some of them didn't even have *that* going for them. The jig was just about up for Bob Gallo.

In 1986, Gallo was brought up on charges of scientific misconduct. During the investigation, he was forced to admit that the electron micrographs he used in his landmark paper on HTLV-III were actually Montagnier's LAV. Also during this investigation, which involved several government organizations, including Congress, the Secret Service, and the Office of Research Integrity, Mikulas Popovic, one of Gallo's co-authors, came forward with an original draft of that same key paper, which he had wisely hidden overseas. In that draft, Popovic gave Montagnier full credit for finding the virus. However, Gallo had crossed out these admissions and written in the margins, "Mika, you are crazy... I just don't believe it. You are absolutely incredible." Popovic was later fired by the NIH. Of course, he was just the scapegoat. *Gallo* was the one falsifying all the information and making claims he had no right to.

Had Gallo gotten away with his scam, he would surely have been awarded the Nobel Prize. Instead, in 1992, he was convicted of scientific misconduct (specifically that he had fabricated his results and then covered it up) by a team of his fellow scientists. The National Academy of Sciences called it "intellectual recklessness" and "essentially immoral" behavior. Gallo appealed the decision, however, and a team of lawyers was able to get him acquitted on the charge by forcing his peers to prove that Gallo had not only made fraudulent claims, but that he had *consciously* planned this whole scam. This was, of course, impossible, so the charges were dropped. Similar charges by other government bodies were dropped due to statute of limitations requirements and other technicalities. Thus, Robert Gallo, the father of human retroviruses and the "co-discoverer of HIV," basically escaped criminal prosecution by a hair's breadth. Nevertheless, his credibility amongst his peers was completely destroyed, and because he was, in fact, guilty of fraud, he was "asked to leave" the NIH in 1995.

Harold Varmus, then head of the NIH, described Gallo as a "thug." Dr. Sam Broder, the one who asked him to leave, reportedly said to one of the senior scientists at the NIH, "Believe me, Bob is going to leave here one way or another. I'm going to tell Bob it is time to retire. And if he doesn't, other things are going to happen. As far as I am concerned, the books can be closed if Bob leaves. But the implications of his leaving will be clear. Bob has beaten a rap. There will be no ticker tape parades." He then told Gallo, "You have degraded the institute. You've degraded the public and you have degraded the reporters by lying to them. I have not forgiven you for this. People are dying of real diseases and this is not a game." [31]

Robert Gallo has also been accused of stealing HTLV-I from Japanese scientists. In 1990, he took part in an illegal experiment on an unapproved AIDS vaccine. Three of the patients died as a result of the vaccine. There are additional cases of his stealing others' work and then lying about it as well, which we will not go into here, but it's very obvious that this "co-discoverer of HIV" and the champion of the HIV-causes-AIDS theory is a very dishonest scientist.

The French scientists, as you might imagine, were not happy that Gallo had stolen their virus and that the HHS had unilaterally announced it to be the cause of AIDS without giving them any credit at all. A three-year international legal battle between the two countries ended in a public meeting between President Reagan and French Prime Minister Jacques Chirac. In the end, the two governments agreed to share the credit for co-discovering the virus. The names HTLV-III and LAV were both dropped and a new name was chosen—the now-familiar Human Immunodeficiency Virus or HIV. Let me remind you now, however, that the virus that created all of this hubbub, originally found in Montagnier's lab and stolen by Gallo, was found in a patient who didn't even have AIDS!

In 2008, Luc Montagnier was awarded half of the Nobel Prize in Physiology or Medicine for his discovery of HIV 24 years earlier. He shared the award, not with Robert Gallo, but with Harald zur Hausen, who discovered that the Human Papilloma Virus supposedly causes cervical cancer.

AIDS Is Not an Infectious Disease

The idea that HIV doesn't cause AIDS is much more prevalent than you might think. In fact, some very big names in AIDS research have come out and said as much, at great risk to their careers. (Visit www.rethinkingaids.com for a list of over 2,600 doctors and scientists who deny the party line that HIV causes AIDS.) One of the most shocking of these declarations occurred in

June 1990 at the Sixth International Conference on AIDS. There, Luc Montagnier, the man who *really* discovered the virus, used his allotted time to announce that HIV *could* not cause AIDS—at least not by itself. Standing at the lectern, he cited many of the same arguments used in this chapter against HIV, namely the low levels of HIV in the bodies of AIDS patients, the long/indefinite latent period, the large number of infected people who never get AIDS, and most importantly, the inability of retroviruses to actually kill cells. Montagnier has also mentioned that after years of monitoring hemophiliacs, he's found the same immune suppression in HIV-negative individuals as he has in HIV-positives.

We've already mentioned the 2006 paper in *JAMA* that reported HIV could not possibly be killing more than 5 percent of the T-cells in AIDS patients, thus indicating that it *could not* be the cause of AIDS.

We've also seen how Robert Gallo has agreed with many other scientists who no longer believe HIV is the (main) cause of Kaposi's sarcoma, the gay cancer.

Kary Mullis, the Nobel Prize laureate mentioned at the start of this chapter, who created the PCR test, which is used to assess viral loads in AIDS patients, is another dissenting voice. When he first started researching AIDS, he discovered that nobody knew what resource or scientist to reference when making the statement "HIV, the virus that causes AIDS." He was told by his colleagues that he didn't *need* to reference that statement because it was common knowledge. He disagreed.

Dr. Mullis did exhaustive literature and computer searches and asked everyone he knew in the field of AIDS research, including Luc Montagnier, what the proof was for making that statement, but nobody could give him a single reference. This eventually led him to the conclusion that there really *is no* proof that HIV causes AIDS, and in the Forward to *Inventing the AIDS Virus,* he states very clearly that he does not believe HIV *is* the cause.

"We have not been able to discover any good reasons why most of the people on earth believe that AIDS is a disease caused by a virus called HIV. There is simply no scientific evidence demonstrating that this is true."

—Kary Mullis, Nobel Prize in Chemistry, 1993

But Peter Duesberg doesn't just believe HIV is innocent, he believes AIDS is not an infectious disease at all. If it were, he argues, it would have spread beyond the original risk groups by now.

To most of us today, it seems obvious that lung cancer and emphysema are caused by long-term cigarette smoking. If someone were to try to blame lung cancer or emphysema on a virus today, they would probably be laughed right out of the room. This is partly because virtually every person diagnosed with these diseases has smoked cigarettes heavily for 10 or 20 years. But even with this evidence, proving that smoking was the causal factor in these diseases was not so easy. It took years and many studies to convince people of what today seems so obvious a child could figure it out.

Scurvy, like AIDS, had many aspects to it that caused men to believe it was contagious, and so the real cause was overlooked or ignored for hundreds of years, even when millions were dying and the cure was staring them in the face. Similar stories are true for pellagra, beriberi, and the like.

Duesberg spends many pages in his book describing a Japanese disease called SMON that plagued the island country for many years. SMON has many parallels to the AIDS story including the fact that almost everyone believed it to be contagious. It was finally proved, much to the embarrassment of the medical establishment there, that SMON was caused by the very medication used to treat the symptoms of SMON!

The point is, first appearances are not always what they seem, and virus hunters like to blame viruses for everything that looks even remotely like it may be contagious, and even things that obviously aren't contagious, like cancer.

Because AIDS is currently *defined* by the presence of HIV, a discussion on the possibility that HIV doesn't cause AIDS can be quite confusing. To minimize this confusion, I'm going to temporarily drop all this HIV malarkey and simply discuss the more common AIDS-defining diseases as they occur in individual AIDS risk groups.

Homosexual AIDS

There are certain things that all AIDS patients have in common, regardless of their risk group. They all suffer from immune deficiency (as demonstrated by the loss of T-cells) and they all develop opportunistic infections because of it. These two things together, more than anything else, define Acquired Immune Deficiency Syndrome.

Candidiasis (a.k.a. systemic yeast/fungal infection, or "thrush" if it's in the oral cavity) occurs almost exclusively in patients who've been on many courses, or long-term use of antibiotics. As was detailed in Chapter 7, antibiotics destroy the beneficial bacteria or "normal flora," which assist in immune function, the metabolism of certain vitamins, etc. The destruction of these good germs allows the overgrowth of yeast throughout the body. This yeast overgrowth further destroys the immune system, which often leads the patient to the doctor for more antibiotics, and a vicious cycle ensues. Eventually, the patient's immune system is so weak that he is susceptible to anything. The patient's body is so sick and infested with fungus at this point that his somatids enter the longer lifecycle (as described in Chapter 6), thus *creating* new germs (like HIV?). All of this can and does happen whether a patient has HIV or not.

Most, if not all fast-track homosexuals are on antibiotics continually to help ward off the urinary tract infections and other sexually transmitted diseases brought on through oral and anal intercourse with multiple partners. There is currently no explanation or even theory (that I am aware of) as to how HIV infection (or any other virus for that matter) could lead to yeast/fungal overgrowth in the body. Even if it *does* destroy T-cells, as they claim, never have I seen or heard any indication that T-cells play a role in controlling the overgrowth of *Candida albicans*. It's *bacteria* that do this, not the immune system proper. Thus, flagrant antibiotic use seems to me the most likely cause of the candidiasis or thrush seen in AIDS patients, just as it is in non-AIDS patients.

Pneumocystis carinii pneumonia (PCP) is another opportunistic infection that occurs in homosexual AIDS. It was the original AIDS disease and was dubbed "the gay pneumonia." Interestingly, it, too, is a fungal infection and this fungus is found in the lungs of just about every person on the planet. It's only when the immune system has been sacked, as in chemotherapy patients, or in someone who's been on antibiotics for years, leading to systemic yeast/*Candida* overgrowth, that it causes any problems. Also, just like with candidiasis, PCP can and does occur in the absence of HIV.

Kaposi's sarcoma (KS) is not a new disease either, but with the onset of AIDS, it's taken on a new presentation. Old KS was very rare and generally only seen in older patients of Italian or Jewish heritage. It was usually found on the skin of the lower extremities, was rarely found in the organs, and was equal in both sexes. New KS, i.e., "the gay cancer," is more common on the face (especially the tip of the nose and ears), head, and upper body. Also, in AIDS patients, KS commonly attacks the organs and one of its favorite sites is the lung. (Hmm, inhaled drugs, lung problems...very interesting.) Unlike candidiasis and Pneumocystis pneumonia, KS is found in a fairly exclusive group: fast track male homosexuals with a long history of heavy drug use—especially nitrite inhalants or poppers. According to *Harrison's Principals of Internal Medicine*

(12th edition, p. 1,408), KS occurs in 34 percent of male homosexuals with AIDS and less than 10 percent of heterosexuals with AIDS.

Remember that Kaposi's sarcoma is a cancer and poppers are known carcinogens. Poppers come in small bottles and are inhaled through the nose before, obviously, reaching the lung. The toxic fumes of these carcinogens also waft across the face, ears, and head as the person breathes them in. Knowing these things, as well as the fact that many scientists, including Robert Gallo, no longer believe KS is caused directly by HIV (owing in part to the many cases of HIV-negative Kaposi's sarcoma), it seems very possible that poppers could be the cause of the gay cancer.

Of course, poppers are not the only drugs consumed by these in-dividuals. Many also use cocaine, marijuana, and methamphetamines (all inhaled drugs), as well as heroin, ecstasy, and just about every other recreational drug on the planet. Each of these drugs carries its own degree of toxicity, which when used long-term can affect the im-mune system. Add in constant antibiotic use and the overgrowth of yeast with concomitant immune system failure and you've got AIDS.

KS, much like all those HIV-negative AIDS cases now called ICL, may soon be pushed out from under the AIDS umbrella. Some scientists are racing to find a new virus to hold responsible, but keep in mind that old KS was not caused by a virus. Why should the new KS be any different? The admission of HIV's innocence in all these cases of ICL and KS can only help in the eventual discovery of the true cause of these diseases.

AIDS in IV Drug Users

If you had never heard of AIDS, would it surprise you to find out that heavy IV drug users such as heroin addicts and intravenous cocaine users often die at an early age and that many of these addicts suffer from immune deficiency problems? Probably not. Not only are these drugs toxic in and of themselves and, therefore, put a heavy strain on the body, they often lead to other problems such as chronic malnutrition and insomnia. These are also potential causes of immune deficiency. These people, who often share needles, are prone to getting infections at the injection site, which causes them to take many doses of antibiotics over a lifetime. This, of course can lead to the same problem it does in the homosexuals—candidiasis, which happens to be one of the more common opportunistic infections in this AIDS risk group.

But besides having candidiasis in common, the AIDS diseases that IV drug users get are very different from the diseases fast-track, male, homosexual, popper users get. Instead of Kaposi's sarcoma, IV drug users get tuberculosis, pneumonia, weight loss, septicemia (a systemic infection of the blood), and endocarditis (inflammation of the heart's valves and/or the lining of the heart's chambers—likely due to infection as well). Most of these can easily be explained by the long-term injection of toxic drugs, often using dirty needles, into the bloodstream. Again, add in a systemic yeast infection brought on by the overuse of antibiotics and you've got AIDS.

HIV is not needed in this hypothesis, nor can it explain the pathogenesis of these problems, or why IV drug users would get different diseases than homosexuals or other AIDS risk groups. In fact, *according to one American study, both HIV-positive and HIV-negative IV drug users die of the exact same conditions.*[32] Also, according to one German study, the average age at death for this sub-group of the population is 29.6 years for HIV-negative individuals and 31.5 for HIV-positive individuals.[33] So again, it's the drug use (to include antibiotics), not HIV, that's the common denominator and thus the most likely cause of AIDS in IV drug users.

Hemophiliac AIDS

Only about one percent of all AIDS cases occur in hemophiliacs. Nevertheless, the fact that hemophiliacs die from AIDS is one of the most commonly held out justifications for the hypothesis that AIDS is infectious. The theory implies that because they've had blood transfusions, and now they're sick, they must have acquired a virus in one or more of those transfusions. Well, let's have a look, shall we?

Hemophilia is a genetic disorder whose victims lack the proteins needed to make their blood clot. Without treatment, hemophiliacs can bleed to death from minor trauma and usually succumb at an early age. In fact, as recently as 1972, hemophiliacs had an average life expectancy of only 11 years.[34] But then scientists developed a truly lifesaving treatment for these people. They discovered a way of extracting what's known as factor VIII (the missing protein) from normal people's blood, and when this donated factor VIII is injected into the bloodstream of a hemophiliac, it gives them the ability to clot their blood and lead a near normal life. With these transfusions of factor VIII, by 1987, hemophiliacs had more than doubled their median life expectancy to 27. (Keep in mind that HIV was not removed from the blood supply until 1984.)

When factor VIII is highly purified, the person's immune system stays strong and the patient remains healthy, but purified factor VIII is expensive and hard to come by, so most hemophiliacs use what is referred to as "commercial factor VIII," or "partially purified factor VIII," which, as the name implies, is not so pure. For one thing, it contains proteins that have nothing to do with the clotting of blood. But what's more, commercial factor VIII is from a mixture of *many* (up to 25,000) different donors' blood and hemophiliacs receive *many* transfusions over the course of a lifetime. This may be why 75 percent of all hemophiliacs test positive for HIV antibodies.

The result of receiving this partially purified factor VIII is that over time, the person's immune system starts to break down and they begin to develop opportunistic infections. The reason for this is currently unknown but may be related to what's seen when patients receive any *other* organ from a donor—the immune system attacks that which has been donated because it is "foreign." If the immune system is constantly being barraged by foreign proteins in the blood, it may just become overwhelmed and eventually can no longer handle any *other* invaders. But whatever the cause, HIV doesn't seem to play a part, because the exact same opportunistic infections occur whether these patients test positive for HIV or not. Even Luc Montagnier agrees with this.

So with hemophiliac AIDS, the common denominator is the long-term use of commercial factor VIII, not HIV. In fact, several doctors from the CDC stated in *JAMA* in 1986 that "Hemophiliacs with immune abnormalities may not necessarily be infected with HTLV-III/LAV [i.e. HIV], since factor [VIII] concentrate itself may be immune suppressive even when produced from a population of donors not at risk for AIDS." [35] Another study done in 1992 found that between 25–40 percent of immunodeficient hemophiliacs (those showing the signs of AIDS) were HIV-negative.[36] Yet another study done in 1992 showed that in HIV-negative hemophiliacs, "with increasing age [and therefore more doses of factor VIII], numbers of CD4+ CD45RA+ cells [types of T-cells] decreased and continued to do so throughout life." [37]

The fact that commercial factor VIII is the common denominator is further born out with the realization that the removal of all HIV tainted blood from the blood supply in 1984 has not improved the plight of this risk group at all. It is further strengthened by the fact that *immune compromised hemophiliac patients who are put on* **purified** *factor VIII are often cured of their "AIDS."* [38]

Another factor that helps disprove the contagiousness of AIDS is a 1984 study from *JAMA* that measured the T-cell counts of the sexual partners of immune deficient hemophiliacs. The average length of relationship was 10 years, with an average of 111 sexual contacts per year, only 12 percent using condoms. At the end of the study, the authors concluded that, "there is no evidence to date for heterosexual or household-contact transmission of T-cell subset abnormalities from hemophiliacs to their spouses..." [39] There is some contention on this matter however. (See box below.)

The CDC says that between 1985 and 1992, 131 wives of American hemophiliacs were diagnosed with AIDS-defining diseases. (That's 16 cases per year out of approximately 5,000 wives of HIV-positive hemophiliacs in the United States.) A 1990 study looked into this tiny subset of the population and found that 81 percent of these "AIDS diseases" were pneumonia, which may or may not have been due to AIDS. They also found that other AIDS-defining diseases like Kaposi's sarcoma, dementia, lymphoma, and wasting syndrome are not found in the wives of hemophiliacs. [40]

Non-Risk Group AIDS

Ninety-four percent of American and European AIDS cases fall into the three risk groups mentioned above (60 percent homosexual, of whom essentially 100 percent admit to being heavy users of inhaled and/or injected drugs; 33 percent IV drug users; and one percent hemophiliacs). The failure of AIDS to spread beyond these risk groups in any significant amount is another one of the major factors that helps disprove the contagiousness of AIDS. But what of the six percent who are not in one of these risk groups?

First, remember that the current definition of AIDS is the diagnosis of any of 30 or so diseases in the presence of HIV antibodies. Also note that the CDC has expanded the number of diseases on the AIDS list on three separate occasions (1985, 1987, and 1993). This expanding definition makes the number of AIDS cases per year appear to be going up and also makes it appear to be spreading into the heterosexual population, but this is merely statistical tomfoolery.

Cervical cancer, for example, is one of the more recently added AIDS diseases. So, as it currently stands, if a woman develops cervical cancer and also tests positive for HIV, she can be listed as having AIDS, whereas before 1993, this same woman would have merely had cervical cancer. See how they play? So now, with a little sleight of hand, just as they predicted in the early 1980s, AIDS is suddenly spreading into the heterosexual population, proving that it is indeed contagious. But did HIV *cause* the cervical cancer? There's absolutely no evidence that it does or even that it *could*. Like Kaposi's sarcoma and other cancers, cervical cancer is neither an infectious disease, nor is it caused directly or primarily by immune deficiency. So the CDC's ever-expanding definition of AIDS is what's responsible for a large portion of non-risk group AIDS.

What about babies born with AIDS? Eighty percent of these children are born to mothers who used IV drugs while they were pregnant. Does this mean they caught a virus from an infected needle their mother used to get high? No, it simply means that IV drug use (i.e., major toxicity) during pregnancy can mess up your baby's immune system and cause disease. What of the other 20 percent in this group? First of all, realize that this is a *very* small number of children; so small in fact that getting statistically significant numbers simply isn't possible. Second, were these children born with AIDS or is their illness a reaction to a vaccination or some hospital-borne infection? Third, some babies are born sick even in the best of situations. Fourth, it's possible that some of these mothers were doing drugs and simply didn't admit to it, or perhaps had some other toxin in their system that affected their baby's immune system. And finally, remember our pitiful numbers in the U.S. regarding infant mortality—a fact that is independent of the infant's HIV status. So this tiny number of

"AIDS babies" may just represent the normal incidence of newborns who are born sick and who also have HIV.

The symptoms of these AIDS babies include low birth weight, mental retardation, and immunodeficiency. These symptoms, as well as the medical findings for this tiny sub-group of the AIDS population, are quite different from those of the homosexual population, the hemophiliacs, or the IV drug users. Most notably, these children suffer from deficiencies of *B-cells* rather than T-cells and they also get certain bacterial infections not seen in other groups. Why would HIV, a virus that supposedly attacks and kills millions of T-cells in adults, decide instead to attack B-cells in infants?

There's one more factor to discuss regarding non-risk group AIDS and this is perhaps the most tragic of them all because these people were actually given AIDS by their doctors. Not through some needle stick or mixing of blood, but by prescription.

AIDS by Prescription

Azidothymidine, or AZT, was created in 1964 as a chemotherapy drug. The drug acts by interrupting the duplication of DNA and thereby stops all new cell production in the body. If these new cells happen to be cancerous, the drug will halt the growth of that cancer. If the cells happen to contain HIV, it will stop the spread of HIV to other cells. But if the cells happen to be muscle, hair, stomach lining, blood cells, or any other tissue, it stops the growth of these, too. The drug is a classic poison. It was tested briefly on cancer-ridden mice, but because it was *so* effective at stopping cell reproduction, all the mice in the experiment died. AZT was such a miserable failure that the researcher never bothered to publish the study. He shelved the drug and never even applied for a patent.

For 20 years, AZT remained blessedly unused. But when AIDS was blamed on HIV, the virus hunters needed something to pacify the panicky public. They had promised a vaccine within two years, but what could be done in the meantime? They needed something that could prevent HIV from infecting new cells. For this, AZT seemed like just the ticket.

In an early test tube experiment, AZT clearly prevented HIV from spreading better than other drugs. This raised some hopes and led to a few shoddy human experiments that were quickly thrown together. These experiments showed some impressive results, but the numerous flaws in each of the studies made those results impossible to trust. Space does not permit a detailed description of these experiments and all their flaws, but suffice it to say that several studies have since debunked the myth that the benefits of AZT are worth the risks. However, lacking these more recent and accurate studies and having nothing else to offer, these early studies were submitted to the FDA drug approval board. Despite many objections by those on the board, AZT was pushed through the "fast-track" approval process (not to be confused with the fast-track *group,* which this drug was intended for) by the head of the FDA and was available for prescription in record time.

It wasn't long before these other studies began showing the real picture though, and it was a bleak one. AZT prevented HIV from spreading to other cells, but it had to kill T-cells in order to do it. Of course, like most chemotherapy drugs, it also killed *other* dividing cells as well, but the end result of killing off T-cells in this fashion was the very same immune deficiency syndrome we were trying to stop. In other words, AZT slows the spread of HIV, but at the same time it *causes* AIDS. This is all the more tragic knowing that HIV is apparently innocent.

While experimenting with AZT on people who already have AIDS is bad enough, giving the drug to those who are merely HIV-positive but showing no signs of illness is downright criminal. And yet this is exactly what's been done, and according to Peter Duesberg, *this* is where most of the non-risk group AIDS has come from—AZT.

Because everyone at the CDC was so quick to believe the fraudulent research put out by Dr. Gallo, doctors were told that finding HIV antibodies in a patient's blood was a sure death sentence. When AZT became available, doctors began giving this AIDS-causing poison to HIV-positive patients in order to prevent the onset of AIDS. Of course, what happened was predictable: The patients developed AIDS. To the true believers, this only helped confirm that HIV was the cause of AIDS. But when some of these patients *stopped* the AZT and made a full recovery, the true story began to surface.

This is exactly what happened to Irvin "Magic" Johnson. While applying for a marriage license in November 1991, Magic was discovered to have HIV antibodies in his blood. Although he was perfectly healthy at the time and still playing professional basketball, his doctors convinced him to go on AZT prophylactically. He quit playing basketball, started taking the drug, and within a month became sick. Newspapers across the country reported the sad story: Magic now had AIDS. Luckily for Magic, the AZT made him feel *so* bad that he stopped taking it. What happened then did *not* make the papers. Magic recovered—completely. He then went on to play in the 1992 Olympics, winning the gold medal as part of the "Dream Team." And as you probably know, Magic is alive and well to this day.

Many healthy HIV carriers, like Magic, have had the virus for well over 10 years. Several studies have been done on these "long-term survivors" (a.k.a. non-progressors) and they all agree on two points: None of them have been convinced by their doctors to go on antiretroviral drugs to prevent AIDS,[41, 42] and they've either given up or never taken recreational drugs.[43] Furthermore, there is no evidence that HIV-positive people, who are not drug users, are sicker or die any sooner than people without HIV.[44]

Magic was smart. Others were not so fortunate. Wimbledon champ Arthur Ashe, for example, was another person who didn't engage in any high-risk activities, but was discovered to have HIV, which he apparently contracted through a blood transfusion during heart bypass surgery. Like Magic, he was put on AZT, ostensibly to try to save his life. Instead, the drug did the exact opposite—it took it. Less than five years after testing positive, he was dead. Interestingly, neither Ashe's wife nor his child, who was born three years after his blood transfusion, ever contracted AIDS.

I've seen a similar tragedy in my own practice. Billy (not his real name) was a happily married young father when he went in for an insurance physical. This included an AIDS test. When he got the results, he was shocked to find out that he was HIV-positive. He confided in me that he had no idea how he had contracted the virus and that he was not a member of any of the risk groups.

Though he was perfectly healthy at the time, Billy's doctors convinced him that prevention was the best route to take. They said his T-cell count was high and his viral load was low, but they wanted to keep it that way. So, he went on a cocktail of several anti-AIDS drugs, including AZT. Within weeks, Billy was sick, and he looked it. His drug cocktail was weakening his immune system so severely that it became obvious to all who knew his HIV status—Billy had AIDS. To make matters even worse, his wife left him because she believed he must have cheated on her, though he swore to me he hadn't. He eventually moved from the area, so I don't know what became of him, but I suspect he's left this plane by now.

You may also remember the story of Dr. David Acer, the homosexual dentist who supposedly gave seven of his patients AIDS. What actually happened was this: One of Dr. Acer's patients, a 19-year-old college student named Kimberly Bergalis, developed an oral yeast infection and later that year she also had some dizziness, nausea, and a brief pneumonia. The pneumonia sent her to the hospital, and because yeast infections and pneumonia are on the AIDS list, the doctor ran a test for HIV. The test came back positive. It was December 1989.

Because she was a virgin, had never received a blood transfusion, and had never done any IV drugs, the CDC became involved in the case. They had to find some way that this young virgin could have contracted a sexually transmitted, contagious disease or the public's perception of AIDS being infectious could become compromised. After a lot of digging they discovered a plausible route of infection. Her dentist, Dr. Acer, had AIDS. Since they could find no other possible cause, they blamed her HIV status on him.

Dr. Duesberg, in *Inventing The AIDS Virus* states:

Before the HIV hypothesis of AIDS, no medical expert in his right mind would ever have entertained the slightest thought that a dentist with a Kaposi's tumor and a patient with a yeast infection had anything in common. But in the era of AIDS, doctors tended to discard common sense. That the dentist and patient both carried a dormant virus was enough.[45]

Bergalis was put on AZT and in a short time, became very sick. Again, to quote Dr. Duesberg:

Her yeast infection worsened and became uncontrollable, she lost more than thirty pounds, her hair gradually fell out, her blood cells died and had to be replaced with transfusions, and her muscles wasted away. Her fevers hit highs of 103 degrees, and by late 1990 her T-cell count had dropped from the average of 1,000 to a mere 43. She looked just like a chemotherapy patient—which she now was.[46]

Because of the media frenzy surrounding the case, by mid-1991 more than 90 percent of the public believed that HIV-positive doctors should be forced to inform their patients of their status and the majority believed these doctors should be banned from practicing at all. By December 1991, just two years after her HIV diagnosis, Ms. Bergalis was dead as a result of AZT. The dentist had nothing at all to do with her getting HIV or AIDS. Kimberly Bergalis was killed by her medical doctors.

Could Bergalis have gotten HIV from her dentist? Theoretically, yes, but Dr. Acer probably would have had to intentionally inject her with a fairly large quantity of his infected blood without her knowledge. Why? According to *Harrison's Principals of Internal Medicine*, "Of the several hundred health care workers who have sustained penetrating injuries with instruments contaminated with HIV-infected blood, less than 0.5 percent have become infected."[47] This is likely because it's so rare to find any active HIV, even in a person with full-blown AIDS. And according to Dr. Duesberg (as of 1996), though over 400,000 AIDS patients have been treated by millions of healthcare workers, there's not a single case in the scientific literature of a healthcare worker actually developing AIDS from a patient.[48]

The victims of AZT-induced AIDS suffer from problems including anemia, leukopenia (too few white blood cells), pancytopenia (too few blood cells in general, including platelets), diarrhea, weight loss, hair loss, impotence, hepatitis, Pneumocystis pneumonia, muscle atrophy, dementia, and cancers such as lymphoma.

HIV Jails?

In the 1990s, tuberculosis made a huge comeback and became epidemic in New York, especially among the poor and homeless, but also in those with psychiatric problems, those who used IV drugs, and, of course, those with AIDS. Many of these people are not very compliant when it comes to staying on a long-term treatment regimen, and patients stopping treatment before they're completely healed has only helped to create antibiotic resistant TB. To combat this problem, the New York Health Department started placing these people on what was known as directly observed therapy, or D.O.T., where healthcare workers would come and administer or watch the patient take their medication. This program helped to bring the number of TB cases in New York down from epidemic proportions to the lowest it's been in decades.

Patients who "failed" D.O.T., however, were taken to Bellevue or Goldwater Hospitals, kept in a locked ward, and forced to take their medicine. Some call this "tough love," but the detainees themselves refer to this forcible detention as "TB jail." According to the *New York Times*, "More than 250 patients were detained between 1993 and 1998, some for as long as two years.[49]

What does this have to do with AIDS? New York's health commissioner, Dr. Thomas Frieden, estimates that the city is host to about 20,000 people with undiagnosed HIV. In response, he has proposed more aggressive screening of HIV and, "tracking HIV in a manner similar to tuberculosis, monitoring patients and trying to ensure that they take their medications properly." [50] The question is, how far will this tracking go? Because the TB program worked so well, there is some fear that patients could be not only forced into unwanted HIV testing, but if positive, forced to take AZT or other AIDS drugs against their will. In other words, we could be facing the possibility of HIV jails.

Jailed For Spreading HIV

According to the International Planned Parenthood Federation, 58 countries have now made spreading HIV a crime and another 33 countries are considering doing the same. One West African country has even made it a crime to *expose* someone to HIV, even if transmission doesn't occur. In Tanzania, *intentional* transmission can lead to life in prison.

The U.S. government has not yet criminalized the transmission of HIV, but 32 U.S. states *have*, and according to experts, thousands have been charged with the crime. Since 2001, 16 people in the U.K. have been prosecuted for spreading the virus. In Canada, a woman was actually charged with criminal negligence and aggravated assault for passing HIV to her baby. How do you think these "criminals" would feel if *they* knew HIV didn't cause AIDS?

It is interesting to note that Robert Gallo, in defending HIV as the causal factor in AIDS, declares that with infectious diseases, most people are "healthy carriers" of the germ and never actually get the disease. In fact, he says, *"Expression of disease is the exception for the majority of microbes."* [51] (Emphasis his.) This seems a far cry from saying that everyone who has HIV antibodies in his/her blood is going to eventually get AIDS and die, which *is* the justification for putting healthy HIV-positive patients on antiretroviral medications.

Inaccuracy of the AIDS Test

Since we're putting people on poisonous chemotherapy medications that destroy the immune system, stop all cell division in the body, and usually kill the patient within two to five years; and given that we're contemplating *forcing* people to take these nasty medications; and in view of the fact that we've convinced everyone on earth that AIDS is a death sentence that begins with an HIV diagnosis and is spread through sexual contact; because we're now actually putting people in jail for spreading HIV, and because we're basing all of this on the so called "AIDS test," perhaps you'd like to know how accurate this test is.

As I've already mentioned, the AIDS test doesn't actually test for HIV, it tests for HIV *antibodies*. Once again, antibodies (in every *other* infectious disease) indicate the body has successfully found a way to fight off the infection. But in the case of AIDS, we're supposed to believe that HIV is the exception to this hard and fast rule, and that the presence of antibodies means the patient *has* the virus. They give no explanation as to why this should be so. We're just expected to take this on faith.

The test they use to screen for AIDS is called the ELISA test (Enzyme-Linked Immunosorbent Assay). According to an article in *JAMA* entitled "HIV Testing: State of the Art," "[D]epending on the population tested, 20–70 percent of...two successive positive ELISAs are confirmed by Western blot [a more accurate antibody test]." [52] In other words, after a patient tested positive twice using the ELISA test, they attempted to confirm the findings using the Western blot method, and using this test, only 20–70 percent of these patients tested positive. The rest (30–80 percent) are deemed false positives. Why such a large range, i.e., 20–70 percent? The accuracy depends on the population being tested. If most of the population truly *is* HIV-positive (such as the hemophiliac population), obviously there will be fewer false positives than if most are truly negative.

Another study, this one found in the *New England Journal of Medicine,* reported that 83 percent (10,000 out of 12,000) of U.S. Army applicants who tested positive on the ELISA test initially, were actually false positives.[53]

Incidentally, the CDC does not require repeatedly positive ELISA tests, nor do they require the confirmation by Western blot to consider someone HIV-positive. One positive ELISA test is enough for them. This means that a large percentage of the HIV-positive patients in their files could actually be false positives. What's more, the CDC's director of the HIV/AIDS division, Harold Jaffe, has stated that 43,606 of the 253,448 cases of AIDS in the U.S. have *never* been tested for HIV![54] (I wonder how they know these patients have AIDS instead of the "less significant" and made up disease they call ICL.)

How accurate is the Western blot test? First, remember, it, too, is only testing for HIV *antibodies*. Again, it depends on the study, but when Western blot is compared with the PCR test (Polymerase Chain Reaction), it shows about a 50 percent accuracy.

And how accurate is the PCR? The PCR was devised by Dr. Kary Mullis and is the test most often used when they test for viral loads. Dr. Mullis won the Nobel Prize for developing this test and *he* has said *repeatedly* that the PCR cannot be used to measure HIV viral loads and that its results in this regard are "meaningless."

Why are the results meaningless? First of all, the PCR measures "viral loads" by detecting genes. Therefore, the only genes that would have meaning in this case would be the ones that are unique to HIV. (A gene that codes for reverse transcriptase, for example, would be meaningless, since all cells make this enzyme and therefore carry this gene.) The problem is, we don't really know what genes are unique to HIV because HIV has never actually been isolated. The genome they are basing this test on is not even HIV itself, but an HIV clone. What is this clone based upon? Apparently on the un-isolated LAV that Luc Montagnier found in his patient with the swollen lymph nodes— remember, the one that didn't even have AIDS. So, we're comparing unknowns with unknowns. In addition to any active HIV there might actually be in the patient, the PCR also measures dormant viruses, defective bits and pieces of HIV (1/40th of the whole genome is often enough to count as a virus), and HIV that's been neutralized by antibodies. And this is considered the Gold Standard in AIDS testing.

As for actual visual detection of the virus in blood, as is routinely done with bacterial infections, this simply isn't done. Dr. Duesberg claims, "leading AIDS researchers have had notorious difficulties in isolating [and by that he means *finding*, not purifying as I've used this word] HIV, even in people dying from AIDS." [55, 56]

Furthermore, according to Dr. Stephen Davis, author of *Wrongful Death: The AIDS Trial*, "no HIV test, whether it's blood or saliva, has ever been approved by the FDA to diagnose HIV infection. In fact, every test kit manufacturer includes an insert in the package—which no one ever sees—that says that the test was not designed to test for the presence or absence of HIV." [57]

Why do the ELISA and Western blot tests show so many false positives? Over 50 scientific studies have shown that there are at least 70 different factors in the human body that can cause a false positive HIV test. These include a recent flu shot, generalized warts, and even prior pregnancies. In one study, seven out of 10 blood donors who had been given the flu shot became HIV-positive on the ELISA test.[58] This is apparently because the proteins used in the test kits are not specific to HIV. To make things even more confusing, there are 10 different criteria for what constitutes a positive test, so you could be considered HIV-positive in one state, and HIV-negative in another.

Now, does this sound like testing worthy of basing such important, life and death decisions on to you?

AIDS in the Third World

Everything we've discussed so far in this chapter has pertained to AIDS in the U.S. and Europe. Many of you by now are saying, okay, so AIDS hasn't spread outside of the risk-groups here, but what about Africa? Over there AIDS is spreading like wildfire. It's equal in both sexes, children are being orphaned, entire villages are being wiped out, economies are being strained... Hospitals can't even handle all the AIDS patients, so don't try to tell me it's not infectious.

When you hear statements like these regarding the Third World, it helps to keep in mind the facts you've learned thus far, especially the all-important difference between being HIV-positive and having AIDS. Thailand, for example, is often cited as an example of how bad things could possibly get here. They say in bold headlines that Thailand has 300,000 people infected with the AIDS virus. Oooh, sounds scary, especially with the booming industry of sex tourism in that country. But stop and think about what these figures actually mean. All that means is that 300,000 Thai people have HIV antibodies in their blood. They may very well have been HIV-positive their entire lives, having received the antibodies from their mothers. Also, keep in mind that 90,000–240,000 (30–80 percent) of those HIV-positive individuals are in fact *false* positives. How many actually have AIDS? As of 1993, there had only been 1,569 cases of AIDS diagnosed in that country. That amounts to only one-half of one percent of the 300,000 supposedly infected with HIV. Half of these cases are male homosexuals or IV drug users; the other half are prostitutes, most or all of whom use drugs.[59]

A similar situation is happening in Africa. In 2007, that continent reported a frightening 23 million HIV-positive individuals.[60] Once again, pretty scary numbers, until one realizes that 30–80 percent of those are false positives.

But there's much more to this story. The reality is that *many* of the reported cases of AIDS in Africa are not AIDS at all. Celia Farber reported in *Spin* magazine:

Many believe that the statistics have been inflated because
AIDS generates far more money in the Third World from
Western organizations than any other infectious disease.
This was clear to us when we were there: Where there
was "AIDS" there was money—a brand-new clinic, a new
Mercedes parked outside, modern testing facilities, high-
paying jobs, international conferences... When [doctors] get
sent to these AIDS conferences around the world, the per
diem they receive is equal to what they earn in a whole year
at home.[61]

On even closer inspection, the entire AIDS epidemic in Africa
appears to be a myth, and this myth seems to have grown largely
out of a report in the late 1980s by two French charity workers
Philippe (whose quote started this chapter) and Evelyne Krynen.
As heads of a large AIDS charity group, they reported villages
being devastated, homes abandoned, growing numbers of orphans,
and an AIDS epidemic that was threatening to depopulate the
Kagera province of northern Tanzania. The press grabbed this
story and ran with it—and they've continued to run with it, in spite
of the fact that the Krynens have since retracted all of their former
statements.

It seems that after spending some more time there, they came to
the bittersweet conclusion that they had reported a falsehood. There
was no AIDS epidemic. They discovered, first of all, that more than
half of their "AIDS" patients were HIV-negative. The "abandoned
homes" could just as easily be considered *second* homes of families
who had moved to the cities. And the "orphans" were simply being
raised by the grandparents because the parents had gone to the city
to earn money—part of the new social structure there. Incredibly,
the prostitutes of the area did not catch this "sexually transmitted
disease" either.

Krynen states:

> If you say your father has died in a car accident it is bad
> luck, but if he has died from AIDS there is an agency to help
> you. The local people have seen so many agencies coming
> called AIDS support programs, that they want to join this
> group of victims. Everybody claims to be a victim of AIDS
> nowadays. And local people working for AIDS agencies have
> become rich... We have...about 17 organizations reportedly
> doing something for AIDS in Kagera. It brings jobs, cars; the
> day there is no more AIDS, a lot of development is going to
> go away... You don't need AIDS patients to have an AIDS
> epidemic nowadays, because what is wrong doesn't need to
> be proved. Nobody checks; AIDS exists by itself.[62]

Then there's another issue. Just as each risk group in the U.S.
and Europe has their own particular AIDS-defining diseases, Africa
has its own set of AIDS-defining diseases. Most of these African
AIDS diseases are different from those seen in AIDS patients in
the U.S. and Europe, and none of these diseases are new to Africa.
In other words, the diseases that are considered AIDS in Africa
are the same indigenous diseases that have always been on that
continent and they occur with or without HIV infection. Just like
cervical cancer in this country, they've simply been renamed or
re-categorized in order to benefit from the influx of AIDS support
from around the world.

In the mid-eighties, it was discovered that a large percentage of
Africans were HIV-positive, but nobody seemed to be getting the
AIDS-defining diseases (thrush, *Pneumocystis carinii*, and Kaposi's
sarcoma) there. This was a major blow to the HIV-causes-AIDS
theory, so the World Health Organization held a meeting in West
Africa where it was decided that Africa would have its own special
criteria for diagnosing AIDS. (It's called the Bangui Clinical Diagnosis

of AIDS.) At this meeting, they decided that being HIV-positive was no longer necessary for the diagnosis to be made! Second, they devised a symptom score-sheet whereby anybody who scored 12 or more could be diagnosed with AIDS. According to this score sheet, weight loss, fever, coughing, weakness, itching, and diarrhea were now all signs of "AIDS," each being worth a certain number of points.[63] These new criteria meant that many of the diseases that are endemic to Africa would meet the diagnosis of AIDS, whether the patient had HIV or not. Presto, instant AIDS epidemic!

As Janine Roberts says in *Fear of the Invisible*:

> With these symptoms, the African AIDS epidemic could be sharply diminished by funding sewage works, clean water supplies, and better nourishment. These are the very same measures that ended the epidemics that ravaged the British poor in the 19th century. But by adopting this definition and calling this AIDS, the international experts had done the contrary. They had created by fiat a massive African AIDS epidemic reportedly caused by promiscuous sex, with death only delayed by powerful chemotherapy type drugs. This has also led to preachers advocating sexual abstinence and to bishops blaming African bigamy. The result is that in Africa some call AIDS the "American Initiative to Destroy Sex." [63]

One long-time African disease that now fits the diagnosis of "African AIDS" is called "slim disease." The symptoms include weight loss, diarrhea, fever, persistent coughing, skin problems, swollen lymph nodes, and opportunistic infections like tuberculosis. Malaria, the number one killer in the Third World, has many symptoms that can easily be considered part of the African AIDS collage and it is frequently diagnosed as such because of what we've just discussed, i.e., the benefits of being an AIDS victim over being merely a malaria victim. It's the same thing with tuberculosis, another common disease in Africa. According to a doctor in Uganda, "A patient who has TB and is HIV-positive would appear exactly the same as a patient who has TB and is HIV-negative." He says, "clinically, I cannot differentiate the two." [64] Several large studies have found that in randomly selected Africans with AIDS-defining diseases, fewer than half of them were HIV-positive.

In 1994, after much criticism of the Bangui definition, the WHO expanded their definition of AIDS. They said that from then on, if HIV antibody testing *could* be done, it should be done, but if not, the Bangui definition would suffice.[65] It should be noted that most of the HIV testing that *is* done there is performed on pregnant women and as we've just seen, pregnancy (or even prior pregnancy) increases the already high number of false positives. These people are now being put on antiretroviral medications en masse.

How bad is this problem of misdiagnosis? It's impossible to say with any accuracy, but it is apparently rampant. As one nurse in Tanzania put it, "If people die of malaria, it is called AIDS. If they die of herpes, it is called AIDS. I've even seen people die in accidents and it's been attributed to AIDS. The AIDS figures out of Africa are pure lies, pure estimate." [66]

The worst thing about all this misdiagnosis is that patients with treatable diseases like malaria, tuberculosis, or even diabetes, who are diagnosed with AIDS, are not being treated properly. They're either given AZT or they get nothing. In either case they're condemned to die. Such was reported in a letter by four Tanzanian doctors in 1989. The letter appeared in the journal *Lancet*. Here is an excerpt:

> In tropical Africa febrile illnesses are frequently attributed to malaria. Now in certain places AIDS is the fashionable diagnosis, made by the public and doctors. Many patients with treatable and curable illnesses may now be condemned without proper assessment.[67]

Besides the diseases that have always been present in Africa, which are now being blamed on AIDS, drugs like cocaine and heroin are on the rise as well. But drugs are more prevalent in the urban areas of Africa, and wouldn't you know it, the AIDS diseases seen in urban drug users are different from those living in more rural or jungle areas of Africa. Also, only the prostitutes who use drugs heavily seem to "catch" this "sexually transmitted disease." This appears to be true all over the world.

Haitian AIDS has certain aspects of both rural and urban AIDS in Africa. Tuberculosis is the most common AIDS-defining disease there. Kaposi's sarcoma is almost nonexistent. Boy, that HIV is sure one crafty bug.

Our impotent answer to all these problems in the Third World, if I may summarize, has been to send public workers to these countries to hand out condoms. Oh, yes, *and* AZT. It's really no different in this country. This is how we're attempting to handle the worldwide AIDS epidemic and why it's been such a colossal failure!

Spending more money on these inane efforts won't help. The only thing that *will* help is to finally admit that there *is* no AIDS. Or rather, that there *is* a syndrome of acquired immune deficiency, but it's not contagious (sexually or otherwise) and has nothing to do with a virus called HIV (or any other virus for that matter). AIDS (the syndrome that was discovered in 1980 in fast-track homosexuals that is; *not* the expanded definition of what we currently consider AIDS or "HIV disease") is caused by heavy, long-term drug use and a lifestyle that's not compatible with health. This is not an anti-*gay* stance; it's an anti-*drug* stance. But even more so, it's a stance *for* the truth. And while this may be (if I can borrow the expression) an *inconvenient* truth for some, it is far better to know that truth and understand the consequences of one's actions than to remain blissfully ignorant and die because of it.

Occam's razor (sometimes called the "law of succinctness") states that all other things being equal, the simplest solution (that is, the one with the fewest assumptions or irrelevancies) is the best solution. HIV, as we've demonstrated throughout this chapter, is irrelevant to AIDS, and in fact the assumption that it *is* relevant is what's led to the confusion and so much mistreatment in AIDS cases. HIV is, in my opinion, the biggest red herring in healthcare history. It's certainly been the most costly in terms of dollars spent. By contrast, drug use is the most common denominator in true AIDS cases and also the most elegant answer to the problem. Thus, by Occam's razor, by Koch's postulates, by research in the most respected journals in the world, by many of the most learned people on the subject, and by good old common sense, HIV *cannot* be the cause of AIDS.

What to Do

If You Have AIDS or Belong To One of the Aforementioned Risk Groups

This should be fairly obvious, but if you're using inhaled drugs, especially poppers or amyl nitrites, stop. In fact, you should really stop using *all* recreational drugs as well as any prescription drugs that aren't absolutely necessary to your survival. In my opinion, this includes antibiotics, unless you have an active bacterial infection, and all antiretroviral medications. This is a decision that must be made between you and your doctor. Simultaneously, you must begin to detoxify your body (slowly) and re-establish your normal flora (see Chapter 7). Pay attention to your T-cell count and how you feel, but ignore your HIV status and your viral load counts, as they are completely irrelevant. Begin to follow a healthy natural lifestyle to include a diet of good organic and free-range foods that's low in sugar content and processed foods. Exercise. Take *whole food* supplements, not synthetic supplements. Use condoms to prevent STDs. Maintain a positive outlook and anticipate your returning health "against the odds."

If You're HIV-Positive

Don't panic! If you're truly at risk for AIDS (meaning you're an active member of one of the risk groups), follow the steps given above. Otherwise, have your T-cells checked on occasion (for your own mental health) and go on living a normal, healthy life. ***Do not*** give in to your doctor's pressure or fear tactics regarding preventative anti-retroviral treatments. These drugs will *make* you sick and will eventually kill you. There is no credible evidence that they actually help HIV-positive people to live longer or that they prevent AIDS. People who are HIV-positive and not part of a risk group who refuse these treatments are living for decades without any sign of disease. People who accept these treatments are succumbing to disease.

Always remember, no matter how many times you've heard the phrase, "HIV, the virus that causes AIDS," there is no proof whatsoever that it does. Worry, whether about your HIV status or anything else, can actually reduce your T-cell count, so ***don't worry***. It doesn't help anyway. If you choose, use your HIV status as a motivating factor for you to be even healthier. Join the Natural Healthcare Revolution and help to prove the status quo wrong. Print T-shirts that say, "HIV≠AIDS!" and give them to everyone you know. Get involved in this movement; after all, you are the proof that their accusations are false.

For More Information:

Books:
Inventing the AIDS Virus, by Peter Duesberg
Fear of the Invisible, by Janine Roberts

Websites:
Virus Myth: http://www.virusmyth.com/
Rethinking AIDS: http://www.rethinkingaids.com/
This website lists many more books, videos, and articles on the subject as well as a list of over 2,600 doctors and scientists who openly reject the HIV-causes-AIDS theory.

Videos:
Deconstructing the Myth of AIDS, by Gary Null, Copyright 2005
AIDS Inc., by Gary Null, Copyright 2007
House of Numbers: Anatomy of an Epidemic, by Brent Leung, Copyright 2009

13

Freedom from Fear:
Bird Flu, the Boogie Man & Beyond

---

*"Those who cannot remember the past
are condemned to repeat it."*

—George Santayana, *The Life of Reason*, 1905

Having tackled AIDS, now I'd like to address all of those *other* killer germs out there—those that have caused us to panic in the past few years, and whatever's lurking around the next corner, too. No doubt the drug companies, the media, and the germ hunters are all on the lookout for the next germ that could be built up enough to scare the ever lovin' fecal matter out of you. It's become standard operating procedure. The drug companies do this, of course, in order to get you to buy their new drug; the media wants you to tune in to their next broadcast; and the germ hunters do it hoping for their 15 minutes of fame, some prestigious award that can be parlayed into more money, or simply to justify their existence and, therefore receive more government funding. Besides, our fear of germs and relative ignorance of them makes these germ hunters seem like heroic geniuses, doesn't it? They're like firefighters with Ph.D.s rushing into a burning building. So, a worldwide pandemic, whether natural *or* manmade, would suit all three of these groups just fine. But short of that, scaring us half to death every couple of years can often reap the same benefits, whether that fear is founded or not.

Thanks in part to these sensationalized news stories, we have become a nation of germophobes. I rarely watch TV, but recently my wife and I were eating at a restaurant where a TV was on and I happened to see an advertisement (designed to look like a public service announcement) giving advice on who should get the flu shot. They then proceeded to list so many different age groups, occupations, and classifications of people that basically everyone on the face of the planet would fall into at least one, if not more of the groups mentioned. In other words, *everyone* needs our shot, and some of you may need two or three. To my wife and me, this was clearly a shameless ploy to sell more drugs, but to many, this is seen as "health advice" from a trusted source—the boob tube.

Of course, I can't predict what the next big killer germ will be, nor can I say with absolute certainty that the next killer germ *won't* become pandemic, but I want to at least convince you that these news stories and ads are *scare tactics* and that a healthy immune system is the only *sane* way to stave off any real "attack bug," especially if that bug is a virus. Vaccines, antibiotics, and antiviral medications are cheap, *cheap* substitutes for the amazing system you have written into your DNA. Think of your immune system as you would a muscle, and the rule with any muscle is: Use it or lose it. So, too, it is with your immune system. And just as building a muscle can sometimes lead to soreness or pain, building your immune system can also have some pain involved. But after the pain is gone, you emerge stronger than you were before.

When I first wrote this chapter, bird flu was all over the news. Currently, as I complete the writing of this book, the H1N1 swine flu is all over the news. By the time you read this book, the swine flu may be a distant memory and there may even be a new killer virus in the news that makes the swine or bird flu viruses sound like cuddly little bunnies. What I'm encouraging you to do is to *not forget* the swine flu, bird flu, or any of the others, because when you remember these outbreaks, you'll start to see the patterns, and next time a virus is in the news, you'll know that it's probably just another scare tactic designed to get more money into Big Pharma's pocket and less in yours. Hopefully then, you won't go rushing right out to get the vaccine or the latest antiviral drug or whatever else they've concocted for the misled and frightened public to buy. And by not doing so, you won't get the antibiotics, chemicals, heavy metals, attenuated, genetically modified, or cancer-causing wild monkey viruses. That means you won't end up with Alzheimer's, Parkinson's, ALS, MS, cancer, yeast infections, or any other side effect of Western medicine. And what's more, you'll be *allowing* your immune system to stay healthy.

Remember what Darwin said about the survival of the fittest? Well, those who keep taking drugs and vaccines, sadly to say, will probably be among the first to go in a true worldwide pandemic. It will be those of us with healthy immune systems who've gained *natural* immunity to germs who will be left to repopulate the planet, just as it's the healthy bacteria who've gained natural immunity to the drugs that are left after a course of antibiotics.

Interesting comparison, isn't it? Have you ever thought about this before? Disease kills off the weak in every species of plant and animal. Weak plants are quickly engulfed in bugs or taken over by fungus. People who make poor health choices tend to have more sickness and disease, including those that are considered "infectious" in nature. Remember, bacteria's job in the eternal cycle is to return unviable and diseased tissue back into soil so that nature can start over. Only the strong are allowed to survive and reproduce. This is nature's way.

Just as antibiotics are helping to create stronger germs, germs are helping the human race to become stronger over time. In this rather Zen way of thinking, the one we think of as our enemy (the germ) is actually our friend, and the one we think of as our friend (the drug/vaccine) is actually our enemy. Rather than concentrating on *killing* the germ, thereby making the human race weaker and the germs stronger, we *should* be concentrating on strengthening our immune systems—*naturally*—and learning to live in symbiosis with our new friends, the germs.

Bird Flu

I'm going to let you in on a dirty little secret: Virtually all of the chickens affected by bird flu are the ones that have been raised in tiny cages (called CAFOs or Concentrated Animal Feeding Operations) and fed hormones, antibiotics, and arsenic (yes, arsenic!) all their lives. These poor chickens get no exercise. They never see the sun. They're exposed to all kinds of toxins and chemicals, and they're highly stressed. They're forced to grow so fast and they get so little exercise that their little chicken legs can barely hold their weight long enough to walk a few steps, which is all the room they have to move anyway. In short, they're raised in very inhumane conditions and because of this, they suffer from almost constant low-level disease; which is why they're fed antibiotics as part of their diet. These antibiotics, of course, don't protect them from viral infections, however, and thus, we have bird flu.

Where do all these bacteria and viruses come from? The stressed out chickens produce them and spread them to their neighbors, much as we humans produce cold and flu viruses in the winter, through the magic of pleomorphism.

Free-range, organic chickens are basically unaffected by bird flu. In fact, scientists in Thailand who studied the epidemic there found that the risks for bird flu infection were 32.4 times higher in commercial birds than backyard chickens.[1, 2]

> Guess what they do with the 26–55 billion pounds of chicken poop produced in all these caged chicken farms. They sell it as fertilizer and fish food for farm-raised fish! Yes, just as arsenic stimulates chicken growth, apparently chicken poop (laced with arsenic) stimulates fish growth. This waste often contains campylobacter, salmonella, parasites, drug residues, lead, cadmium, mercury, and of course, the bird flu virus.

Here's a refresher on what Dr. Joseph Mercola called "The Great Bird Flu Hoax." Julie Gerberding, the head of the CDC said, "there is no evidence that [bird flu] will be the next pandemic." She stated that the human victims of this disease (about 200 people in all) were in intense daily contact with sick flocks, often sharing the same living space. Only two people had been reported to have spread the virus from person to person and she said there was "no reason to think it ever will" pass easily from person to person.[3] In fact, the real experts thought it *very* unlikely or even impossible. Dr. Shiv Chopra, a veterinarian and microbiologist stated:

> Infectious diseases in animals, including bird flu, can occasionally transmit to humans... But it does not then spread from a thus infected person to the next person to the next person. For example, people handling cattle

or sheep carcasses can get anthrax but anthrax does not spread from people to people to cause human epidemics... Any microbiologist who tells you otherwise is lying. This is an absolute lie. It has not happened, it will not happen, it cannot happen. We know that from science.[4]

So, the whole bird flu scare was founded on one giant lie and supplemented by several smaller lies. Who has the clout to perpetrate such lies on the public, and why would they do it?

Follow the Money

Despite the complete lack of evidence that a bird flu pandemic was even possible, let alone likely, on November 1, 2005, President George W. Bush announced the "Pandemic Influenza Strategic Plan" and ordered Congress to approve $7.1 billion in emergency funding to prepare for one. This included $1.5 billion for the purchase of flu vaccines and $1 billion to stockpile antiviral medication.

The government then announced that they planned to buy 75 million doses of Tamiflu, which set the stage for other countries to do likewise. Following suit, the U.K. ordered 14.5 million doses; Germany ordered 6 million doses; Canada stockpiled 35 million doses; and France, New Zealand, and Norway all planned to buy enough to treat 20–25 percent of their populations. That's a *lot* of Tamiflu!

One of the people who just happened to benefit from this deal was our then Secretary of Defense, Donald Rumsfeld. Rumsfeld was on the board of Gilead Sciences (makers of Tamiflu) from 1988 right up until he joined the Bush administration in 2001. When he left, he retained his stockholdings, which were then valued at $7.00/share. When his boss announced his plan for dealing with the fabricated bird flu threat, Rumsfeld's Gilead stocks suddenly jumped in value to

$50.00/share. "Rummy" then sold off some of those shares, making himself more than $5 million in the trade. As of October 2005, he still retained at least $25 million dollars worth of Gilead stocks.[5]

Donald Rumsfeld was also CEO of G.D. Searle in the early 1980s when its toxic artificial sweetener NutraSweet was finally approved. He used his political connections, namely with newly elected president, Ronald Reagan, to have the head of the FDA fired and replaced with someone more friendly to the food poisoning industry. You'll read more about this infuriating story in a future *Why We're Sick*™ book.

Tamiflu, which is an oral antiviral medication that costs over $100.00 per prescription, has been shown to shorten the effects of *seasonal* flu by about one day, as per their website. As of 2006 (a year *after* Bush's announcement), there were no published studies showing that Tamiflu was effective *at all* for *bird* flu. One independent study showed that in order for it to be as effective on bird flu as it is against the seasonal flu (which is not very effective), it would take *30 times* the normal dose to do so![6] That would mean spending $3,000.00 in the hopes of shortening your bird flu crisis by 1.3 days—assuming of course that you live through the attack.

Many researchers working in Thailand and Vietnam, including some from the World Health Organization, have concluded that Tamiflu is "useless" and that it did *not* reduce the mortality of their patients or indeed have any beneficial effect at all.[7-13] In fact, there are reports that Tamiflu may actually make the virus mutate more quickly and become more aggressive, leading some to fear that the drug could actually *cause* the very pandemic government officials are trying to avoid.[14] Finally, and most tragically, in 2005, 11 million Japanese kids were given Tamiflu to treat the seasonal flu. Twelve of these children died from the drug and 32 others reported neuropsychiatric symptoms including seizures, loss of consciousness, hallucinations, and delirium.[15, 16]

Seventy-five million doses? Does this sound like a billion dollars in tax money well spent to you? By the way, the FDA refuses to list any of these serious adverse events as potential side effects.

Preparedness or Paranoia?

As anyone who lived through the Y2K scare can attest, there is sometimes a fine line separating preparedness and paranoia. During these times of anxiety and trepidation, it's best to look at the evidence as objectively as possible before making one's decisions. Making wise decisions is especially important when one is entrusted with spending other people's money to safeguard the public. However, it's equally important in these matters to safeguard the people's *trust*. When the CDC and other government organizations are constantly crying, "Wolf!" or telling us the sky is falling, we have only two choices: Live in constant fear of non-existent threats (the stress of which can weaken the immune system) or simply tune out the cries. This issue was discussed in an editorial in *Maclean's* magazine in May 2006.

> ...in recent years the World Health Organization has frequently allowed preparedness to mutate into paranoia. You'd think it would have learned from the SARS debacle, during which it issued a warning for foreign tourists to avoid Toronto, even though the outbreak was minuscule and quickly contained. Ebola and West Nile raised similar panics. When our guardians of global health tilt at every windmill on the epidemiological landscape they erode their own credibility. One day, there will be a genuine crisis. We

can only hope that the public won't have tuned out the constant alarms.[17]

Between 1999 and 2007, West Nile Virus killed 1,086 people in the United States. That's about 120 people per year. Most, if not all of them were elderly and/or immune-compromised. The virus is spread by a mosquito bite and causes encephalitis (brain inflammation), which can result in death. The current plan to control the spread of West Nile Virus is the spraying of insecticides including those containing DEET. Ironically, one of the more common side effects of DEET poisoning is *encephalitis*. (Hmm. Sounds an awful lot like the story connecting DDT and polio, doesn't it?) Anvil, another pesticide used to control mosquitoes, is known to cause brain tumors in children and birth defects in animals. Other problems associated with these pesticides include respiratory illnesses, seizures and other neurological disorders, immune system dysfunction, cancer, reproductive problems, and learning disorders. In a 2001 study conducted by the National Audubon Society, scientists discovered that in birds collected because of suspected West Nile Virus, more had actually been killed by pesticides and other toxins than were killed by the virus.[18] If these toxins are killing birds, they're certainly killing bees, bats, and butterflies too, and with the loss of these creatures, our entire ecology hangs in the balance. As for humans, even if we don't actually inhale these pesticides while they're in the air, they land in the trees, on our crops, and on our grass. Our pets and children then roll around on that grass and track them into our houses. They contaminate the ground water and the soil we grow our food with. They accumulate in domestic feed animals... All of this to control a virus that kills 120 people per year. What makes this practice seem even *more* insane is that in countries where West Nile Virus has been around for some time, most of the population is completely immune to it by the age of 40. So, is it worth poisoning everyone in America and destroying our entire ecology to save 120 immune-compromised people per year? Wouldn't strengthening our collective immune system be the wiser choice?

From Animal Farm to 1984

Besides the drug companies and our former Secretary of Defense, who else is benefiting from the hysteria brought about by bird flu, mad cow, etc.? Oddly enough, even though it's meant the slaughter of millions of animals, in the long run, the big agribusinesses will likely *benefit* from these scares.

Over 200 million chickens were destroyed during the 2006 bird flu scare. Many, if not most, of these birds were not even sick, but merely "at risk." Similar "culls" of healthy cows and sheep occurred a few years prior during the mad cow and foot and mouth disease scares.

In 2002, the mad cow scare led the National Institute for Animal Agriculture (NIAA) to call for a nationwide livestock registration tracking system. The members of the NIAA include the major U.S. meat producers and manufacturers of high-tech animal identification equipment. This small interest group managed to sell their idea to the USDA, who published their plan, called the National Animal Identification System (NAIS), in 2005. This plan would require farmers to radio tag or microchip all of their animals and put them into a database so their every move can be tracked.

The government claims it wants this done so that it can track diseased animals back to their source, which may be a good idea. The problem is, the costs for installing the survey equipment will likely be put on the farmers, which may be cost prohibitive to the small farmer and much more difficult for those who raise their animals humanely in open pastures rather than the inhumane stalls and cages of "conventional farms," which are the real breeding grounds for these diseases. The cost of this technology for the big meat producers like Monsanto, Tyson, and Cargill Meat, will be minuscule compared to their profits. The end result may be that the small farmer is driven out of business, or at the very least, the cost of organic, free-range meat, poultry, and eggs may increase to the point that it's out of reach for most people. This loss of competition works gloriously to increase the growing monopoly of big agribusiness. The huge irony of this is, the organic, free-range animals raised on small, independent farms are considerably healthier than the "conventional" animals and are almost never the ones who have the diseases (like mad cow or bird flu) that need to be tracked.

If the USDA were truly interested in preventing these types of illnesses, instead of simply creating a whole new branch of government bureaucracy to track our nation's feed animals, they would create a mandate whereby farmers were forced or enticed to raise their animals in healthy, humane conditions. Not only would this tactic virtually eliminate such diseases in animals, it would also have the happy side effect of creating a healthier human population at the same time.

Domestic animals are now being tagged with RFID chips. In 2004, the FDA approved their use in humans, and as of this writing, about 2,000 people have voluntarily undergone the procedure. The tags, which are about the size of a grain of rice, can be simple "beacons" that make the person or animal easy to find, or they can be programmed to contain any information that can be digitized, such as bank account numbers or medical information. How long will it be before the government wants all children tagged with a microchip—for their safety? How long after that before all adults will want/need to be tagged? How long before having your wrist scanned replaces your having to pull out your debit card or having to fill out medical forms in triplicate? How long before the government knows exactly where you are, what you're buying, and what you're doing every moment of the day—no matter where you go? The chips will likely be marketed to the public as both a safety and a convenience item. Convenience sells itself, but it takes a fearful public to sell safety, which is where the media comes in.

The cows that died of mad cow disease were also the ones who were *not* being fed their natural diet of green grass, but rather corn, ground up animal parts, antibiotics, hormones, etc. Likewise, animals in the wild do not suffer the same diseases as we humans because they're simply not smart enough to try to improve upon nature. It took good old human ingenuity to figure out how to make a Twinkie® after all.

It's almost always when humans get a little too involved that we create some monster that we end up needing to be saved from. Why do we refuse to learn this lesson? Why do we continue to pursue the "better living through chemistry" lie rather than getting back to nature, as we all inherently know we should? Buying the cheaper, "conventionally farmed" and processed food leads to paying more in healthcare bills later on. So, do we pay now and remain healthy or pay later and suffer through all manner of disease? Is the convenience or the taste of the food you're about to ingest worth the abuse it will put your body through? Are the benefits of your current eating habits worth the misery of the disease you are creating with each mouthful? The choice is yours.

Seasonal Flu

What about seasonal flu? The CDC tells us that 36,000 Americans die every year from the flu. *Really?* Thirty-six *thousand*? It's an impressive number, but is it true? Whenever I've heard this, I've always found that number *staggering*, especially since with all my years in healthcare, I don't think I've ever actually heard of *anyone* (patients, their friends, their grandparents, etc.) dying of the flu.

Shedding some much-needed light on the subject, the *British Medical Journal* published a letter from Harvard grad student Peter Doshi entitled, "Are U.S. flu death figures more PR than science?" [19] The letter listed the actual numbers (acquired from the National Center for Health Statistics), which showed an average of only 1,348 yearly deaths from the flu between 1979 and 2002, with a range between 257 and 3,006. (Okay, 3,006; 36,000; it's easy to see how you could get those numbers mixed up, I guess—if you're a moron.) But what you find when you look a little closer is that the bulk of these people supposedly dying of the "flu" are actually dying of *pneumonia*, which is a completely different disease caused by completely different germs. And by the way, the flu shot does absolutely *nothing* to prevent pneumonia.

If you're wondering why the CDC would inflate their flu figures so drastically, go back and read Chapter 4 again. Just like the FDA, these government researchers are highly paid to create statistics that scare Americans into getting the flu vaccine every year.

Whenever someone is brave enough to doubt the kill factor of the flu virus, people always bring up the great Spanish flu pandemic of 1918, which killed millions of people worldwide and more than half a million Americans. The thing they neglect to mention, however, is that *that* flu happened during the famously harsh conditions of World War I, when thousands upon thousands of soldiers were packed into filthy trenches under *highly* stressful conditions and worldwide sanitation was horrible compared to what we have today. It's also been reported by Yale Professor Emeritus of Epidemiology and Public Health, Robert E. Shope that the severe illness and deaths from the 1918 "flu" were not caused by a flu virus at all, but rather the bacteria *haemophilus influezae suis*.[20] This theory, however, has been largely ignored.

Professor Shope took mucus and fluids from the lungs of infected pigs. He then filtered out all bacteria, including the one mentioned above, then introduced this fluid (still containing the flu virus) to both pigs and humans. These test subjects only got a mild flu. However, he also reported, "Mixing the filtrate with the bacterium reproduced the severe disease." [21] He also found that those who survived the great flu of 1918 were immune to this bacteria, indicating they had been exposed and survived.

The Flu Shot

As with many other vaccines, originally, the flu shot was recommended for a select group of people. Now it's more or less recommended for everyone. And since it requires a yearly update at a cost of $15–35, it gives the drug companies a permanent stream of income, even if only for a few months out of the year. So does it actually work? Let's see:

The flu is caused by any one of a dozen or so influenza viruses. These viruses have the ability to mutate many times within a single season. They can even mutate within an individual. In fact, the sicker the patient, or the greater the number of people with the virus, the faster the virus mutates. This is known as gene amplification and it makes permanent immunity to the flu an impossibility. I'm sure you can see the problem with this vaccine already: How do they know which virus and which form it will be in when it infects you? Answer: They don't. To add to the complications, the vaccine goes into production about 11 months before it's distributed. This means the best they can possibly do is *guess* at which three bugs to include into the shot. With all this guesswork and constant mutation going on, it's pretty easy to see why the flu shot doesn't work most of the time. And yet when there's a shortage (which seems to be almost every year, thus creating a false demand and more media coverage), you'll see people standing in line for hours, climbing over one another trying to be one of the "lucky ones" to receive his/her shot.

So, is the flu shot effective? A 1993 Dutch study performed on nursing home residents showed that 48 percent of the non-vaccinated population got the flu, while 50 percent of those who *were* vaccinated got it.[22] This study is in line with many others I've seen, which show a slight statistical advantage to *not* getting the shot over getting it. In January 2004, the CDC and the *New York Times* reported that the flu shot had either no or very low effectiveness that season. Depending on how one interpreted the data, the shots were only 0–14 percent effective.[23] I'd dare to say that a placebo would probably work better. The journal *Archives of Pediatric & Adolescent Medicine* stated in October 2008 that, "significant influenza vaccine effectiveness could not be demonstrated for any season, age, or setting."[24] In 2006, the *British Medical Journal* published a review of 51 studies by the renowned Cochrane Collaboration, whose reviews are considered the gold standard for determining the effectiveness of healthcare interventions. The review involved 260,000 children 6–23 months of age and showed that the flu shot is no more effective than a placebo for kids under two years old—one of the major groups the shot is recommended for.[25] *The Lancet* has stated that for those over 65 years of age (the other major group marketed these shots), the flu shot is perhaps 30 (ranging from 25–45) percent effective and reported that no studies have ever shown the flu shot to reduce or prevent flu-related deaths in this group.[26] The flu shot given in the 2007–08 season only contained one virus out of three that was considered a "good match," making the shot almost worthless—again.

Then there are the dangers. Remember the swine flu debacle of 1976? That spring, we were warned that the swine flu was going to be especially deadly and there was a huge push by the CDC and the federal government to get every man, woman, and child in the United States vaccinated. This included a televised message by President Ford and public service announcements showing patriotic citizens lined up like cattle to get their herd-strengthening shots. About 45 million U.S. citizens (22 percent of the population) received the shot before the program was discontinued.[27]

This entire swine flu campaign was based on the death of *one* Army recruit at Fort Dix, a Private David Lewis, who reportedly died of the swine flu. The CDC panicked when they realized that this flu strain was related to the one that caused the 1918 flu pandemic and decided that it *must* be contained. Four other soldiers at Fort Dix were also confirmed to be carrying the swine flu, but they all recovered without issue. There were no other confirmed cases of swine flu anywhere in the world, but something as minor as *that* wasn't about to stop the CDC from completely freaking out over this very scary germ.

The flu shot that year, *which was never field-tested*, ended up paralyzing 565 infants with Guillain-Barré syndrome (GBS) and at least 25 people died. (Some authors give higher numbers including Janine Roberts who reports 52 deaths.[28] Mike Wallace of CBS's *60 Minutes* reported on November 4, 1979 that there had been 300 alleged deaths from the vaccine and 4,000 cases of GBS.[29] Many of these cases were apparently dismissed by the Justice Department as not having indisputable claims to having been caused by the vaccine.) Hundreds more suffered from other serious side effects. As Dr. Mercola reports, "Even healthy twenty-year-olds ended up as paraplegics in wheelchairs." [30] In the end, there was not a single case of swine flu outside of Fort Dix reported as being passed from person-to-person and no one else died from the flu itself. It was later discovered that the recruit this whole campaign was based upon died as a result of a forced march he participated in while sick rather than the flu. Oops!

The lawsuits resulting from the swine flu shot totaled $1.3 billion[31] (*60 Minutes* reported 3.5 billion[32]). The government eventually paid out more than $400 million in damages when it was proven that *they knew the shot was dangerous beforehand.* J. Anthony Morris, a top research scientist at the FDA's Division of Biologic Standards (the agency in charge of vaccine safety), was fired just before the vaccine was released for trying to warn the public that there was really no evidence that there was a swine flu epidemic coming and that the vaccine had dangerous side effects.[33] Dr. Michael Hattwick, director of the surveillance team for the swine flu program at the CDC also reported complications associated with the shot to his superiors. In particular, he noted neurological disorders as potential problems. These warnings were ignored.[34]

"There is no evidence that any influenza vaccine thus far developed is effective in preventing or mitigating any attack of influenza. The producers of these vaccines know that they are worthless, but they go on selling them anyway."

—J. Anthony Morris, former chief vaccine control officer of the FDA.

Today, there are probably hundreds of cases of GBS that occur every year just after the flu shots are given out, most of which go unreported. Most of these cases are mild and self-limiting, but some are permanently crippling. A bad case can cause permanent nerve damage, including severe weakness, pain, paralysis, or even death. Guillain-Barré is *remarkably* similar to what *used* to be called polio (but which is now given names like acute flaccid paralysis because, *remember*, the polio vaccine wiped out polio).

Research published in the December 17, 1998 issue of the *New England Journal of Medicine* showed a 70 percent increase in Guillain-Barré paralysis in people who had received the flu shot.[35] According to the CDC's website, on average, one to two persons in a million gets Guillain-Barré from the flu shot,[36] though some years (like 1976) are worse than others and some flu shot manufacturers are apparently worse than others. Remember though, it has been estimated that only one to 10 percent of the adverse reactions to vaccines ever get reported. If we take the more conservative estimate of 10 percent, this would make your chances of contracting GBS more like one or two in 100,000.

It is now thought that Franklin D. Roosevelt's paralysis, long attributed to polio, was actually caused by Guillain-Barré syndrome.[37]

Perhaps all this post-vaccine Guillain-Barré has something to do with the fact that the flu shot (just like other vaccines) contains toxic chemicals like formaldehyde, aluminum, polyethylene glycol, and 25 mcg/dose of mercury. Hmm. Remember that wacky theory about polio being caused by heavy metal toxins and formaldehyde?

Hugh Fudenburg, M.D., a leading immunogeneticist who has published at least 850 peer-reviewed articles, has said, "If an individual had five consecutive flu shots between 1970 and 1980 [the years studied], their chances of [contracting] Alzheimer's Disease was 10 times greater than for those getting zero, one, or two shots." [38]

Even though the Environmental Protection Agency and the Food and Drug Administration recommended removing thimerosal from children's vaccines in 1999 and the Institute of Medicine recommended removing thimerosal from all vaccines and over-the-counter drugs in 2001, as of this writing (2010), some flu shots still contain the full dose of mercury. Flulaval, for example, contains 25 mcg of mercury per dose. Fluarix contains "trace amounts" of mercury, plus formaldehyde and polysorbate 80. Each of these shots is produced by Glaxosmithkline and is recommended for those 18 years and older. Each was studied *for a total of three days* following vaccination and has not been studied for whether or not it causes cancer or birth defects or whether or not it's safe to take while nursing.[39] Sanofi Pasteur has a single-dose mercury-free shot called Fluzone, which is recommended to anyone over six months of age. But be warned: This shot *does* contain formaldehyde and polyethylene glycol p-isooctylphenyl ether. Also, the *multi-dose* version of Fluzone *does* contain 25 mcg of mercury,[40] so ask your doctor for the single-dose version if you decide to take this shot or allow your child to be vaccinated. The American Academy of Pediatrics' website, however, still encourages parents not to worry about the thimerosal content of the flu shot and just take whatever their doctor has on hand. They even brashly state that "this includes high-risk children with underlying central nervous system disorders." [41] The nasal-spray flu vaccine (FluMist) does *not* contain mercury. Instead, *it* contains weakened live flu viruses. (It also contains sucrose, monosodium glutamate (MSG), and the antibiotic Gentamicin.) FluMist is also contraindicated in patients with asthma, one of the population subsets most at risk for the flu. The nasal-spray is also not recommended for those under two or over 49 years of age. The clinical study on FluMist lasted *10 days*.[42]

So the question is, are you willing to gamble with your life and limbs for a zero to 30 percent chance that you *might* avoid the flu? Do you really want to have toxic chemicals and heavy metals injected into your bloodstream every year, increasing your chances of getting Alzheimer's disease, paralysis, or even death, especially when the statistics show that the shots do not decrease mortality from the flu? Talk about a no-brainer.

The Solution

While I'm sure there are exceptions, the vast majority of those who are affected by germs (colds, flu, *e-coli*, SARS, bird flu, swine flu, West Nile virus, etc.) are affected because of a compromised immune system. These people eat low quality foods, don't exercise, live with constant stress, assume that every bug that comes down the pike is going to get them, and take every vaccine that's offered. Then when their self-fulfilling prophecy comes to pass, they run to the doctor for more drugs. These hapless victims are caught in the wheels of a massive propaganda machine designed to sell them chemicals, and, thereby, keep them sick and reliant on the machine. If you are one of these people, you *must* get out.

Your escape starts with understanding the machine you've unwittingly become a part of. By this point in the book, you should have a good working knowledge of that machine. The next step is to wean yourself off of drugs, taking only the ones you absolutely need to live, with the goal of not needing *those* as soon as possible.

Next, you *must* start eating properly. This means eating food the way nature intended it—in other words: organic, free-range, and little or no processing, pasteurizing, or preserving. The vegetables should be raw or lightly steamed. If you can get food that's locally grown, or better yet, grown by you, by all means do it. A good rule of thumb is, you want to primarily shop the *perimeter* of the grocery store, avoiding going down the aisles as much as possible. The perimeter is usually where the "real food" is. The aisles are where all the boxed, preserved, processed, junk food resides.

Instead of getting the flu shot, work on enhancing your immune system naturally. You can take echinacea all winter long if you're prone to the flu, despite what you may have heard. (Statements that say echinacea should only be taken for 15 days at a time were born out of a mistranslation of German research on the herb.) Echinacea *does* need to be balanced with real whole vitamin C complex (not just ascorbic acid) to be effective, however. (Standard Process has two great supplements with this combination: Cataplex AC, which also contains vitamin A, and Echinacea C.)

Vitamin D (the sunshine vitamin) has also been shown to help prevent the flu. The cholesterol in our skin converts the sun's ultraviolet rays into vitamin D, which is really a hormone. Vitamin D helps us absorb calcium from our food, thus raising our blood calcium levels. Calcium buffers our blood, keeping our pH neutral to slightly alkaline. Without this buffering effect of calcium, especially when we're eating more sugar, our blood can become acidic, which creates a friendly environment for germs. Since there are fewer hours of sun and less exposed skin in the winter, this may very well help to explain why there's more flu in the winter. So, going to a safe tanning salon and staying away from sugar in the winter can bolster your immune system and help prevent the flu. Cataplex D (a natural, absorbable, food-based form of vitamin D) from Standard Process may also help.

Many studies have shown that spinal adjustments help improve immune system function. (For a list of 109 references on spinal manipulation strengthening immunity, check out the World Chiropractic Alliance website.[43]) In the early 1990s, a series of studies was performed by Patricia Brennan, Ph.D., et al. at the National University of Health Sciences (then called the National College of Chiropractic). Dr. Brennan and her cohorts analyzed the white blood cell response of patients following either a spinal adjustment or a "sham" adjustment (these being the control group). (I'm honored to say that I took part in one of these experiments while in chiropractic college.) The results of these studies indicated that an adjustment to either the thoracic or lumbar spine "primes" at least three of the five types of white blood cells (neutrophils, monocytes, and lymphocytes) for battle.[44, 45, 46] When these white blood cells are primed and circulating, germs can't get a foothold in the body. This is natural immunity at its best.

The Great Flu Pandemic of 1918 is estimated to have killed 25–40 million people worldwide, and about half a million in the United States. That year, Palmer College of Chiropractic ran a study on the flu. In 1919, they published *The Flu and You*, which showed their results. Patients who received *medical* care for the flu that year died at a rate of one out of 17. Patients who received *osteopathic* care died at a rate of one out of 36. Those who received *chiropractic* care died at a rate of one out of 886.[47] Not a perfect study perhaps, but interesting nonetheless.

A more recent study at Florida Atlantic University showed patients who were under chiropractic care had a 15 percent lower incidence of the flu than those not under chiropractic care.[48] Although prevention is difficult to prove, I have had *many* patients tell me that while under chiropractic care, they and their kids get sick less often.

The above are some specific steps to help you prevent colds and flus, but don't wait until late October before implementing them. The ideal solution is to live a healthy lifestyle all year long. With this in mind, I've come up with 20 different steps one can take to help return the body and all its systems, including the immune system, to perfect health. I call these, The 20 Steps to Perfect Health™. Some of the steps are meant to be done continuously, while others may only need to be done occasionally. Depending on how sick you are, you may need to do all of the steps or you may be able to skip certain ones. I suggest ranking all 20 of them in the order of importance for *you*, then start working your way through the list. By following these steps, you will make yourself practically impervious to whatever the next wave of germs may be, as well as cancer, heart disease, diabetes, stroke, etc.

All of these steps will be explained fully throughout the *Why We're Sick*™ series, so if you don't understand the rationale for a certain step right now, rest assured that it will be covered later in this series. In fact, if one simply wanted to be healthy without understanding why, s/he could just follow all these steps and do very well. So, here are the concrete steps you can take to help you improve your health right now.

The 20 Steps to Perfect Health™ Checklist

☐ 1. Eat a Natural Foods Diet of Meat, Fish, Eggs, Nuts, Seeds, Vegetables, and Fruit
    ☐ The pHIL Up & Slim Down Diet™
☐ 2. Take Whole Food Supplements—Need Determined By:
    ☐ Nutrition Response Testing/Applied Kinesiology
    ☐ Hair Analysis
    ☐ Symptom Survey
☐ 3. Wean Yourself Off All Non-Essential Prescription & Non-prescription Drugs
    ☐ Have Your Doctor Help You with This
☐ 4. Take a Good Essential Fatty Acid Supplement Daily
    ☐ Flax Seed Oil (1–2 TBSP/day)
    ☐ Olive Oil (Good for Cooking)
    ☐ Fish Oil, Borage Oil, Coconut Oil, Macadamia Nut Oil, Black Currant Seed Oil, Evening Primrose Oil, etc.
☐ 5. Hydrate Your Body Daily
    ☐ Drink ½ Your Body Weight in Ounces of High Quality Water Daily
    ☐ Minimize Alcohol and Caffeine
☐ 6. Avoid Toxins
    ☐ Air Filter (If Necessary)
    ☐ Water Filter (Shower and Drinking Water)
    ☐ Buy Organic, Locally Grown Foods as Much as Possible
    ☐ Use Natural Cleaners, Soaps, Deodorants, Toothpaste, Cosmetics, etc.
    ☐ Don't Smoke or Second Hand Smoke
    ☐ Avoid Processed, Radiated, or Genetically Modified Foods
    ☐ Avoid Trans Fats
    ☐ Don't Drink to Excess

☐   7. Do a Full Body Detoxification 1–2 Times/Year
-      ☐ Detoxification/Purification Program (Supplements/ Herbs, etc.)
-      ☐ Colonics/Coffee Enemas
-      ☐ Gall Bladder Flush
-      ☐ Fasting
-      ☐ Infrared Saunas, Sweating, Skin Brushing
-      ☐ Deep Breathing Exercises

☐   8. Heavy Metal Detoxification
-      ☐ Remove Silver/Mercury Amalgams
-      ☐ Oral Chelation
-      ☐ IV Chelation

☐   9. Remove Pathogenic Organisms
-      ☐ Anti-Fungal (Caprylic Acid, Goldthread, Garlic, Pau d'Arco)
-      ☐ Anti-Bacterial/Anti-Viral (Colloidal Silver, Echinacea)
-      ☐ Anti-Parasitic (Digestive Enzymes, Garlic, Wormwood, Black Walnut)

☐ 10. Re-inoculate Bowel Flora With Probiotics
-      ☐ Acidophilus, Bifidus Supplements
-      ☐ Probiotic Yeasts (Zymex, Lactic Acid Yeast)
-      ☐ Yogurt, Kefir, Sauerkraut & Other Fermented Foods

☐ 11. Correct Biomechanics & Remove Nerve Interference
-      ☐ Chiropractic Adjustments
-      ☐ Orthotics/Heel Lift
-      ☐ Massage/Rolfing/Physical Therapy/Rehab
-      ☐ Good Supportive Bed, Pillows
-      ☐ Good Posture and Ergonomics

☐ 12. Exercise Daily (Stretching/Cardio/Resistance/Breathing)
-      ☐ Yoga/Pilates
-      ☐ Hiking/Walking
-      ☐ Weight Lifting
-      ☐ Swimming, Biking
-      ☐ Rebounder or Vibration Plates
-      ☐ Sports

- [ ] 13. Support Glands/Balance Hormone Levels
  - [ ] Protomorphogens/Glandulars
  - [ ] Bioidentical Hormone Replacement
  - [ ] Get Some Sun (Vitamin D is a Hormone Derived from Sunshine)
- [ ] 14. Balance the Body's Energy Systems
  - [ ] Reconnective Healing
  - [ ] Acupuncture
  - [ ] Cranio Sacral Therapy/Reiki/Polarity
  - [ ] Chakra/Aura Work
  - [ ] Homeopathy
  - [ ] Applied Kinesiology/Muscle Testing/Total Body Modification
- [ ] 15. Electromagnetic Field Protection (Cell Phones, Computers, Microwaves, TV)
  - [ ] Multipolar Magnet
  - [ ] Q Link
  - [ ] Crystals
- [ ] 16. Eliminate All Allergies/Sensitivities
  - [ ] Nambudripad's Allergy Elimination Technique (NAET)
  - [ ] BioSET
  - [ ] Total Body Modification
- [ ] 17. Get Eight Hours of Restful Sleep/Night
  - [ ] Make Sure Your Room is Totally Dark
- [ ] 18. Remove Abnormal Emotional Patterns
  - [ ] Emotional Freedom Technique
  - [ ] Neuro Emotional Technique
  - [ ] Callahan Technique
  - [ ] Total Body Modification/Applied Kinesiology
  - [ ] Inner Child Work/Counseling
- [ ] 19. Replace Undesired Thought Patterns with Desired Patterns
  - [ ] Emotional Freedom Technique
  - [ ] Affirmations/Anchors
  - [ ] Visualization
  - [ ] Goal Setting
  - [ ] Self Help Books/CDs/Seminars

❑ 20. Nurture Your Spirit
- ❑ Commune with Your Creator
- ❑ Meditate/Pray
- ❑ Spend Time Reveling in Nature
- ❑ Make Love
- ❑ Get/Give Lots of Hugs
- ❑ Do the Things You Truly Love to Do
- ❑ Take Vacations
- ❑ Follow Your Passion

By doing all of these things, your body will respond by giving you your health back. The examples given below the steps are not meant to be an all-inclusive list. There are many valuable techniques I've not included here and I encourage you to explore any other natural healthcare options that appeal to you.

Many of the steps will require the guidance or help of a healthcare practitioner. Finding the right person or persons to help you with this may actually be the hardest step in whole the process of getting well. Much of your getting well will be determined by your practitioner's skill and by the products s/he recommends.

I have explored countless supplement companies and tested thousands of products in the clinical setting. My experience has led me to the conclusion that one company stands head and shoulders above all the rest. That company is Standard Process. Standard Process was founded in 1929 by Dr. Royal Lee. Dr. Lee was a dentist and a Renaissance man who studied with the greatest nutritional minds of his day, including Weston A. Price (another dentist). Standard Process has their own organic farm in Palmyra, Wisconsin, where they grow all their own produce under ideal conditions. This produce is then made into whole food concentrates, which are the genuine replacement parts for bodies. They also have a line of herbal products called MediHerb. These products are top-of-the-line herbs as well. Because the results one achieves as a healthcare practitioner are so dependent upon the products one uses, I strongly suggest finding a practitioner who uses Standard Process. (I have no affiliation with Standard Process whatsoever. Like many of my colleagues, I just really like their products because unlike many nutritional supplements, their products actually work.)

Standard Process's website (www.standardprocess.com) has a referral function that will help you to find a practitioner in your area who understands and carries their products. I suggest using this as your starting place, then checking out each practitioner in your area through their website, Yellow page ad, phone calls, or personal consultations. Many doctors who use Standard Process are also chiropractors and many of them use muscle testing. Specific techniques I look for in a nutritional doctor include Nutrition Response Testing, Applied Kinesiology, Contact Reflex Analysis, Electro-acupuncture According to Voll (EAV) (a.k.a., electro-dermal testing), and hair mineral analysis. These techniques will be explained in future books, but all are ways of testing for exactly what nutrients the body needs.

Not only will the doctors/practitioners who use these techniques be able to determine the exact supplements you need to take and coach you on your diet, they can also help guide you through any crisis that *does* come up like a cold, flu, etc. I suggest using a traditional medical doctor only to help you manage your current (hopefully lessening) drug need, for any crisis management or emergency situations, and for certain diagnostic procedures you can't get elsewhere.

Always do the most conservative thing that will handle a problem. If changing your diet will fix something, do that. Don't just start taking the latest drug simply because your doctor offers it. If it takes a supplement or an herb to fix a problem, do *that*. Remember, overkill kills. If you really *must* take an antibiotic, follow the advice given in Chapter 7. And when you hear about the next killer germ on the evening news, don't panic. Remember, it's only dangerous to the people who haven't been giving their bodies and minds what they need. In fact, I suggest every time you hear about *any* bug that's going around, you say to yourself, "I'm immune," and don't give it another thought. By focusing on your immunity rather than the germ, you attract immunity and sustained health into your life.

In short, ignore the thugs, say "no" to the drugs, and for God's sake, focus on the health of your immune system, not on the bugs.

14

Viruses: Message in a Bottle, Or Attack of the Living Dead?

"In my opinion, the greatest error which I have committed has been not allowing sufficient weight to the direct action of the environment, i.e. food, climate, etc., independently of natural selection."

—Charles Darwin

By this point in the book, you've heard a lot of theories that probably don't jibe with what you thought you knew about medicine, healthcare, and the germ theory. But since you're still with me, allow me to reveal one more new idea about germs before we close the book on the topic. The latest research indicates that viruses are not really germs at all, nor do they cause disease (as we've alluded to at several points in this book). They're actually messenger molecules used in intercellular communication, and they're intimately involved with the evolution of life on earth.

As you know by now, viruses are not actually living creatures; they're merely tiny bits of DNA or RNA surrounded by a protein shell called a "capsid." They cannot "reproduce" without the help of a cell. They have no organelles (mitochondria, nucleus, golgi body, etc.). They do not "eat" and, therefore, do not produce or consume energy. They have no sensory or nervous systems and, therefore, lack any intelligence—at least as far as we can tell. They're incredibly tiny, *much* smaller than bacteria. In fact, they're about a billion times smaller than a cell. Amazingly, at less than 200 nanometers in diameter, they're actually shorter than a light wave!

As you've now read, viruses have been implicated in a number of deadly diseases (polio, AIDS, West Nile Virus, cervical cancer, etc.). When the research is viewed with an objective mind, however, we've discovered that these scourges are not caused by viruses at all, but by drugs, pesticides, and other toxins. In other instances, such as in the cases of pellagra and scurvy, viruses have been accused of causing diseases that were later discovered to be nutritional deficiencies. We've also seen leukemia blamed on a virus when it was actually caused by nuclear radiation. We've seen how the government spent billions of dollars in the War on Cancer trying in vain to prove that any or all cancer was caused by a virus. There's evidence that the majority of the deaths from worst "flu" in history may have actually been caused by bacteria. And, of course, we've seen how the body *creates germs,* including viruses, *in response* to illness. In light of all of this, the question that begs to be asked is, do viruses cause any disease at all?

When discussing viruses, most virologists describe them as cunning little creatures with reproductive habits that border on the suicidal. They usually start by saying that a virus "infects" a cell. That is, these tiny, non-living, non-intelligent molecules of foreign genetic material are somehow able to *con* their way through the cell's membrane. (By the way, this membrane *does* have intelligence, including self-protective mechanisms.) They then hijack that cell's "machinery" (use its organelles) and force it to produce more viruses—so many viruses, in fact, that they eventually burst forth, killing the host cell. (Most biologists now feel this bursting out of the cell is inaccurate and probably impossible.) Those viruses then go on to infect other cells in like manner.

This is the basic story of how viruses supposedly operate and cause ill health. And while many people tend to think of modern science as being almost infallible, we must remember that because of the tiny size of viruses, most of this story is based on *indirect* testing methods. Because of this, assumptions have been piled upon assumptions, which have been piled upon other assumptions, until eventually the original assumptions are *assumed* to be fact. When pet theories regarding viruses haven't panned out, magical characteristics have been invented and ascribed to them, whereby they can now cause disease without being present, or be present and not cause disease. Or, they can lie in wait for decades before finally launching their deadly attack. After reading some of these magical theories, it begins to sound like viruses can do whatever virologists *say* they can do, and that, my friends, sounds more like mythology than science. You might as well just say your disease is a curse from God.

As a review, here's a quick rundown of the most common tests used in virology, along with each of their bigger problems: Viral "isolates" are not really isolated viruses at all. Remember the SV40 contamination of poliovirus "isolates" we've been injecting into our kids for several decades now? The PCR test detects bits and pieces of genetic code, which must be compared to a *known, unique* genetic code of whatever you're looking for. The problem is, since no virus has ever been truly isolated (and even if it had, we've only studied a handful of viruses in any depth), we don't know what's unique to *any* virus. Plus, viruses supposedly mutate very rapidly, meaning these codes are constantly in a state of flux. Antibody tests, as we've discussed, are very non-specific, leading to rampant false positives. They don't detect the virus at all, but immune components in the blood, which merely indicate a possible past exposure. And though it's rarely used in virology, the occasional still picture taken through an electron microscope often carries considerable disagreement amongst experts as to what is actually a virus and what is merely cellular debris, artifact, or something called an "exosome," which we will be discussing shortly. The detailed, colored pictures you may have seen of viruses are merely artists' depictions of them. So, the story on viruses is mostly *theory* arrived at through the active imagination and educated guesses of some highly educated germophobes.

Virologists are not only fully indoctrinated (i.e., brainwashed) themselves, they're also completely dependent on everyone else whole-heartedly believing in the germ theory of disease. These scientists, with decidedly invested interests in the topic, quite paradoxically believe and report that a virus is at once an inert, non-living entity, which could have no survival instinct or desire to propagate the species, let alone could it take the initiative to attack a cell or hijack its well-protected DNA; and also that they're a cunning and ruthless foe. (In fact, they make viruses sound a lot like the subject of a bad B movie: *Virus—Attack of the Living Dead*.) We hold these people with their white coats and microscopes in such high regard that we never question their information or their motives. These entities, which we call viruses, are so shrouded in mystery and science that is "over our heads" that most of us have never noticed that the story we've been told simply doesn't make sense. So, kindly allow me to demystify the subject for you a little.

DNA and RNA (even full chains of human DNA) are merely molecules of genetic code—at least, this is our current understanding. (See box below.) They are the blueprints to the building, nothing more. They are not the contractor or the materials, and they're *certainly* not the brains of the operation. Blueprints are passive. They don't make decisions and, therefore, they *cannot* be ruthless (though they *can* be defective). They are tools to be used, or not used (90 percent of our DNA is supposedly unused and has been rather arrogantly labeled "junk DNA") by the cells they inhabit. In other words, *the cell controls and regulates the genes*, not the other way around. This is stated very conclusively in Bruce Lipton's book *The Biology of Belief.* He says that the cell's *membrane* is analogous to its brain. DNA is more like the *gonads* of the cell—that is, its primary function is reproduction. But *it* doesn't decide when it's time to reproduce. So again, viruses are nothing more than very short strands of DNA or RNA wrapped in protein shells.

Bruce Lipton and others have alluded to the idea that DNA, with its double-helix shape, can also act like a radio antenna, picking up on information coming from the brain, other cells, and elsewhere in the universe. Research indicates this DNA-DNA communication happens *instantly*, that is, faster than nerve transmission and even faster than the speed of light, and that distance is not a factor. This discovery could potentially explain the phenomena of synchronicity, which sometimes borders on the telepathic, as well as true psychic abilities. It could also explain distance healing, how praying for someone without their knowledge seems to help, and many other metaphysical phenomena. It's well known, for example, that twins, with their identical DNA, share an inexplicable psychic connection, even when separated at birth and raised thousands of miles apart. It also explains how our thoughts can affect our physiology. This is the basic premise of *The Biology of Belief*—that what we believe affects what genes are, or are *not*, expressed.

> Unlike bacteria, which at the very least eat dead and decaying matter, thus returning it to soil and allowing life to continue on earth, viruses (according to the story we've been told) have no purpose in "life" other than to create more viruses and leave a path of sickness and death in their wake. This seems to me a violation of natural law.

Since viruses cannot reproduce without cells, we must assume that every virus on earth was produced by a cell, including the very first virus. Now, why would a cell, which *does* have intelligence, as well as multiple layers of protective mechanisms, produce something that was harmful or even deadly to it? Some would say that first virus was an accident, a fatal mistake of epic proportions, but what if it wasn't? What if that cell *needed* that virus?

As Janine Roberts says in her book *Fear of the Invisible*, "...cells apparently consider retroviruses [like HIV and HTLV] so harmless that they will trustingly incorporate codes brought by them into their very genomes, into the protected centers of their being." She then states, "Why do we presume that viruses take the initiative when they enter a cell, when viruses are universally recognized to be inert? What if it's the other way around? What if cells actively attract the passing retrovirus because they need the information they carry?" [1] When you think about it, why else would we have virus receptor sites on the membrane of every cell? This is an intriguing thought, is it not? Let us delve a little deeper.

Cells are individual living organisms. A typical cell performs about 100,000 chemical reactions per second. Human beings are made up of about 10 trillion of these cells all working together as a community in cooperation with each other. Every cell has to know what every other cell in our body is doing at every second of the day, not to mention the fact that they are also tracking the motion of our planet, the sun, and the stars. One can't even begin to imagine the complexity of it all.

Our ability to grow, heal, and live is completely dependent on the cooperation and communication between these cells. This means that there must be *lots* of intercellular communication, which there is. One way cells communicate with each other is by sending out thousands of little packets of "information" inside tiny hollow vesicles (called "microvesicles" or "exosomes") along a system of interconnecting microtubules and actin filaments. These exosomes are carried by special molecules (the most studied of these is called "kinesin"), which literally "walk" along these tubules and filaments like tiny little porters, complete with "hands" and "feet" carrying their cargo.

One type of information that's transferred from cell to cell is genetic material, which helps cells to "learn" from one another. Of course, the "original" (DNA) isn't sent; a duplicate, called messenger RNA or mRNA is. (It was described in Chapter 12 how retroviruses are basically identical in structure to mRNA.)

Cells also make molecules called "transposons" and "retrotransposons." These molecular-sized engineers are used to alter our genetic code in response to stressful environmental stimuli. Transposons alter DNA; retrotransposons alter RNA. Thus, transposons and retrotransposons help our cells to evolve. This same process is used by bacteria to become "superbugs" in response to the environmental stressor we call "antibiotics," which, of course, are toxic to them.

Like mRNA, retrotransposons can also bud out of one cell via an exosome and be exported to another cell. Upon arrival, they pass through the cell's membrane, find their way to the nucleus, and enter it. Once inside the nucleus, they "teach" that cell how to evolve, just as the original cell did, by incorporating themselves right into the DNA. (This process can be likened to using a USB flash drive or memory stick to carry bits of coded information between computers. For those of you less technologically oriented, retrotransposons are like tiny little messages in *very* small bottles.)

If you've been paying attention, this process may sound kind of familiar. That's because this is the exact same process a virologist would describe as a retroviral infection. And that's because retrotransposons are precisely what retroviruses *are*. (Though all scientists may not accept this as fact, they would be hard pressed to distinguish one from another.) Scientists from the Department of Biological Chemistry at Johns Hopkins University School of Medicine have said, "[an] intracellular, non-infectious retrotransposon [becomes] a budding, infectious retrovirus merely by appending a retroviral MA domain," in other words, by adding a protein shell. [2, 3] Janine Roberts says, "In summary: retroviruses, like retrotransposons and messenger RNA (mRNA), carry information encoded into double-stranded RNA. They are formed inside cells on membranes. They are then budded out through the cell wall, which on the way through, donates to them their protective coating of proteins. On arrival at another cell, their RNA is passed inside, converted, and incorporated into that cell's library of DNA." [4]

So while the virologist, viewing the world through germ theory glasses, sees a cell being "invaded" by a virus, and that virus then incorporating itself into the DNA of the cell, s/he can be forgiven for the mistake. However, if the "messenger theory" is right, to stop this process with anti-viral or anti-retroviral medication is also to prevent cell-to-cell communication and our very evolution as a species, without even mentioning these drugs' *other* dangers!

In electron micrographs, viruses and retroviruses are indistinguishable from "normal" exosomes. As such, several HIV specialists have now reported in well-respected journals that HIV is "an exosome in every sense of the word." [5, 6, 7, 8, 9] Furthermore, we now know that even healthy cells produce retroviruses. They're called endogenous retroviruses (ERV) and there are thousands of them in the human genome. In fact, they make up a large part of the so-called "junk DNA." [10]

> Shockingly, about 8 percent of the human genome is due to retroviral infection. If we include fragments and derivatives of retroviruses, we can raise the tally to 50 percent! [11]

Interestingly, the way virologists (including Luc Montagnier and Robert Gallo in their infamous HIV experiments) induce cells to make viruses or retroviruses is not to introduce viruses to their culture, but to *expose the cells to toxic chemicals and stress*! And different chemicals produce different viruses.[12] Though this may be new information to you, it's hardly breaking news. The fact that toxins induce normal cells to produce viruses has been known since at least 1928! [13]

Likewise, when cells are sick, injured, or dying, as is caused by chemical toxicity, nutritional deficiency, trauma, radiation, heavy metals, etc., they produce clouds of hundreds of exosomes (viruses?) as a means of communicating this danger and what to do about it with other cells. Immune cells, like T-cells, are naturally a big part of this communication system. (This may be why T-cells are sometimes "infected" with HIV in patients with AIDS.) There are also large numbers of exosomes surrounding tumor cells, which is probably why scientists tried for years to blame retroviruses (like HTLV) for cancer.

Harkening back to Chapter 6 when we discussed pleomorphism and the new germ theory, we said that viruses are produced when cells are stressed, and that stress is usually caused by a lack of proper nutrition, toxins, psychological/emotional stress, radiation, or trauma. Sloan-Kettering Institute for Cancer Research actually stated in 1963 that viruses are formed after cells are exposed to X-ray, ultraviolet light, or certain mutagenic chemicals.[14] Thus, it seems likely that all the diseases we think of as being viral in origin (colds, flus, AIDS, measles, mumps, rubella, polio, smallpox, etc.,) are actually caused by one or more of these stressors and that the viruses that doctors find in association with these diseases are merely the body's way of dealing with the stress. In other words, the viruses are secondary. When the stress becomes *too much* and cells begin to sicken and die, *bacteria* are produced in order to clean up the mess and start the recycling process. These "secondary bacterial infections" are often the justification for giving antibiotics in what are normally considered "viral diseases." When the problem gets even worse, fungi are created leading to systemic yeast overgrowth or candidiasis.

Could viruses cause disease? Perhaps, but the evidence suggests that if they do, they only cause mild forms of rather benign diseases such as colds, the flu, uncomplicated chickenpox, measles, etc. Furthermore, these "infections" generally only happen if the person's immune system has already been compromised by some other factor. When people have *severe* forms of these diseases, it's always because of other factors, such as malnutrition, toxins, stress, radiation, etc. So these "other factors" are much more important than the virus is.

In 1990, The *New York Times* reported on a study conducted in South Africa that found vitamin A supplementation in measles cases reduced the risk of death by half, and the duration of serious complications such as pneumonia and diarrhea by a third.[15] This study led to the World Health Organization distributing vitamin A to those with measles, especially in areas known to be deficient in the vitamin. A 1996 study reported in *Pediatric Nursing* showed that 72 percent of the hospitalized measles cases in America are deficient in vitamin A. The more deficient the patient was, the worse their case of measles.[16]

It's widely accepted that lysine helps prevent or lessen the severity of herpes outbreaks. Vitamin C and zinc have been recommended for colds for ages, and recently vitamin D has been getting similar attention. It's likely the same with other viral diseases and other nutrients as well. So, is it the deficiency or the virus that's the true cause of the disease?

What if viruses/exosomes/retrotransposons are truly our bodies' means of adapting to the increasingly toxic and nutritionally deficient environment that we're creating for ourselves? We know that cells produce viruses/exosomes in response to stress, radiation, toxic chemicals, and nutritional deficiency. We further know that these little bits of genetic code are a means of communicating with other cells. We know that retroviruses enter our DNA and that we currently have thousands of human endogenous retroviruses making up a large portion of our genome. And we know that retrotransposons, which are indistinguishable from retroviruses, help in the evolution of the species by altering our DNA in response to stress.

So here's the theory in a nutshell: Exposure to heavy metals, chemical toxins, drugs, vaccines, radiation, nutritional deficiencies, etc. causes stress on cells. These cells either evolve, sicken, or die. The ones that learn to evolve send out little packets of genetic code to their neighboring cells to "teach" them how to evolve too. These cells then pass the information on to their neighbors and on down the line until the threat ceases or all cells have "learned" how to handle the threat. Immune cells, which circulate freely, help this information to spread through the body more quickly. The body has certain symptoms during these times of stress and forced, rapid evolution. The death, clean-up, and rebuilding of many cells, including millions of white blood cells and bacteria, are prevalent reasons for these symptoms. Scientists see areas of diseased tissue, take a sample, filter out all the cells and bacteria, and are left with these tiny bits of genetic code. They point an accusatory finger at them, name them "viruses" (poisons) and declare them our mortal enemies. Then they spend billions of dollars trying to find ways of killing them (knowing they aren't even alive) or preventing our cells from making more of them—thus slowing the evolutionary process. In an effort to do this, they inject us with more drugs, toxins, heavy metals, and modified viruses, then sit back and wonder why we have all these chronic diseases. When some start to get wise and blame *them* for the diseases, they turn around and blame genetics! Isn't *this* our current healthcare crisis?

As we've alluded to throughout this book, this new germ theory would explain why fast-track homosexuals and IV drug users are frequently "infected" with HIV, despite HIV's innocence in causing AIDS. It would explain why so many people "catch the flu" during times of high stress, poor sanitation, or poor nutrition like we had in 1918. It explains why polio happened around harvest time each year in areas sprayed with chemical/heavy metal pesticides. It explains why chickens who are fed arsenic, hormones and antibiotics as part of their normal diet and who are raised in highly stressful and inhumane conditions get the bird flu, while those raised on free-range farms do not. It explains the outbreak of the 2009 swine flu, which occurred shortly after the huge economic meltdown of the previous year. It explains why people get sick at holiday time and why some (i.e. those who eat right, detoxify, and handle their stress with exercise or meditation) are seemingly immune to germs, even after massive exposure to them. The old germ theory cannot explain *any* of this.

Undoubtedly, more research into this area is needed, but until that happens, I have a suggestion. There's an old Arabic saying that goes, "Trust in Allah, but tie your camel." My personal variation on this is, "Trust in pleomorphism, but wash your hands." This is my advice to you as we close this first book on *Why We're Sick*™.

Good luck and good health.

Epilogue

If you're like most people, once you learn about an injustice or something that is horribly wrong in the world, you want to do something about it, or at least you want *someone* to do something about it. It's not enough that you know and can discuss the healthcare conspiracy fluently with your friends; you want to do something that will actually help to change the situation. Also, if you're like most people, there is a relatively short window in which you're actually motivated enough to do something and after that, life creeps back in. Therefore, I strongly encourage you to go to our website www.HealthIsNatural.com and click on the "Get Involved" tab right *now*, while you're still fired up about this. You'll find all kinds of resources there that will help you to get involved in The Natural Healthcare Revolution.

I urge you to spread the word about this important issue far and wide. Only by making this information universally known and widely accepted will things begin to change, so make sure everyone you know and care about reads this book. If your library doesn't carry it, buy one and donate it to them. Give them out as gifts, blog about it, anything you can do to help get the word out.

The most important people we need to educate on this situation, however, are our nation's politicians. If we're ever going to effectively take on the multi-billion dollar Big Pharma machine, we *must* make sure that every member of the U.S. House of Representatives and Senate is aware of the information contained in this book. For that reason, I am asking you to donate $15.00 toward this issue. For that contribution, we will mail a copy of *Thugs, Drugs and the War On Bugs* to the U.S. representative of your choice. We have ordering information at the back of this book. When you do so, we will mail your representative a book along with a letter from you urging him or her to read the book and then vote in accordance with the principals and philosophy of natural healthcare. If you can't make the $15.00 donation, you can also find this same letter on the website (urging them to buy their own copy), which you can copy and paste into an email and send that to your representatives.

Remember, the pharmaceutical companies have more lobbyists in Washington than there are members of Congress, but they don't have more lobbyists than there are of us. Let your representatives know that you're mad as hell about this and that you demand things get fixed.

We also have many other things on the site that will enhance this book for you. For example, we have things you can download or purchase that will help you incorporate a healthier lifestyle including the diet we recommend, a list of the seven primary causes of disease, and a downloadable version of The 20 Steps To Perfect Health™. One of the best resources we have on there right now is our *Guidelines For Healthy Living* e-book. This is completely free, as is our e-newsletter. By signing up for our e-newsletter, you'll not only learn more about the topics discussed in this and future books, but you'll be the first to know when the next book in the *Why We're Sick*™ series is coming out and any other breaking news in healthcare. Things are always changing at www.HealthIsNatural. com, so check back frequently.

Thanks for your help, and welcome to The Natural Healthcare Revolution!

Appendix A

How Big Business Took Over Medicine

Though he is perhaps best known as an oil magnate, John D. Rockefeller also invested heavily in the pharmaceutical industry. Rockefeller rarely, if ever, invested in something he and perhaps his allies, couldn't take over and control, i.e., monopolize. With that goal in mind, he carefully and patiently went about creating a self-perpetuating system of healthcare—that is, one that creates sickness with one hand and treats it with the other. This ingenious system, once created, would support his pharmaceutical investments forever.

> Interestingly, though he invested heavily in pharmaceuticals, J. D. Rockefeller knew enough about the poisonous effects of drugs not to take them himself. According to Kenny Ausubel, writing in *When Healing Becomes a Crime*, Rockefeller "was a stalwart devotee of homeopathy, shunning medical doctors and refusing to consult anyone but a homeopath well into his robust nineties." [1]

One of the things he did toward this goal was to establish the General Education Board around the turn of the century. The first publication put out by this board described its objective, which was not to improve the level of education, as most thought, but to turn the American public into a docile herd of contented workers with no ambition of upward mobility. Thus began the "dumbing down" of Americans.

He then began donating large sums of money to universities who would then roll over on their backs and allow him to direct things through personally appointed presidents and faculty members. Eventually, Rockefeller and others like him, through these "philanthropic foundations," had essentially created a national system of education with a tightly controlled curriculum.

By controlling what we are taught in school, controlling the media, including newspapers, radio, TV news, and other television content, as well as what is advertised in the media, these filthy rich men control, to a large degree, our entire base of knowledge. This is why the Internet *must* be kept free from such control.

But public education was not the big prize in this game; *medical* education was. So, in 1901, he created the Rockefeller Institute for Medical Research. Meanwhile, Andrew Carnegie also had *his* eyes on medical education (as well as other professions) and had set up the Carnegie Foundation for the Advancement of Teaching. As is true of all international cartelists, Rockefeller and Carnegie often worked together in an effort to further their mutual goals. This was one of those times.

Prior to 1910, medical schools were unregulated and the education received there often left much to be desired. Some schools were still known to have mail order medical degrees and many doctors received marginal training at best. Because of this and the fact that their treatments for disease were often deadly and considerably worse than the disease itself, the medical profession was suffering from a bad reputation, and had been for a very long time. (This was long before the miracle of antibiotics, remember.) There were also too many schools producing too many M.D.s, which was over-saturating the market. This, not to mention the competition they were receiving from natural healthcare practitioners such as homeopaths, osteopaths, naturopaths, herbalists, and chiropractors, was making things very difficult for the medical profession to survive. The result of all of this was that allopathic physicians were starving. According to Harris Coulter, the average allopath in 1900 was only earning about $750 annually. They also suffered the shortest life expectancy of any profession and about 40 physicians committed suicide every year because of poverty or financial insecurity.[2]

The AMA recognized these problems and stated in the *Journal of the American Medical Association* in 1902, "What the medical profession needs is a leader, to take it out of the valley of poverty and humiliation..."[3] They found this leader in Dr. George Henry Simmons, a former homeopath, who eventually became the head of the AMA. Dr. Simmons stated that the two key sources of the profession's woes were the oversupply of doctors and competition from "quackery."[4]

To solve the quackery problem, he offered his opponents a Trojan horse. He opened the doors of the AMA to these "quack sectarians," as he called them, and offered them membership in their elite club. Not sensing the trap, large numbers of homeopaths, osteopaths, and "eclectics" (see box below) joined the AMA in order to gain professional acknowledgment. The result of this, however, was that the lines between the two schools of thought began to blur. Rather than gaining influence, the "sectarians" ended up losing political leverage along with their identity as natural, drugless healers. In other words, the AMA swallowed them whole.

Eclectic medicine was an organized school of herbal medicine that thrived for over a hundred years from around 1827–1939. It was based on early American herbal traditions.

The next thing Simmons did was to design medical standards that strongly favored the allopaths. In 1907, he created the Council on Medical Education, which was to evaluate the education at medical schools throughout the United States and Canada and then make specific recommendations for their improvement. Because the AMA now encompassed these natural healers, however, the homeopathic, osteopathic, and eclectic schools were evaluated right alongside with medical schools.

By 1908, the AMA's council was running into friction (partly due to the fact that they were evaluating their competitors) and also running out of money. At that point, the Carnegie Foundation offered to take the whole project over and the AMA gladly passed the buck on to this seemingly objective body.

The AMA, however, had already done the bulk of the research and they also kept their hand in the pie by sending an AMA official to help direct and guide the project to fruition. Because the illusion of objectivity was more important to the AMA than taking credit, the Carnegie Foundation only invested $10,000 into the project and received full credit.

Carnegie put a man by the name of Abraham Flexner in charge of the operation. In 1910, he released his report entitled *Medical*

Education in the United States and Canada, known popularly as "the Flexner Report." To its credit, this report *did* do much to improve upon the inadequacies of medical education at the time, which served to improve the ailing reputation of medical doctors. This was surely one of the goals of this "philanthropy" because, as was noted earlier, the pharmaceutical industry (and their major investors) could not afford to have their "sales force" (M.D.s) be seen as snake oil salesmen with mail order medical degrees.

The Flexner Report recommended the closing of approximately half of the nation's medical schools, and graduates of those schools were excluded from practicing. But it also recommended the closing of *all* the homeopathic and eclectic schools. As Kenny Ausubel puts it, "in practical terms the report served as a political hatchet to chop away the competition that the AMA had been seeking to eliminate for sixty years." [5]

Knowing who was backing the Flexner Report, it should come as no surprise that one of its key recommendations was the strengthening of courses in pharmacology and also encouraging the addition of research departments at all "qualified" medical schools. Osteopathy survived the culling by adopting these ideas, thus abandoning the anti-drug tenets of its founder. The report also guided the state medical examining boards in setting up their standards. The AMA Council on Medical Education saw it as their duty to enforce the Flexner Report and took on the air of a self-appointed national accrediting agency with all the force of law behind it.

Rockefeller and Carnegie then began to give millions of dollars to the medical schools that were susceptible to their control. By 1936, Rockefeller's General Education Board by itself had donated $91 million to select medical schools. The schools that did not conform to the Flexner Report's recommendations were not given these grants and eventually were closed down or forced out of business. By 1927, the number of medical schools in existence had dropped from 162 to 80, and all 80 of these were now firmly under the AMA's control. But the AMA was already being controlled by the pharmaceutical companies (through advertising in their journals etc.), which were, in turn, controlled by these international cartelists.

During this same time, the 22 homeopathic colleges previously in existence were reduced to seven; and the nine eclectic schools were reduced to one. The last eclectic school closed its doors in 1939. Thus, in less than 30 years, these international cartelists had completely taken control of the medical profession and could now use it as a vast money-making machine. What's more, they had virtually wiped out the competition that the allopaths had been struggling with for decades.

> It's ironic that Rockefeller, a staunch homeopathic believer and user himself, was to a large degree responsible for the closing of all of these homeopathic schools and nearly destroying the profession.

Since 1910, the Rockefeller and Carnegie foundations have invested over $1 billion into the medical schools of America. The primary criterion for receiving this money has always been a willingness to accept a curriculum centered on drug research. This virtually guarantees that medical students learn the "all-for-drugs-and-drugs-for-all" approach to healthcare. It also guarantees the Rockefellers, the Carnegies, and all of their ilk continued profits.

Rockefeller's foundations and others involved in the business of pharmaceuticals have also been a major source of support to the Association of American Medical Colleges. This is the organization that produces the Medical College Admission Test (MCAT) and determines the criteria for selecting medical students. It also helps determine and standardize the medical curriculum and regulates what continuing education courses will be accepted.

The MCAT is one of the requirements to satisfy before applying to medical school. The main focus of this eight-hour exam is to test one's knowledge and problem-solving skills in chemistry, physics, and biology. (Reading for comprehension and writing samples also play a part, but are given much less weight by the medical schools.) The questions on the exam have absolutely nothing to do with ones aptitude for being a good doctor, though they *may* indicate ones aptitude for being a good scientist. Still, only those who do extremely well on this exam and have outstanding GPAs (especially in the sciences) are invited to sit for interviews at medical schools.

The Rockefellers and the other "philanthropic" foundations also control the medical schools' faculty through funds appropriated for fellowships and scholarships for the training of medical instructors. Also, the students of today become the instructors of tomorrow, and instructors are likely to teach what they themselves were taught. Thus, teaching pharmaceutical medicine to the exclusion of all other things becomes a self-perpetuating cycle.

G. Edward Griffin describes the situation nicely in *World Without Cancer*. He says:

And so it has come to pass that the teaching staffs of our medical schools are a special breed. In the selection and training process, emphasis has been put on finding individuals who, because of temperament or special interest, have been attracted by the field of research, and especially by research in pharmacology. This has resulted in loading the staffs of our medical schools with men and women who, by preference and by training, are ideal propagators of the drug-oriented science that has come to dominate American medicine. And the irony of it is that neither they nor their students are even remotely aware that they are products of a selection process geared to hidden commercial objectives.[6]

Finally, just as was done at the public universities, Rockefeller and his cronies hand-selected individuals and placed them on the boards of these medical institutions, extending their pharmaceutical influence even further.

In all of these ways and more, those with vested interests in the ever-increasing sales of pharmaceuticals are controlling the education and the shaping of medical students into medical doctors.

Appendix B

A Comparison of Medical & Chiropractic Education

Here's a comparison of the classroom hours in the basic sciences based on a survey of chiropractic colleges and medical schools: [1]

Subject:	Chiropractic College Hours	Medical School Hours
Anatomy	540	508
Physiology	240	326
Pathology	360	401
Chemistry	165	325
Microbiology	120	114
Diagnosis	630	324
Neurology	320	112
X-ray	360	148
Psychology/Psychiatry	60	144
Obstetrics & Gynecology	60	148
Orthopedics	210	156
TOTAL HOURS	**3,065**	**2,706**

As you can see, Doctors of Chiropractic are very well trained in the basic sciences. In fact, the majority of the training of Doctors of Chiropractic and Doctors of Medicine are identical. (The same can be said for Naturopathic Doctors and Doctors of Osteopathy.)

The minimum undergraduate requirements for both professions are also identical. Both professions require a minimum of 60 credit hours of accredited college courses emphasizing the sciences, to include: biology, chemistry, psychology, and physics. (My alma mater, the National University of Health Sciences, now requires a bachelor's degree to matriculate. This means that their minimum requirements are actually higher than almost every medical school in the country.)

The first two years of medical school and chiropractic college are where the basic sciences are taught. You can see how the two professions compare during years one and two in the chart above. And lest you think the quality or intensity of chiropractic college courses is less than that of medical school, most of the professors teaching the basic sciences at my alma mater were either Ph.D.s, M.D.s, or D.C., Ph.D.s. John Mennell, M.D., (who was mentioned in Chapter 2 for having testified for the chiropractors in the Wilk v. AMA trial), has taught at eight different medical schools and visited dozens more as a guest lecturer. At the time of the Wilk trial, Dr. Mennell was a professor of physical medicine at the University of Connecticut. He visited my alma mater and said that it had the finest department of anatomy he had ever seen.[2]

It isn't really until the last two years of training (out of 8 years total), referred to as the "clinical" years, that chiropractic and medical school begin to differ significantly. At that point, medical students enter a hospital setting and begin doing clerkships in the various specialties. This is where they begin to really learn about pharmacology and surgery. Chiropractic students, on the other hand, begin (or in many cases, continue) intensive training in adjusting techniques, orthopedics, and physiotherapy. They also learn about nutrition, how to take and read X-rays, and they do internships in chiropractic clinics. (Some chiropractic colleges, like the National University of Health Sciences, have relationships with local hospitals, and chiropractic interns actually go on rounds with medical students.)

However, besides the differences between the two schools during the clinical years, there are many things that are the same. Namely, both professions receive hands-on training in diagnostic and physical exam procedures such as pulse, blood pressure, eyes, ears, nose, and throat exams, they learn to perform thorough neurological exams, how to order, read, and interpret blood and urine labs, etc. Although rarely done in practice, chiropractors also learn CPR, to read EKGs, perform blood draws, and do breast, gynecological, and rectal exams. We also learn to read MRIs, CTs, and bone scans. So chiropractors are trained to be able to diagnose a wide variety of healthcare problems.

Both professions require the passing of rigorous National Board exams before graduation and State Board exams before being licensed. Both also require yearly continuing education courses in order to stay current and maintain their licenses. The only other major difference between the two professions' educational processes is that medical doctors are required to go through a residency after graduation and before going into practice in order to learn a specialty. This is not a requirement to practice chiropractic, although some D.C.s do go through a residency and obtain specialties in things like radiology, orthopedics, neurology, or family practice.

In other words, although the two professions have slightly different standards as far as emphasis goes, the overall intensity and length of the training processes for Doctors of Chiropractic and Doctors of Medicine are equal. Again, the same can be said for Doctors of Naturopathy or Doctors of Osteopathy. The truth is, other than philosophy, there is very little difference between a newly graduated chiropractor, allopath, naturopath, or osteopath. All are graduates of accredited doctoral programs and each can perform as a primary care or family practice physician. So regardless of what the Morris Fishbeins of the world may say, there are no shortcuts or "back door" routes to becoming a doctor. There are only differences in philosophy.

My choice to become a Doctor of Chiropractic was based solely on my resonating with the more natural, drugless approach to healthcare. "And," to quote Robert Frost, "that has made all the difference."

Notes

Chapter 1: Genesis of the Medical Monopoly

1. *The Holy Bible, New International Version*, Zondervan Publishing House, 1986, p. 3.
2. Stephen Barrett, M.D. "Quackery, Fraud and 'Alternative' Methods: Important Definitions." www.quackwatch.org.
3. *Reformed Medical Journal*, Vol. I, No. 1, 1832, p. 6; Harris L. Coulter, Ph.D., *Divided Legacy: The Conflict Between Homeopathy and the American Medical Association: Science and Ethics in American Medicine: 1800–1914*, North Atlantic Books, Berkeley, California, 1973, pp. 90–91.
4. D. W. Bates, D. J. Cullen, N. Laird, et al., "Incidence of adverse drug events and potential adverse drug events. Implications for prevention," ADE Prevention Study Group, *Journal of the American Medical Association*, 5 July 1995;274(1):29–34.
5. Richard Smith, "Where is the Wisdom…? The Poverty of Medical Evidence," *British Medical Journal*, 303 (6806), 5 October 1991, pp. 798–799; David Eddy and J. Billings, "The Quality of Medical Evidence and Medical Practice," (Washington: National Leadership Commission on Health Care, 1987).
6. Beverly Rubik, Ph.D., "The Quest of the Frontier Scientist," *Creation* magazine, November/December 1989 issue.
7. Chester A. Wilk, *Medicine, Monopolies, and Malice*, Avery Publishing Group, Garden City Park, New York, 1996, p. 121; Harris L. Coulter, *Divided Legacy: Twentieth-Century Medicine: The Bacteriological Era: A History of the Schism in Medical Thought Volume IV*, North Atlantic Books, Berkeley, California, 1994, pp. 22–3.

Chapter 2: The American Medical Association's War on the Competition

1. *Journal of the American Medical Association*, Vol. XLI, 1903, p. 263, and Vol. XXXIX, 1902, p. 1,061.
2. David Noonan, "Doctors Who Kill Themselves," *Newsweek*, 19 April 2008, www.newsweek.com/id/132887.
3. Eva S. Schernhammer, M.D., D.P.H., and Graham A Colditz, M.D., D.P.H., "Suicide Rates Among Physicians: A Quantitative and Gender Assessment (Meta-Analysis)," *The American Journal of Psychiatry*, 161:2295–2302, December 2004, http://ajp.psychiatryonline.org/cgi/content/full/161/12/2295.
4. Howard Wolinski and Tom Brune, *The Serpent on the Staff*, p. 122, Tarcher/Putnam, 1994.
5. Terry Rondberg, D.C., *Chiropractic First*, pp. 8–9.
6. Ibid.
7. John S. Haller, Jr., *The History of American Homeopathy*.
8. *Journal of the American Medical Association*, Vol. 39, 25 October 1902, p. 1,061.
9. Terry Rondberg, D.C., *Chiropractic First*, pp. 11–12.
10. Morris Fishbein, *The Medical Follies*, New York: Boni & Liveright, 1925, 61.
11. Ibid, 98.
12. Robert B. Throckmorton, legal counsel, Iowa Medical Society, "The Menace of Chiropractic," an outline of remarks given to the North Central Medical Conference, Minneapolis, 11 November 1962, plaintiff's exhibit 172, *Wilk, et al. v. AMA et al.* trial.
13. Howard Wolinski and Tom Brune, *The Serpent on the Staff*, p. 126.
14. Memo from Robert Youngerman to Robert Throckmorton, 24 September 1963, plaintiff's exhibit 173, *Wilk, et al. v. AMA et al.* trial.
15. The Committee on Quackery stated in a memo that "since its formation in 1964 [the Committee] has considered its mission to be, first the containment of chiropractic, and, ultimately, the elimination of chiropractic as a recognized health-care provider."

16. American Medical Association House of Delegates, official policy statement on chiropractic, adopted November 1966, in American Medical Association, *Opinions and Reports of the Judicial Council* (Chicago, IL: American Medical Association, 1971), p. 15. Quoted in William Trever, *In the Public Interest*, p. 56.

17. Howard Wolinski and Tom Brune, *The Serpent on the Staff*, pp. 127, 129.

18. For the whole story, read Chapter 7 in Howard Wolinski and Tom Brune's book *The Serpent on the Staff*, pp. 144–173.

19. Chester A. Wilk, *Medicine, Monopolies, and Malice*, pp. 35–36.

20. Samuel R. Sherman, M.D., member, Health Insurance Benefits Advisory Council, U.S. Department of Health, Education, and Welfare (San Francisco, CA), letter to H. Doyl Taylor, Director, Department of Investigation, American Medical Association (Chicago, IL), 11 March 1968. Also Plaintiff's Exhibit 1414 in *Wilk v. AMA*.

21. William M. Lees, M.D., "Snap, Crackle, and Pop!" *Illinois Medical Journal* 480.2, April 1971, pp. 326–332.

22. Notes taken at the Michigan State Medical Society Chiropractic Workshop, 10 May 1973 (Lansing, Michigan: Michigan State medical Society, 1973), p. 2. Also Plaintiff's Exhibit 1288 in *Wilk v. AMA*.

23. Chester A. Wilk, *Medicine, Monopolies, and Malice*, pp. 38, 50, 90–91.

24. American Medical Association Committee on Quackery, memorandum to the American Medical Association Board of Trustees, 4 January 1971. Quoted in William Trever, *In the Public Interest*, Los Angeles: Scriptures Unlimited, 1972, pp. 4, 29. Also Plaintiff's Exhibit 1338 in *Wilk v AMA*.

25. William Trever, *In the Public Interest*, Los Angeles: Scriptures Unlimited, 1972.

26. Chester A. Wilk, *Chiropractic Speaks out: A Reply to Medical Propaganda, Bigotry and Ignorance*, Park Ridge, IL: Wilk Publishing, 1973.

27. Howard Wolinski and Tom Brune, *The Serpent on the Staff*, pp. 134–35; Chester A. Wilk, *Medicine, Monopolies, and Malice*, p. 70.

28. Ibid., p. 81.

29. Howard Wolinski and Tom Brune, *The Serpent on the Staff*, p. 137.

30. Ibid.

31. Testimony of Dr. Chester A. Wilk in transcript of the proceedings, *Wilk et al. v. AMA et al.*, 21 May 1987, 1014.

32. John McMillan Mennell, M.D., testimony entered as evidence in *Wilk, v. AMA*, 6–7 May 1987. From transcript of proceedings before District Judge Susan Getzendanner, pp. 2,090–2,093.

33. Transcript of the proceedings, *Wilk et al. v. AMA et al.*, 26 May 1987 3132.

34. Transcript of the proceedings, *Wilk et al. v. AMA et al.*, 2 July 1987, 3396.

35. Getzendanner, Memorandum Opinion and Order, 5.

36. Howard Wolinski and Tom Brune, *The Serpent on the Staff*, p. 140.

37. S. Getzendanner, "Permanent injunction order against AMA," *Journal of the American Medical Association*, 1998;259:81–82.

38. Michael Briggs, "Chiropractors' Victory over AMA Ban Is Upheld," *Chicago Sun-Times*, 27 November 1990, p. 6.

39. Settlement figures come from AMA financial statements, Wolinsky, "After 15-Year Fight, AMA Gives OK to Chiropractors," *Chicago Sun-Times*, 9 January 1992, p. 3.

Chapter 3: The Drugging & Brainwashing of America

1. Public Citizen Congress Watch, "2002 Drug Industry Profits: Hefty Pharmaceutical Company Margins Dwarf Other Industries," June 2003, www.citizen.org/documents/Pharma_Report.pdf. The data are drawn mainly from the Fortune 500 lists in *Fortune*, 7 April 2003 and 5 April 2004, and drug company annual reports.

2. U.S. Centers for Medicare & Medicaid Services, Office of the Actuary, National Health Statistics Group, Baltimore, Maryland. Summarized by Cynthia Smith, "Retail Prescription Drug Spending in the National Health Accounts," *Health Affairs*, January–February 2004, 160.

3. Marcia Angell, M.D., *The Truth About the Drug Companies, How They Deceive Us and What to Do About It*, p. 5.

4. Joseph Mercola, D.O., www.mercola.com.

5. Angell, *The Truth About the Drug Companies*, p. 85.

6. Thomas B. Newman and Stephen B. Hulley, "Carcinogenicity of lipid-lowering drugs," *Journal of the American Medical Association*, 275:55–60, 1996.

7. Richard A. Willis, Karl Folkers, J. Lan Tucker, Chun-Qu Ye, Li-Jun Xia and Hiroo Tamagawa, "Lovastatin decreases co-enzyme Q levels in rats," *Proceedings of the National Academy of Sciences*, USA 87:8928–8930, 1990.

8. Angell, *The Truth About the Drug Companies*, p. 86.

9. Ibid, p. 88.

10. Ibid, p. 182.

11. See the FDA website: www.fda.gov/cder/about/smallbiz/patent_term.htm or www.fda. gov/cder/about/smallbiz/generic_exclusivity.htm.

12. Angell, *The Truth About the Drug Companies*, p. 204.

13. Liz Kowalczyk, "Use of Drug Soars Despite Controversy," *Boston Globe*, 25 November 2002, A1; Melody Petersen, "Suit Says Company Promoted Drug in Exam Rooms," *New York Times*, 15 May 2002, C1.

14. Joseph Mercola, D.O., www.mercola.com.

15. Ibid.

16. Susannah Markandya and James Love, "Timeline of Paclitaxel Disputes," 23 August 2001, Consumer Project on Technology, www.cptech.org. Public Citizen Health Research Group's Health Letter, "Taxol: How the NIH Gave Away the Store," August 2003, 12; Peter Landers, "U.S. Recoups Modest Sum on Taxol," *Wall Street Journal*, 9 June 2003, B7; Common Cause, "Prescription for Power: How Brand-Name Drug Companies Prevailed over Consumers in Washington," June 2001, 13, www.commoncause.org; Eliot Marshall, "Universities, NIH Hear the Price Isn't Right on Essential Drugs," *Science*, 27 April 2001, 614, www.sciencemag.org.

17. Angell, *The Truth About the Drug Companies*, p. 119.

18. Ibid, p. 120.

19. Ibid, p. 11.

20. Ibid, p. 48.

21. Families USA, "Profiting from Pain: Where Prescription Drug Dollars Go," July 2002, www.familiesusa.org/site/DocServer/PReport.pdf?docID=249.

22. Angell, *The Truth About the Drug Companies*, p. 219.

23. Public Citizen Congress Watch, "The Other Drug War 2003: Drug Companies Deploy an Army of 675 Lobbyists to Protect Profits," June 2003, www.citizen.org.

24. Sheryl Gay Stolberg and Gardiner Harris, "Industry Fights to Put Imprint on Drug Bill," *New York Times*, 5 September 2003, A1.

25. See the report from Common Cause, "Prescription for Power: How Brand-Name Drug Companies Prevailed over Consumers in Washington," June 2001, www.commoncause.org.

26. Patricia Barry, "Why Drugs Cost Less up North," *AARP Bulletin*, June 2003, 8; also Abigail Zuger, "Rx: Canadian Drugs," *New England Journal of Medicine*, 4 December 2003, 2188, www.nejm.org.

27. Common Cause, "Prescription for Power: How Brand-Name Drug Companies Prevailed over Consumers in Washington," 13 June 2001, www.commoncause.org.

Chapter 4: Big Pharma & the FDA, An Unhealthy Alliance

1. Comments in federal testimony by Elmer M. Nelson, M.D., head of U.S. Food and Drug Administration, Division of Nutrition, *Washington Post*, 26 October 1949.

2. Wolfe, M. M.D., Lichtenstein, D. M.D., and Singh, Gurkirpal, M.D., "Gastrointestinal Toxicity of Non-steroidal Anti-inflammatory Drugs," *The New England Journal of Medicine*, 17 June 1999, Vol. 340, No. 24, pp. 1888–1889; Singh, Gurkirpal, M.D., "Recent Considerations in Non-steroidal Anti-Inflammatory Drug Gastropathy," *American Journal of Medicine*, 27 July 1998, p. 318.

3. Testimony of David J. Graham, M.D., M.P.H., Associate Director for Science and Medicine in FDA's Office of Drug Safety, before a special Congressional Committee regarding Vioxx, 18 November 2004.
4. Joseph Mercola, D.O., www.mercola.com.
5. Testimony of David J. Graham, M.D., M.P.H., Associate Director for Science and Medicine in FDA's Office of Drug Safety, before a special Congressional Committee regarding Vioxx, 18 November 2004.
6. "Drug Advertising Skyrockets," 13 February 2002, p. 1, www.cbsnews.com/stories/2002/03/13/health/main329293.shtml.
7. Testimony of David J. Graham, M.D., M.P.H., Associate Director for Science and Medicine in FDA's Office of Drug Safety, before a special Congressional Committee regarding Vioxx, 18 November 2004.
8. Ibid.
9. Ibid.
10. Marcia Angell, M.D. *The Truth About the Drug Companies, How They Deceive Us and What to Do About It*, Random House, 2004, p. xviii.
11. Congressman Dan Burton, *Congressional Hearing on Autism and Vaccines*, 6 April 2000, U.S. House of Representatives, www.c-span.org.
12. Ibid.
13. Dennis Cauchon, "FDA Advisors Tied to Industry," *USA Today*, 25 September 2000, 1A.
14. *San Francisco Chronicle*, 2 January 1970.
15. Angell, *The Truth About the Drug Companies*, p. 35.
16. David Willman, "FDA Post-Mortem Finds Drug Approval Problems," *Los Angeles Times*, 16 November 2001, A1.
17. Laurence Landow, M.D., "FDA approves drugs even when experts on its advisory panel raise safety questions," *British Medical Journal*, 3 April 1999; 318 (7188): 944.
18. Justin E. Bekelman et al., "Scope and Impact of Financial Conflicts of Interest in Biomedical Research," *Journal of the American Medical Association*, 22–23 January 2003; 289 (4): 454–65.
19. Angell, *The Truth About the Drug Companies*, p. 36.

Chapter 5: Bad Medicine
1. L. L. Leape, "Error in medicine." *Journal of the American Medical Association*, 21 December 1994;272(23):1851–7.
2. T. A. Brennan, L. L Leape, N. M. Laird, et al., "Incidence of adverse events and negligence in hospitalized patients Results of the Harvard Medical Practice Study I," *New England Journal of Medicine*, 7 February 1991;324(6):370–6.
3. Gary Null, Ph.D., Carolyn Dean, M.D., N.D., Martin Feldman, M.D., Debora Rasio, M.D., Dorothy Smith, Ph.D., "Death by Medicine," *Life Extension*, www.lef.org/magazine/mag2004/mar2004_awsi_death_01.html.
4. Jason Lazarou, M.Sc., Bruce H. Pomeranz, M.D., Ph.D., Paul N. Corey, Ph.D., "Incidence of Adverse Drug Reactions in Hospitalized Patients," *Journal of the American Medical Association*, 1998;279:1200–1205.
5. R. A. Weinstein, "Nosocomial Infection Update," *Emerging Infectious Diseases*, 1998 Jul–Sept;4(3):416–20.
6. W. J. Watkins, "The epidemic of medical malpractice," *Gallery*, 1976.
7. Harvard Medical Practice Study Group, "A Measure of Malpractice," Harvard University Press, 1993.
8. J. Ritter, *Chicago Sun Times*, 10 February 1992.
9. D. W. Bates, D. J. Cullen, N. Laird, et al., "Incidence of adverse drug events and potential adverse drug events. Implications for prevention," ADE Prevention Study Group, *Journal of the American Medical Association*, 5 July 1995;274(1):29–34.
10. Jerry H. Gurwitz, M.D., Terry S. Field, D.Sc., Jerry Avorn, M.D., Danny McCormick, M.D., M.P.H., Shailavi Jain, R.Ph., Marie Eckler, R.N., M.S., Marcia Benser, R.N., M.S., Amy C. Edmondson, Ph.D., David W. Bates, M.D., "Incidence and preventability of adverse drug events in nursing homes," *American Journal of Medicine*, 2000;109(2):87–94.

11. Linda T. Kohn, Janet M. Corrigan, Molla S. Donaldson, editors; Committee on Quality of Health Care in America, *To Err is Human: Building a Safer Health System*, Washington, D.C., Institute of Medicine, 1999.

12. C. A. Bond, C. L. Raehl, T. Franke, "Clinical pharmacy services, hospital pharmacy staffing, and medication errors in Unites States hospitals," *Pharmacotherapy*, February 2002;22(2):134–47.

13. K. N. Barker, E. A. Flynn, G. A. Pepper, D. W. Bates, R. L. Mikeal, "Medication errors observed in 36 health care facilities," *Archives of Internal Medicine*, 9 September 2002;162(16):1897–1903.

14. N. M. LaPointe, J. G. Jollis, "Medication errors in hospitalized cardiovascular patients," *Archives of Internal Medicine* 23 June 2003;163(12):1461–6.

15. D. Phillips, N. Christenfeld, L. Glynn, "Increase in U.S. medication-error deaths between 1983 and 1993," *The Lancet*, 351:643–644.

16. Linda T. Kohn, Janet M. Corrigan, Molla S. Donaldson, editors; Committee on Quality of Health Care in America, *To Err is Human: Building a Safer Health System*, Washington, D.C., Institute of Medicine, 1999.

17. C. Zhan, M. Miller, "Excess length of stay, charges, and mortality attributable to medical injuries during hospitalization," *Journal of the American Medical Association*, 8 October 2003;290:1868–1874; also S. N. Weingart, L. I. Lezzoni, "Looking for medical injuries where the light is bright," *Journal of the American Medical Association*, 8 October 2003;290(14):1917–9.

18. Injuries in hospitals pose a significant threat to patients and a substantial increase in health care charges [press release], Rockville, MD: Agency for Healthcare Research and Quality, 7 October 2003.

19. U.S. Congressional House Subcommittee Oversight Investigation, *Cost and Quality of Health Care: Unnecessary Surgery*, Washington, D.C., Government Printing Office; 1976; also L. L. Leape, "Unnecessary surgery," *Health Services Research*, August 1989 ;24(3):351–407.

20. Gary Null, Ph.D., Carolyn Dean, M.D., N.D., Martin Feldman, M.D., Debora Rasio, M.D., Dorothy Smith, Ph.D., "Death by Medicine," *Life Extension*, www.lef.org/magazine/ mag2004/mar2004_awsi_death_01.html, p. 14.

21. W. J. Watkins, Consumer Watch, *Reserve*, July/August 1976.

22. L. L. Leape, "Unnecessary Surgery," *Health Services Research*, August 1989;24(3):351–407.

23. M. R. Chassin, J. Kosecoff, R. E. Park, et al., "Does inappropriate use explain geographic variations in the use of health care services? A study of three procedures," *Journal of the American Medical Association*, 13 November 1987;258(18):2533–7.

24. *Understanding Acute Low Back Problems*, Consumer Version, Clinical Practice Guideline Number 14, AHCPR Publication No. 95-0644 (Rockville MD: Agency for Health Care Policy and Research, Public Health Service, U.S. Department of Health and Human Services, December 1994).

25. Julian Whitaker, M.D., Special report, *Health and Healing*, p. 11.

26. J. W. Gofman, *Radiation from Medical Procedures in the Pathogenesis of Cancer and Ischemic Heart Disease: Dose-Response Studies with Physicians per 100,000 Population*, San Francisco, CA: CNR Books; 1999.

27. J. W. Gofman, *Preventing Breast Cancer: The Story of a Major, Proven, Preventable Cause of This Disease*, 2nd ed. San Francisco, CA: CNR Books; 1996.

28. Gary Null, Ph.D., Carolyn Dean, M.D., N.D., Martin Feldman, M.D., Debora Rasio, M.D., Dorothy Smith, Ph.D., "Death by Medicine," *Life Extension*, www.lef.org/magazine/ mag2004/mar2004_awsi_death_01.html, p. 16.

29. Russ Kick, 50 *Things You're Not Supposed to Know*, The Disinformation Company Ltd., New York, NY, 2003, p. 84.

30. Gary Null, Ph.D., Carolyn Dean, M.D., N.D., Martin Feldman, M.D., Debora Rasio, M.D., Dorothy Smith, Ph.D., "Death by Medicine," *Life Extension*, www.lef.org/magazine/ mag2004/mar2004_awsi_death_01.html.

31. L. L. Leape, "Error in medicine," *Journal of the American Medical Association,* 21 December 1994;272(23):1851–7; H. Wald, K. G. Shojania, Incident reporting. In: K. G. Shojania, B. W. Duncan, K. M. McDonald, et al., editors; *Making Health Care Safer: A Critical Analysis of Patient Safety Practices.* Rockville, MD: Agency for Healthcare Research and Quality; 2001: Chap 4; Evidence Report/Technology Assessment No. 43. AHRQ publication 01-E058; C. Vincent, N. Stanhope, M. Crowley-Murphy, "Reasons for not reporting adverse incidents: an empirical study," *Journal of Evaluation in Clinical Practice,* February 1999;5(1):13–21.

32. C. Vincent, N. Stanhope, M. Crowley-Murphy, "Reasons for not reporting adverse incidents: an empirical study," *Journal of Evaluation in Clinical Practice,* February 1999;5(1):13–21; Kolata G., New York Times News Service, "Who cares when our drugs fail?" *San Diego Union-Tribune,* 15 October 1997: E-1,5.

33. M. J. Grinfeld, "The debate over medical error reporting," *Psychiatric Times,* April 2000.

34. J. G. Dickinson, "FDA seeks to double effort on confusing drug names," *Dickinson's FDA Review,* March 2000;7(3):13–4.

35. J. S. Cohen, *Overdose: The Case Against the Drug Companies,* New York, NY: Tarcher-Putnam; 2001.

36. D. W. Bates, "Drugs and adverse drug reactions: how worried should we be?" *Journal of the American Medical Association,* 15 April 1998,279(15):1216–7.

Chapter 6: A New Germ Theory

1. Joseph Mercola, "100 Trillion Bacteria in Your Gut: Learn How to Keep the Good Kind There," www.Mercola.com.

2. Wikipedia, article on Abiogenesis.

3. Wikipedia, article on Prions.

4. Christopher Bird, *The Persecution and Trial of Gaston Naessens,* p. 5.

5. Ibid. p. 8.

6. Ibid. p. 14–15; also Ralph Moss, *The Cancer Chronicles* #24 & 25, December 1994, "Two Odd Experiments," www.ralphmoss.com.

7. Ibid. p. 12.

8. Barry Lynes, *The Cancer Cure That Worked.*

9. Antoine Béchamp, *The Blood and its Third Element,* p. 223.

10. Wikipedia, article on Pleomorphism.

Chapter 7: Antibiotics & the Yeast Connection

1. M. Mellon et al., *Hogging It!: Estimates of Antimicrobial Abuse in Livestock,* (2002) 1st ed. Cambridge, MA: Union of Concerned Scientists.

2. P. Little, et al., "Open Randomized Trial of Prescribing Strategies in Managing Sore Throat," *British Medical Journal,* 8 March1997; 314 (7082): 722–7.

3. H. C. Bucher, et al., "Effect of amoxicillin-clavulanate in clinically diagnosed acute rhinosinusitis: a placebo-controlled, double-blind, randomized trial in general practice," *Archives of Internal Medicine,* 11–25 August 2003;163(15):1793–8.

4. "Sinus Bug Antibiotics 'No Good,'" *BBC News,* http://news.bbc.co.uk/go/pr/fr/-/2/hi/health/7294244.stm, 14 March 2008; also, J. Young, et al., "Antibiotics for adults with clinically diagnosed acute rhinosinusitis: a meta-analysis of individual patient data," *Lancet,* 15 March 2008;371(9616):908–14, Review.

5. S. S. Braman, "Chronic cough due to acute bronchitis: ACCP evidence-based clinical practice guidelines," *Chest,* January 2006; 129 (1 Suppl.): 95S–103S.

6. T. G. Phillips, et al., "Calling acute bronchitis a chest cold may improve patient satisfaction with appropriate antibiotic use," *The Journal of the American Board of Family Practice,* Nov–Dec 2005;18(6): 459–63.

7. R. Gonzales, "Uncomplicated acute bronchitis," *Annals of Internal Medicine,* 6 November 2001;135(9):839–40.

8. R. Gonzales, et al., "Principles of appropriate antibiotic use for treatment of uncomplicated acute bronchitis: background," *Annals of Internal Medicine,* 20 March 2001; 134(6):521–9.

9. J. Froom, et al., "Antimicrobials for acute otitis media? A review from the International Primary Care Network," *British Medical Journal*, 12 July 1997, 315: 98–102.
10. L. Culpepper, J. Froom, "Routine antimicrobial treatment of acute otitis media: is it necessary?" *Journal of the American Medical Association*, 26 November 1997; 278: 1643–1645.
11. J. Froom, et al., "Antimicrobials for acute otitis media? A review from the International Primary Care Network," *British Medical Journal*, 12 July 1997, 315: 98–102.
12. J. Froom, et al., "Diagnosis and antibiotic treatment of acute otitis media: a report from the International Primary Care Network," *British Medical Journal*, 3 March 1990, 300(6724): 582–6.
13. T. Lehnert, "Acute otitis media in children. Role of antibiotic therapy," *Canadian Family Physician*, October 1993, 39:2157–62.
14. D. Mackinnon, "The sequel to myringotomy for exudative otitis media," *The Journal of Laryngology and Otology*, August 1971; 85(8):773–94.
15. S. E. Stangerup, M. Tos, "Etiologic role of suppurative otitis media in chronic secretory otitis," *The American Journal of Otology*, March 1985; 6(2):126–31.
16. Media Advisory, Henry Ford Health System, Sept. 30, 2003.
17. Barbara J. Stoll, et al., "Changes in Pathogens Causing Early-Onset Sepsis in Very-Low-Birth-Weight Infants," *New England Journal of Medicine*, 25 July 2002;347(4):240–7.
18. W. Wilson, et al., "Prevention of infective endocarditis: guidelines from the American Heart Association: a guideline from the American Heart Association Rheumatic Fever, Endocarditis and Kawasaki Disease Committee, Council on Cardiovascular Disease in the Young, and the Council on Clinical Cardiology, Council on Cardiovascular Surgery and Anesthesia, and the Quality of Care and Outcomes Research Interdisciplinary Working Group," *Journal of the American Dental Association*, June 2007; 138(6):746; also, *Circulation*, 9 October 2007;116(15):1736–54.
19. Ibid.
20. The World Health Organization's annual report following its 49th annual session in the Palais des Nations, Geneva, 20–25 May 1996.
21. Paul G. H. Wolber, M.D., *Drug Notes*, May 1971.
22. "Stop Squandering Antibiotics," Center for Science in the Public Interest, 28 May 1998.
23. Gary Null, Ph.D., Carolyn Dean, M.D., N.D., Martin Feldman, M.D., Debora Rasio, M.D., Dorothy Smith, Ph.D., "Death by Medicine," *Life Extension*, www.lef.org/magazine/mag2004/mar2004_awsi_death_01.html, p. 2.

Chapter 9: Vaccines: Are They Safe? Do They Work?

1. AAP Immunization Schedule; American Academy of Pediatrics, www.aap.org.
2. J. Drazen, M.D., "Smallpox and Bioterrorism," *New England Journal of Medicine*, 25 April 2002, 346:17, pp. 1,262–3.
3. U.S. National Institutes of Health database on cowpox and smallpox, www.ncbi.nlm.nih.gov.
4. J. Baron, *The Life of Edward Jenner*, Volume 2, London, 1888.
5. Douglas E. Hume, *Béchamp or Pasteur? A Lost Chapter in the History of Biology*, 1929.
6. Edward Jenner, M.D., *An Inquiry into the Causes and Effects of The Variolae Vaccinae*, London, 1798, p. xv.
7. A. R. Wallace, "Vaccination A Delusion – Its Penal Enforcement a Crime," London, 1898.
8. Genevieve Miller, ed., "To Doctor Alexander J. G. Marcet, London, 11 November 1801," *Letters of Edward Jenner and Other Documents Concerning the Early History of Vaccination*, London, England: The Johns Hopkins Press, 1983, p. 13.
9. William White, *The Story of a Great Delusion*, London: E. W. Allen, 1885, p. xvii.
10. Ibid., p. xxxii.
11. S. Frey, et al., "Clinical responses to undiluted and diluted smallpox vaccine," *New England Journal of Medicine*, 25 April 2002, 346:17 p. 1,265.
12. William White, *The Story of a Great Delusion*, London: E. W. Allen, 1885, p. xxxv.
13. Eleanor McBean, *The Poisoned Needle*, Mokelumne Hill, CA: Health Research, 1957, pp. 5–85.

14. Ibid., p. 13.
15. Gary Null, Ph.D., "Vaccines: Are They Really Safe?" Part I, II, III, and IV, www.garynull. com/Documents/vaccines3.
16. Eleanor McBean, *The Poisoned Needle*, Mokelumne Hill, CA: Health Research, 1957, pp. 12–20.
17. Trevor Gunn, *Mass Immunisation: A Point in Question*, England: Cutting Edge Publications, 1992, pp. 14–15.
18. Walter Hadwen, M.D., Verbatim report of an address given at Goddard's Assembly Rooms, Gloucester, England, 25 January 1896.
19. Neil Miller, *Immunization Theory vs. Reality*, p. 28.
20. H. B. Anderson, "The Facts against Compulsory Immunization," Citizens Medical Reference Bureau, New York, 1929.
21. Robert Mendelsohn, M.D., *How to Raise A Healthy Child in Spite of Your Doctor*, Ballantine, New York, 1984, p. 232.
22. H. B. Anderson, "The Facts against Compulsory Immunization," Citizens Medical Reference Bureau, New York, 1929.
23. Tim O'Shea, D.C., *The Sanctity of Human Blood: Vaccination Is Not Immunization*, North Woods, San Jose, CA, p. 25.
24. Burnet & White, *The Natural History of Infectious Disease*, Cambridge U Press, New York, 1972, p. 93.
25. Stephanie Cave, M.D., F.A.A.F.P., *What Your Doctor May Not Tell You about Children's Vaccinations*, p. 162.
26. Janine Roberts, *Fear of the Invisible*, Impact Investigative Media Productions, 2008, p. 46.
27. Ibid., p. 47.
28. John Cooke, *A Treatise on Nervous Diseases*, 1824.
29. Janine Roberts, *Fear of the Invisible*, Impact Investigative Media Productions, 2008, p. 56.
30. C. S. Caverly, *Yale Medical Journal*; 1:1, 1894. Also C.K. Mills, *Boston M & S Journal*, 108: 248–250, 15 March 1883.
31. *Australian Medical Gazette*, 24 August 1897.
32. D. Bodian, *American Journal of Hygiene*, 60, 339, 1934.
33. Janine Roberts, *Fear of the Invisible*, Impact Investigative Media Productions, 2008, p. 58.
34. Albert Sabin, *Journal of the American Medical Association*, June 1948.
35. Janine Roberts, *Fear of the Invisible*, Impact Investigative Media Productions, 2008, p. 58.
36. M. S. Biskind and I. Bieber, "DDT poisoning: A new syndrome with neuropsychiatric manifestations," *American Journal of Psychotherapy*, p. 261, 1949.
37. M. S. Biskind; Statement on clinical intoxication from DDT and other new insecticides, presented before United States House of Representatives to investigate the use of chemicals in food products; *Journal of Insurance Medicine*, May 1951.
38. D. Dresden, "Physiological Investigations into the Action of DDT," G. W. Van Der Wiel & Co., Arnhem, 1949.
39. Dr. Ralph R. Scobey, "The Poison Cause of Poliomyelitis," *Archives of Pediatrics*, vol. 69, p. 172, April 1952.
40. http://www.agius.com/hew/resource/toxicol.htm.
41. M. S. Biskind, Statement on clinical intoxication from DDT and other new insecticides, presented before United States House of Representatives to investigate the use of chemicals in food products, *Journal Of Insurance Medicine*, May 1951.
42. I. S. Eskwith, *American Journal of Diseases of Children*, 81: 684–686, May 1951.
43. F. R. Klenner, *Journal of Southern Medicine and Surgery*, pp. 211–212, July 1949.
44. Janine Roberts, *Fear of the Invisible*, Impact Investigative Media Productions, 2008, p. 61.
45. Ibid.
46. Ibid., p. 62.
47. Ibid., p. 21.
48. Joshua Lederberg, Letter to the Editor, *Science*, October 1967.
49. Janine Roberts, *Fear of the Invisible*, Impact Investigative Media Productions, 2008, p. 25.
50. Bookchin & Schumacker, "The Virus and the Vaccine," *Atlantic Monthly*, February 2000.

51. Stephanie Cave, M.D., F.A.A.F.P., *What Your Doctor May Not Tell You about Children's Vaccinations*, p. 174.
52. Tim O'Shea, D.C., *The Sanctity of Human Blood: Vaccination Is Not Immunization*. North Woods, San Jose, CA, p. 65.
53. Neil Miller, *Immunization Theory vs. Reality*, p. 37, 55.
54. Leonard Horowitz, *Emerging Viruses: AIDS and Ebola*, Tetrahedron, Inc., 1999, p. 493.
55. Stephanie Cave, M.D., F.A.A.F.P., *What Your Doctor May Not Tell You about Children's Vaccinations*, p. 174–75.
56. Ibid.
57. Neil Miller, *Immunization Theory vs. Reality*, p. 37, 55.
58. Stephanie Cave, M.D., F.A.A.F.P., *What Your Doctor May Not Tell You about Children's Vaccinations*, p. 174–75.
59. Ibid.
60. Bernice E. Eddy, "Tumors Produced in Hamsters by SV40," 21 *Fed'n Proc* 930, pp. 930–35, 1962; also, Bernice E. Eddy et al., "Identification of the Oncogenic Substance in Rhesus Monkey Kidney Cell Cultures as Simian Virus 40," 17 *Virology*, pp. 65–75, 1962.
61. Edward Shorter, Ph.D., *The Health Century*, Doubleday, New York, 1987, p. 67.
62. Second International Conference on Live Poliovirus Vaccines, Pan American Health Organization and the World Health Organization, Washington, D.C., 6–7 June 1960, pp. 79–85; also, B. H. Sweet and M. R. Hilleman, "The Vacuolating Virus, SV40," *Proceedings of the Society of Experimental Biology and Medicine*, Oct.–Dec. 1960, Vol. 105, pp. 420–427.
63. Janine Roberts, *Fear of the Invisible*, Impact Investigative Media Productions, 2008, p. 26.
64. Edward Shorter, Ph.D., *The Health Century*, Doubleday, New York, 1987, p. 67–69; 195–204.
65. Bookchin & Schumacker, *The Virus and the Vaccine*, St. Martins Press, 2004, p. 105.
66. Leonard Horowitz, *Emerging Viruses: AIDS and Ebola*, Tetrahedron, Inc., 1999, p. 486–487.
67. Stephanie Cave, M.D., F.A.A.F.P., *What Your Doctor May Not Tell You about Children's Vaccinations*, p. 172.
68. Ibid.
69. W. S. Kyle, "Simian retroviruses, polio vaccine, and origin of AIDS," *Lancet* 1992;339(8793):600.
70. T. Curtis, "The origin of AIDS: a starling new theory attempts to answer the question 'was it an act of God or an act of man?'" *Rolling Stone*, 19 March, 1992, p. 54.
71. Stephanie Cave, M.D., F.A.A.F.P., *What Your Doctor May Not Tell You about Children's Vaccinations*, p. 173.
72. Neil Miller, *Immunization Theory vs. Reality*, p. 37.
73. Richard de Long, "A possible cause of acquired immune deficiency syndrome (AIDS) and other new diseases," *Med Hypotheses*, 1984;13(4):395.
74. Stephanie Cave, M.D., F.A.A.F.P., *What Your Doctor May Not Tell You about Children's Vaccinations*, p. 166.
75. H. R. Paul, *History of Poliomyelitis*, New Haven, Conn., Yale University Press, 1971, pp. 373–74.
76. Janine Roberts, *Fear of the Invisible*, Impact Investigative Media Productions, 2008, p. 63–64.
77. *New York Times*, 11 May 1956.
78. Janine Roberts, *Fear of the Invisible*, Impact Investigative Media Productions, 2008, p. 64.
79. Walene James, www.vaccinetruth.org/polio_vaccines.htm.
80. *Journal of the American Medical Association*, 25 February 1961.
81. Robert Gallo, *Virus Hunting: AIDS, Cancer, & the Human Retrovirus*, Harper Collins, 1991, pp. 28–29.
82. "Vaccine Safety Committee Proceedings [Transcripts]," *Institutes of Health*, Washington DC: National Academy of Sciences, 11 May 1992, p. 13.
83. Christopher Kent, D.C., F.C.C.I., "Monkey Business," *The Chiropractic Journal*, December 1997, p. 22.
84. Hearings before the Committee on Interstate and Foreign Commerce, House of Rep., 87th Congress, 2nd Session on HR 10541, May 1962, pp. 94–112.

85. Stephanie Cave, M.D., F.A.A.F.P., *What Your Doctor May Not Tell You about Children's Vaccinations*, p. 163.
86. Christopher Kent, D.C., F.C.C.I., "Monkey Business," *The Chiropractic Journal*, December 1997, p. 22.
87. Hearings before the Committee on Interstate and Foreign Commerce, House of Rep., 87th Congress, 2nd Session on HR 10541, May 1962, pp. 94–112.
88. Stephanie Cave, M.D., F.A.A.F.P., *What Your Doctor May Not Tell You about Children's Vaccinations*, p. 163.
89. Janine Roberts, *Fear of the Invisible*, Impact Investigative Media Productions, 2008, p. 66.
90. Ibid.
91. Ibid., p. 67.
92. Stephanie Cave, M.D., F.A.A.F.P., *What Your Doctor May Not Tell You about Children's Vaccinations*, p. 162.
93. P. Strebel et al., "Epidemiology of Poliomyelitis in the U.S.," *Clinical Infec Dis* CDC, February, 1992, p. 568.
94. AAP Immunization Schedule; American Academy of Pediatrics, www.aap.org.
95. Jonas Salk, M.D., quoted in *Science Abstracts*, 4 April 1977.
96. Stephanie Cave, M.D., F.A.A.F.P., *What Your Doctor May Not Tell You about Children's Vaccinations*, pp. 160–161.
97. 2002 *Physicians' Desk Reference*, 56th Edition, p. 809.
98. Albert Sabin, M.D., La Stampa, Torino, Italy, 7 December 1985.
99. C. Christie, et al., "The 1993 epidemic of pertussis in Cincinnati. Resurgence of disease in a highly immunized population of children," *New England Journal of Medicine*, 7 July 1994; 331(1): pp. 16–21.
100. *Physicians' Desk Reference*, 63rd Edition, 2009, p. 1,479.
101. Harris Coulter, Ph.D., Barbara Loe Fisher, *A Shot In The Dark*, Avery Press, 1991, p. 11.
102. http://us.gsk.com/products/assets/us_pediarix.pdf, Website of GlaxoSmithKline.
103. C. Cody, et al., "Adverse Reactions Associated with DPT Immunizations in Infants and Children," *Pediatrics*, 5 November 1981, 68;5: p. 650; Information based on a UCLA-FDA study, "Pertussis Vaccine Project: Rates, Nature and Etiology of Adverse Reactions Associated with DPT Vaccine," Prepared for the Bureau of Biologics, Food and Drug Administration, 18 March 1980.
104. C. P. Howson, C. J. Howe, H. V. Fineberg, "Adverse Effects of Pertussis and Rubella Vaccines," Institute of Medicine, Washington, D.C., National Academy Press, 1991.
105. G. T. Stewart, et al., "Pertussis vaccine and acute neurological disease in children," *British Medical Journal*, 13 June 1968–69.
106. J. M. Fine and L. C. Chen, "Confounding in Studies of Adverse Reactions to Vaccines," *American Journal of Epidemiology*, Vol. 136, No. 2, 1992,: pp. 121–35.
107. *Physicians' Desk Reference*, 63rd Edition, 2009, p. 1482–1483.
108. Michael Odent, et al., "Pertussis Vaccination and Asthma: Is There a Link?" *Journal of the American Medical Association*, August 1994, 272(8): 592–93.
109. M. Alderson, *International Mortality Statistics*, Facts on File, Inc., 1981.
110. R. Mendelsohn, M.D., *How to Raise a Healthy Child in Spite of Your Doctor*, Ballantine New York, 1984, p. 238.
111. Ibid.
112. L. Garrett, *The Coming Plague*, Penguin, 1994, p. 511.
113. *The Arizona Republic*, 26 May 1990.
114. Tim O'Shea, *The Sanctity of Human Blood: Vaccination Is Not Immunization*, Central Horizons, 11th Edition, 2007, p. 91.
115. W. Orenstein, M.D., et al., "Rubella Vaccine and Susceptible Hospital Employees," *Journal of the American Medical Association*, 20 February 1981; 245(7), pp. 711–713.
116. H. Petola, et al., "Hemophilus influenzae type capsular polysaccharide vaccine in children: a double-blind field study of 100,000 vaccinees 3 months to 5 years of age in Finland," *Pediatrics*, Vol. 60, 1977, p. 730.

117. D. Granoff, et al., "Hemophilus influenzae type b disease in children vaccinated with type b polysaccharide vaccine," *New England Journal of Medicine*, 18 December 1988, (315)25 p. 1,584.

118. 2002 *Physicians' Desk Reference*, 56th Edition, p. 2,202.

119. Ibid.

120. Robert Berkow, M.D., Andrew Fletcher, M.D., *The Merck Manual*, Sixteenth Edition, pp. 814–815.

121. A. Bridges, "FDA: Rotavirus Vaccine May Harm Infants," *The Associated Press*, 13 February 2007.

122. D. McNeil "Africa: W.H.O. Approves Rotavirus Vaccine," *New York Times*, 13 February 2007.

123. M. Benjamin, "UPI Investigates: The Vaccine conflict," *United Press International*, Investigations Editor, 21 July 2003.

124. Kalb and Foote, "Necessary Shots?" *Newsweek*, 13 September 1999, p. 75.

125. A. Bridges, "FDA: Rotavirus Vaccine May Harm Infants," *The Associated Press*, 13 February 2007.

126. T. Vesikari, M.D., et al., "Safety and Efficacy of a Pentavalent Human-Bovine Reassortant Rotavirus Vaccine," *New England Journal of Medicine*, 5 January 2006, Vol. 34, p. 23.

127. D. McNeil "Africa: W.H.O. Approves Rotavirus Vaccine," *New York Times*, 13 February 2007.

128. M. Horwin, "Prevnar: A Critical Review of a New Childhood Vaccine," www.jabs.org.uk/forum/topic.asp?TOPIC_ID=75.

129. A. Schuchat, et al., "Bacterial Meningitis in the United States in 1995," *New England Journal of Medicine*, 2 October 1997, Vol. 337, p. 970.

130. *Physicians' Desk Reference*, 56th Edition, 2002, p. 1,874.

131. Ibid.

132. Robert Berkow, M.D., Andrew Fletcher, M.D., *The Merck Manual*, Sixteenth Edition, p. 899–904.

133. *Physicians' Desk Reference*, 56th Edition, 2002, p. 1,545.

134. Ibid.

135. Tim O'Shea, *The Sanctity of Human Blood: Vaccination Is Not Immunization*, Central Horizons, 11th Edition, 2007, p. 104.

136. Robert Berkow, M.D., Andrew Fletcher, M.D., *The Merck Manual*, Sixteenth Edition, pp. 899–904.

137. Stephanie Cave, M.D., F.A.A.F.P., *What Your Doctor May Not Tell You about Children's Vaccinations*, p. 112.

138. Robert Berkow, M.D., Andrew Fletcher, M.D., *The Merck Manual*, Sixteenth Edition, p. 899–904.

139. Stephanie Cave, M.D., F.A.A.F.P., *What Your Doctor May Not Tell You about Children's Vaccinations*, p. 108.

140. Ibid.

141. *Physicians' Desk Reference*, 56th Edition, 2002, p. 2,179.

142. *CDC Prevention Guidelines: A Guide to Action*, 1997.

143. www.cdc.gov/vaccines/pubs/pinkbook/downloads/hepb-508.pdf, p. 19.

144. http://www.merck.com/product/usa/pi_circulars/r/recombivax_hb/recombivax_pi.pdf, p. 7.

145. *Physicians' Desk Reference*, 56th Edition, 2002, p. 2,178.

146. http://www.epa.gov/mercury/reportover.htm.

147. *Physicians' Desk Reference*, 63rd Edition, 2009, Twinrix, p. 1,628; Comvax, p. 1,966; Energix B, p. 1,409; Recombivax HB, p. 2,107.

148. Michael Belkin testimony to Congress, 18 May 1999, http://www.whale.to/vaccines/belkin.html.

149. P. Biron, et al., "Myasthenia gravis after general anesthesia and hepatitis B vaccine," *Archives of Internal Medicine*, December 1988, 148(12), p. 2,685.

150. H. D. Birley, O. P. Arya, "Hepatitis B immunisation and reactive arthritis," *British Medical Journal*, 3 December 1994; 309(6967): 1514.

151. P. A. Fraser, J. D. Wilson, "Reiter's syndrome attributed to hepatitis B immunisation," *British Medical Journal*, 3 December 1994; 309(6967): 1513.
152. P. Tudela, et al., "Systemic lupus erythematosus and vaccination against hepatitis B," *Nephron*, 1992; 62(2): 236.
153. L. Herroelen, et al., "Central-nervous-system demyelination after immunisation with recombinant hepatitis B vaccine," *Lancet*, 18 January1992, 339(8786): pp. 178–9.
154. "Adverse Events Associated with Childhood Vaccines: Evidence Bearing on Causality," Institute of Medicine, 1994.
155. J. Orient, M.D., Statement of the Association of American Physicians & Surgeons to the U.S. House of Representatives, 14 June 1999.
156. "NVIC Hepatitis B Reaction Report," Townsend Letter for Doctors #205/206, p. 148, Aug/Sep 2000, pp. 148–50.
157. *Physicians' Desk Reference*, 61st Edition, 2007, p. 1,984.
158. Ibid.
159. Robert Berkow, M.D., Andrew Fletcher, M.D., *The Merck Manual*, Sixteenth Edition, p. 1,824.
160. L. Smitherman, "Drug firm pushes vaccine mandate: Merck lobbies on HPV," *Baltimore Sun*, 29 January 2007.
161. L. Peterson, "Vaccine order upsets some, but Perry stands firm," *Associated Press*, 6 February 2007.
162. G. Lopes, "Vaccine center issues warning," *The Washington Times*, 3 February 2007.
163. *Physicians' Desk Reference*, 61st Edition, 2007, p. 1,986.
164. G. Lopes, "Vaccine center issues warning," *The Washington Times*, 3 February 2007.
165. http://www.cbsnews.com/htdocs/NVICGardasilvsMenactraVAERS ReportFeb2009.pdf.

Chapter 10: Autism: How Incompetence, Greed & the Fear of Germs Led to the Biggest Healthcare Cover-up in History

1. M. King, P. Bearman, "Diagnostic change and the increased prevalence of autism," *International Journal of Epidemiology*, 2009 October; 38(5), pp. 1,224–34.
2. Centers for Disease Control and Prevention, "Prevalence of autism spectrum disorders—autism and developmental disabilities monitoring network, 14 sites, United States, 2002," *Morbidity and Mortality Weekly Report Surveillance Summaries*, 9 February 2007, 56(1), pp. 12–28.
3. M. King, P. Bearman, "Diagnostic change and the increased prevalence of autism," *International Journal of Epidemiology*, 2009 October; 38(5): 1224–34.
4. Ibid.
5. http://articles.mercola.com/sites/articles/archive/2009/01/29/what-really-causes-autism.aspx.
6. M. King, P. Bearman, "Diagnostic change and the increased prevalence of autism," *International Journal of Epidemiology*, October 2009; 38(5), pp. 1,224–34.
7. Robert F. Kennedy, Jr., "Deadly Immunity," *Salon.com*, 16 June 2005, http://www.salon.com/news/feature/2005/06/16/thimerosal/index.html.
8. Ibid.
9. E. A. Nelson, R. Y. Gottshall, "Enhanced toxicity for mice of pertussis vaccines when preserved with Merthiolate,"[Merthiolate is Eli Lilly's trade name for thimerosal], *Applied Microbiology*, 1967 May; 15(3): pp. 590–3.
10. http://autismfacts.com/services.php?page_id=177.
11. Ibid.
12. Mukhtarova, "Late After-Effects of The Nervous System Pathology Provoked by The Action of Low Ethyl-Mercuric-Chloride Concentrations," *Gig Tr Prof Zabol*, March 1977, (3), pp. 4–7.
13. http://autismfacts.com/services.php?page_id=177.
14. R. Gosselin, R. Smith, H. Hodge, J. Braddock, *Clinical Toxicology of Commercial Products*, Williams & Wilkins, Copyright 1984.

15. Chervonskaia, Kravchenko, Runova, "Cytotoxic Action of the Chemical Substances Found as Admixtures in Medical Immunobiological Preparations," *Zh Mikrobiol Epidemiol Immunobiol*, December 1988,(12), pp. 85–90.
16. C. Howson, C. Howe, H. Fineberg, Editors, "Adverse Effects of Pertussis and Rubella Vaccines," Institute of Medicine, National Academies Press, Washington, D.C., 1991, http://www.nap.edu/openbook.php?record_id=1815&page=R1.
17. http://autismfacts.com/services.php?page_id=177.
18. FDA advisory, "Mercury in Fish: Cause for Concern?" September 1994.
19. An FDA internal "point paper" for the Maternal Immunization Working Group written by Marion F. Gruber, Ph.D., at the FDA and sent to Drs. Hardegree and Baylor.
20. V. Stejskal, J. Stejskal, "The role of metals in autoimmunity and the link to neuroendocrinology," *Neuro endocrinology Letters*, 1999;20(6): 351–364.
21. http://autismfacts.com/services.php?page_id=177.
22. Ibid.
23. Ibid.
24. Committee on the Toxicological Effects of Methylmercury, Board on Environmental Studies and Toxicology, Commission on Life Sciences, National Research Council, *Toxicological Effects of Methylmercury*, National Academies Press, Washington, D.C., 2000, http://www.nap.edu/openbook.php?record_id=9899&page=R11.
25. William Slikker, Jr., Division of Neurotoxicology, National Center for Toxicological Research/FDA, "Developmental Neurotoxicology of Therapeutics: Survey of Novel Recent Findings," *Neurotoxicology*, 21 (1–2):2000, p. 250, http://www.nomercury.org/science/documents/slikker_abstract.pdf.
26. http://autismfacts.com/services.php?page_id=177.
27. Scientific Review of Vaccine Safety Datalink Information, 7–8 June 2000, Simpsonwood Retreat Center, Norcross, Georgia, http://www.safeminds.org/government-affairs/foia/Simpsonwood_Transcript.pdf.
28. Robert F. Kennedy, Jr., "Deadly Immunity," *Salon.com*, 16 June 2005, http://www.salon.com/news/feature/2005/06/16/thimerosal/index.html.
29. Ibid.
30. Ibid.
31. Kathleen Stratton, Alicia Gable, Marie McCormick (Editors), Institute of Medicine, Immunization Safety Review Committee, Board on Health Promotion and Disease Prevention, *Immunization Safety Review: Thimerosal-Containing Vaccines and Neurodevelopmental Disorders*, National Academy Press, Washington D.C., 2001, p. 4, http://www.nap.edu/openbook.php?record_id=10208&page=4.
32. S. Bernard, A. Enayati, L. Redwood, H. Roger, T. Binstock, "Autism: A Novel Form of Mercury Poisoning," *Medical Hypotheses*, April 2001; 56(4), pp. 462–71.
33. http://autismfacts.com/services.php?page_id=177.
34. Centers for Disease Control and Prevention, "Prevalence of autism spectrum disorders—autism and developmental disabilities monitoring network, 14 sites, United States, 2002," *Morbidity and Mortality Weekly Report Surveillance Summaries*, 9 February 2007 , 56(1), pp. 12–28.
35. F. L. Lorscheider, C. C. W. Leong, N. I. Syed, University of Calgary, Faculty of Medicine, Department of Physiology and Biophysics, "How Mercury Causes Brain Neuron Degeneration," 2001, http://movies.commons.ucalgary.ca/mercury/.
36. *Physicians' Desk Reference*, 57th Edition, 2003.
37. Congressman Dan Burton, Chairman of the Subcommittee on Human Rights and Wellness, Committee on Government Reform, United States House of Representatives, "Mercury in Medicine – Taking Unnecessary Risks," May 2003, http://www.vaccinationnews.com/DailyNews/2003/May/05/MercuryMed5.htm.
38. A. S. Holmes, M. F. Blaxill, B. E. Haley, "Reduced Levels of Mercury in First Baby Haircuts of Autistic Children," *International Journal of Toxicology*, Jul–Aug 2003, 22(4), pp. 277–85.
39. M. Geier, D. Geier, "Thimerosal in Childhood Vaccines, Neurodevelopment Disorders, and Heart Disease in the United States," *Journal of American Physicians and Surgeons*, Vol. 8, No. 1, Spring 2003, p. 9, http://www.jpands.org/vol8no1/geier.pdf.

40. J. Bradstreet, D. Geier, J. Kartzinel, J. Adams, M. Geier, "A Case-Control Study of Mercury Burden in Children with Autistic Spectrum Disorders," *Journal of American Physicians and Surgeons*, Vol. 8, No. 3, Fall 2003.

41. California Environmental Protection Agency, Office of the Environmental health Hazard Assessment, "Response to the Petition of Bayer Corporation For Clarification of the Proposition 65 Listing of 'Mercury and Mercury Compounds' as Chemicals Known to Cause Reproductive Toxicity," February 2004, http://www.nomercury.org/science/documents/OEHHA.pdf.

42. M. Waly, et al., "Activation of Methionine Synthase by Insulin-like Growth Factor-1 and Dopamine: A Target for Neurodevelopmental Toxins and Thimerosal," *Molecular Psychiatry*, April 2004, 9(4), pp. 358–70.

43. S. Havarinasab, et al., "Immunosuppressive and Autoimmune Effects of Thimerosal in Mice," *Toxicology and Applied Pharmacology*, 15 April 2005, 204(2), pp. 109–21.

44. Institute of Medicine, Immunization Safety Review Committee, Board on Health Promotion and Disease Prevention, *Immunization Safety Review: Vaccines and Autism*, National Academy Press, Washington D.C., 14 May 2004, http://www.nap.edu/openbook.php?record_id=10997&page=R1.

45. T. Verstraeten, et al., "Safety of Thimerosal-Containing Vaccines: A Two-Phased Study of Computerized Health Maintenance Organization Databases," *Pediatrics*, Vol. 112, No. 5, November 2003, pp. 1,039–1,048.

46. http://www.iom.edu/~/media/Files/Activity%20Files/PublicHealth/ImmunizationSafety/GeierandGeierslides.ashx.

47. M. Geier, D. Geier, *Epidemiology, Clinical Medicine, Molecular Biology, and Atoms, to Politics: A Review of the Relationship between Thimerosal and Autism*, Institute of Medicine, U.S. National Academy of Sciences, January 2004.

48. "Public Readiness and Emergency Preparedness Act Questions and Answers," http://www.hhs.gov/disasters/emergency/manmadedisasters/bioterorism/medication-vaccine-qa.html.

49. David Kirby, "Government Concedes Vaccine-Autism Case in Federal Court – Now What?" *The Huffington Post*, 5 February 2008, http://www.huffingtonpost.com/david-kirby/government-concedes-vacci_b_88323.html. For the full text: http://www.ageofautism.com/2008/02/full-text-autis.html.

50. Alison Young, "Georgia Girl Helps Link Autism to Vaccines," *Atlanta Journal-Constitution*, 6 March 2008.

51. David Kirby, "The Vaccine-Autism Story: Trust Your Government or Be a Patriot and Get on Google," *The Huffington Post*, 7 March 2008, http://www.huffingtonpost.com/david-kirby/the-vaccineautism-story-t_b_90431.html.

52. Ibid.

53. http://en.wikipedia.org/wiki/Thimerosal.

54. Jim Carrey, "The Judgement on Vaccines Is In???" *The Huffington Post*, 22 April 2009.

55. Tim O'Shea, *The Sanctity of Human Blood*, Central Horizons, 2007.

56. Eli Lilly, Material Safety Data Sheet for Thimerosal, 13 June 1991, http://www.nationalautismassociation.org/pdf/thimerosalmsds.pdf.

57. EMD Chemicals, Inc., Material Safety Data Sheet for Thimerosal, 4 March 2003, http://www.setonresourcecenter.com/msds/emd/docs/wcd00026/wcd026b4.pdf.

58. Harris Coulter, Barbara Loe Fisher, *A Shot in the Dark*, Avery Trade, 1991.

59. Dan Olmsted, "The Age of Autism: The Amish Anomaly," UPI, 18–19 April 2005, http://www.whale.to/vaccine/olmsted.html.

60. A. J. Wakefield, et al., "Ileal-Lymphoid-Nodular Hyperplasia, Non-specific Colitis, and Pervasive Developmental Disorder in Children," *Lancet*, 28 February 1998, 351(9103), pp. 637–41.

61. V. Singh, S. Lin, E. Newell, C. Nelson, "Abnormal Measles-Mumps-Rubella Antibodies and CNS Autoimmunity in Children with Autism," *Journal of Biomedical Science*, July–August 2002, 9(4), pp. 359–64.

62. M. N. Megson, "Is Autism a G-alpha Protein Defect Reversible with Natural Vitamin A?" *Medical Hypotheses*, June 2000, 54(6), pp. 979–83.

Chapter 12: AIDS: Should You Be Worried?

1. N. Hodgkinson, "African AIDS Plague 'a Myth,'" *Sunday Times of London*, 3 October 1993; N. Hodgkinson, "The Plague that Never Was," *Sunday Times of London*, 3 October 1993.
2. Nicholas Regush, *The Virus Within*, Copyright 2000, p. 25.
3. Peter Duesberg, *Inventing the AIDS Virus*, Copyright 1996, pp. 410–11. (Duesberg gives a long list of references to back up this quote.)
4. Edward Hooper, *The River, A Journey to the Source of HIV and AIDS*, Copyright 1999, p. 149.
5. Duesberg, *Inventing the AIDS Virus*, Copyright 1996, p. 52.
6. Regush, *The Virus Within*, Copyright 2000, p. 30.
7. Duesberg, *Inventing the AIDS Virus*, Copyright 1996, p. 190.
8. V. Beral, T. A. Peterman, R. L. Berkelman, H. W. Jaffe, "Kaposi's sarcoma among persons with AIDS: a sexually transmitted infection?" *Lancet*, 20 January 1990, 335(8682), pp. 123–8.
9. Geoffrey Cowley, "Is a new AIDS virus emerging?" *Newsweek*, 27 July 1992; p. 41.
10. Hooper, *The River, A Journey to the Source of HIV and AIDS*, Copyright 1999, p. 150.
11. A. S. Fauci, "CD4+ T-Lymphocytopenia Without HIV Infection—No Lights, No Camera, Just Facts," *New England Journal of Medicine*, 328,1993, pp. 429–443.
12. Hooper, *The River, A Journey to the Source of HIV and AIDS*, Copyright 1999, p. 150.
13. Janine Roberts, *Fear of the Invisible*, Impact Investigative Media Productions, 2008, p. 190.
14. Y. Chang et al., "Identification of Herpesvirus-Like DNA Sequences in AIDS-Associated Kaposi's Sarcoma," *Science*, 1994, 266, 1865–1869; Y. Chang, et al., "Human Herpesvirus-Like Nucleic Acid in Various Forms of Kaposi's Sarcoma," *Lancet*, 1995, 345, 759–761; N. Dupin, et al., "Herpesvirus-Like DNA Sequences in Patients with Mediterranean Kaposi's Sarcoma," *Lancet*, 1995, 345, 761–762; D. Whitby, et al., "Detection of Kaposi's Sarcoma Associated Herpesvirus in Peripheral Blood of HIV-Infected Individuals and Progression to Kaposi's Sarcoma," *Lancet*, 1995, 346, 799–802; A. E. Friedman-Kien, T. A. Peterman, et al., "Kaposi's Sarcoma in HIV-Negative Homosexual Men" (letter), *Lancet*, 1990, 335, 168–169.
15. N. Regush, "AIDS Risk Limited, Studies Suggest," *Montreal Gazette*, 15 August 1987, B1, B4.
16. Benigno Rodriguez, et al., "Predictive Value of Plasma HIV RNA Level on Rate of CD4 T-Cell Decline in Untreated HIV Infection," *Journal of the American Medical Association*, 27 September 2006, Vol. 296., No. 12, pp. 1,498–1,506.
17. J. A. Jacquez, et al., "Role of the Primary Infection in Epidemics of HIV Infection in Gay Cohorts," *Journal of Acquired Immune Deficiency Syndromes*, 7 (1994), pp. 1,169–1,184.; P. H. Duesberg, "AIDS Acquired by Drug Consumption," pp. 201–277.
18. P. H. Duesberg, "AIDS Acquired by Drug Consumption."
19. Ibid.
20. Duesberg, *Inventing the AIDS Virus*, Copyright 1996, p. 180.
21. Duesberg, "AIDS Acquired by Drug Consumption."
22. Ibid.
23. Ibid.
24. Duesberg, *Inventing the AIDS Virus*, Copyright 1996, p. 119.
25. R. Gallo, et al., "Isolation of human T-cell leukemia virus in acquired immune deficiency syndrome (AIDS)," *Science*, 20 May 1983, 220(4599), pp. 865–7.
26. M. Essex, et al., "Antibodies to human T-cell leukemia virus membrane antigens (HTLV-MA) in hemophiliacs," *Science*, 9 September 1983, 221(4615), pp. 1,061–4.
27. J. L. Lauritsen, 1995, NIDA meeting calls for research into the poppers-Kaposi's sarcoma connection; P. H. Duesberg, "AIDS: Virus or Drug Induced," pp. 325–330.
28. E. P. Gelmann, M. Popovic, D. Blayney, H. Masur, G. Sidhu, R. E. Stahl, and R. C. Gallo, "Proviral DNA of a retrovirus, human T-cell leukemia virus, in two patients with AIDS," *Science*, 20 May 1983, Vol. 220. No. 4,599, pp. 862–865.
29. Gallo, et al., "Antibodies reactive with human T-lymphotropic retroviruses (HTLV-III) in the serum of patients with AIDS," *Science*, 4 May 1984, 224(4648), pp. 506–8; Gallo, et al., "Serological analysis of a subgroup of human T-lymphotropic retroviruses (HTLV-III)

associated with AIDS," *Science*, 4 May 1984, 224(4648), pp. 503–5; Gallo, et al., "Frequent detection and isolation of cytopathic retroviruses (HTLV-III) from patients with AIDS and at risk for AIDS," *Science*, 4 May 1984, 224(4648), pp. 500–3; Gallo, et al., "Detection, isolation, and continuous production of cytopathic retroviruses (HTLV-III) from patients with AIDS and pre-AIDS," *Science*, 4 May 1984, 224(4648) pp. 497–500.

30. Duesberg, *Inventing the AIDS Virus*, Copyright 1996, p. 158.

31. John Crewdson, *Science Fictions: A Scientific Mystery, a Massive Cover-up and the Dark Legacy of Robert Gallo*, Back Bay Books, February 2003, p. 515.

32. Stoneburner, Des Jarlais, Benezra, Gorelkin, Sotheran, Friedman, Schultz, Marmor, Mildvan, and Maslansky, "A Larger Spectrum of Severe HIV-I-Related Disease in Intravenous Drug Users in New York City," *Science* 11 November 1988, 242(4880), pp. 916–9.

33. U. Lockemann, F. Wischhusen, K. Puschel, et al., "Vergleich der HIV-I Praevalenz bei Drogentodesfaellen in Deutschland sowie in verschiedenen europaeischen Grosstaedten (Stand: 31.12.1993)," *AIDS-Forschung*, 10, 1995, pp. 253–256.

34. Duesberg, *Inventing the AIDS Virus*, Copyright 1996, p. 286.

35. J. M. Jason, et al., "HTLV-III/LAV antibody and immune status of household contacts and sexual partners of persons with hemophilia," *Journal of the American Medical Association*, 255, pp. 212–215, 1986.

36. H. Prince, "The significance of T lymphocytes in transfusion medicine," *Transfusion Medicine Reviews*, 16, pp. 32–43, 1992.

37. M. A. Fletcher, et al., Transfusion Safety Study Group, "Effect of Age on Human Immunodeficiency Virus Type I—Induced Changes in Lymphocyte Populations Among Persons with Congenital Cloning Disorders," *Blood* 80,pp. 831–840, 1992.

38. S. Schulman "Effects of factor VIII concentrates on the immune system in hemophilic patients," *Annals of Hematology*, 63, pp. 145–151, 1991.

39. J. K. Kreiss, et al., "Nontransmission of T-cell subset abnormalities from hemophiliacs to their spouses," *Journal of the American Medical Association*, 16 March 1984, Vol. 251, No. 11, pp. 1,450–1,454.

40. D. N. Lawrence, et al., "HIV transmission from hemophilic men to their heterosexual partners," *Heterosexual Transmission of AIDS*, pp. 35–53; N. J. Alexander, H. L Gabelnick & J. M. Spieler (eds.), New York, Wiley-Liss, 1990.

41. Cao, Quin, Zhang, Safrit, and Ho, "Virologic and immunologic characterization of long-term survivors of human immunodeficiency virus type 1 infection," *New England Journal of Medicine*, 26 January 1995, 332(4), pp. 201–8.

42. A. Munoz, "Disease Progression 15 Percent of HIV-Infected Men Will Be Long-Term Survivors," *AIDS Weekly (News Report)*, 15 and 29 May 1995: 5–6, 3–4.

43. B. Gavzer, "What We Can Learn from Those Who Survive AIDS," *Parade*, 10 June 1990, pp. 4–7; J. Wells, "We Have to Question the So-Called 'Facts'," *Capital Gay*, 20 August 1993, pp. 14–15; B. Gavzer, "Love Has Helped Keep Me Alive," *Parade*, 16 April 1995, pp. 4–6; R. S. Root-Bernstein, "Five Myths About AIDS that Have Misdirected Research and Treatment," *Genetica*, 95, 1995, pp. 111–132.

44. Duesberg, "The Duesberg-Phenomenon," p. 313.

45. Duesberg, *Inventing the AIDS Virus*, Copyright 1996, p. 349.

46. Ibid., p. 350.

47. *Harrison's Principles of Internal Medicine*, 12th Edition; McGraw Hill, p. 1,404.

48. Duesberg, *Inventing the AIDS Virus*, Copyright 1996, p. 183.

49. Barron H. Lerner, M.D., "'Tough Love' Lessons From a Deadly Epidemic," *New York Times*, 27 June 2006.

50. Ibid.

51. Robert Gallo, *Virus Hunting, AIDS, Cancer & the Human Retroviruses: A Story of Scientific Discovery*, Copyright 1991, p. 279.

52. E. M. Sloand, et al., "HIV testing: State of the Art," *Journal of the American Medical Association*, 27 November 1991, 266 (20), pp. 2861–2866.

53. D. S Burke, et al., "Measurement of the false positive rate in a screening program for human immunodeficiency virus infections," *New England Journal of Medicine*, 13 October 1988, 319(15), pp. 961–4.

54. Duesberg, *Inventing the AIDS Virus*, Copyright 1996, p. 644. (The author cites personal communication with Harold Jaffe in 1993.)

55. R. Weiss, "Provenance of HIV Strains," *Nature*, 31 January 1991, 349 (6308), p. 374.

56. J. Cohen, ""HHS: Gallo guilty of misconduct," *Science*, 8 January 1993, 259 (5092), pp. 168–70.

57. "An Interview with Stephen Davis," *The Chiropractic Journal*, January 2007, p. 34.

58. W. R. MacKenzie, et al., "Multiple false-positive serologic tests for HIV, HTLV-1, and hepatitis C following influenza vaccination, 1991," *Journal of the American Medical Association*, 1992; 268,pp. 1,015–1,017.

59. Duesberg, *Inventing the AIDS Virus*, Copyright 1996, p. 289.

60. http://data.unaids.org/pub/EPISlides/2007/2007_epiupdate_en.pdf.

61. C. Farber, "Out of Africa, Part I," *Spin*, March 1993, pp. 61–63, pp. 86–87.

62. N. Hodgkinson, "African AIDS Plague 'a Myth," *Sunday Times of London*, 3 October 1993; N. Hodgkinson, "The Plague that Never Was," *Sunday Times of London*, 3 October 1993.

63. F. X. Keou, et al., "World Health Organization clinical case definition for AIDS in Africa: an analysis of evaluations," *East African Medical Journal*, October 1992, 69(10) pp. 550–553, http://en.wikipedia.org/wiki/1985_World_Health_Organization_AIDS_surveillance_case_definition.

64. "AIDS and Africa," Meditel, 24 March 1993.

65. http://en.wikipedia.org/wiki/1994_expanded_World_Health_Organization_AIDS_case_definition.

66. Farber, "Out of Africa, Part I," *Spin*, March 1993, pp. 61–63, pp. 86–87.

67. Konotey-Ahulu Fl., "HIV-2 in West Africa," *Lancet*, 11 March 1989, 1(8637), p. 553; Konotey-Ahulu, *What is AIDS?*, p. 119.

Chapter 13: Freedom from Fear: Bird Flu, the Boogie Man & Beyond

1. Dr. Mae-Wan Ho, "Fowl Play in Bird Flu," Institute of Science in Society, 5 May 2006, www.i-sis.org.uk/Fowl-Play-in-Bird-flu.pdf.

2. T. Tiensin, et al., "Highly Pathogenic Avian Influenza H5N1, Thailand, 2004," *Emerging Infectious Disease*, 11, 2005, pp. 1,664–72.

3. M. Alexander Otto, "Bird Flu Threat Not So Grave, CDC Chief Says," *News Tribune*, 15 April 2006, www.thenewstribune.com/health/story/5663764p-5080102c.html.

4. Joseph Mercola, D.O., *The Great Bird Flu Hoax*, Nelson Books, Copyright 2006. p. 10. Personal communication with Dr. Chopra.

5. "Rumsfeld's Growing Stake in Tamiflu," CNN, 31 October 2005, money.cnn.com/2005/10/31/news/newsmakers/fortune_rumsfeld/.

6. Dr. Sherri Tenpenny, *Fowl: Bird Flu, It's Not What You Think*, Sevierville: Insight, 2006.

7. Menno D. de Jong, M.D., et al., "Oseltamivir Resistancce During Treatment of Influenza A (H5N1) Infection," *New England Journal of Medicine*, Vol. 353, No. 25, December 2005, pp. 2,667–72.

8. Q. M. Le, et. al., "Avian Flu: Isolation of Drug-Resistant H5N1 Virus," *Nature*, Vol. 437, No. 7062, October 2005, p. 1,108.

9. R.K. Gupta and J.S. Nguyen-Van-Tam, "Oseltamivir Resistance in Influenza A (H5N1) Infection," *New England Journal of Medicine*, Vol. 354, No. 13, 30 March 2006, pp. 1,423–24.

10. A. Moscona, "Oseltamivir Resistance—Disabling Our Influenza Defenses," *New England Journal of Medicine*, Vol. 353, No. 25, 22 December 2005, pp. 2,633–36.

11. T. Jefferson, et. al., "Anti-virals for Influenza in Healthy Adults: Systemic Review," *Lancet*, Vol. 367, No. 9507, 28 January 2006, pp. 303–13.

12. Sarah Boseley and Jonathan Watts, "Flu Drugs 'Will Not Work' If Pandemic Strikes," *Guardian*, 19 January 2005.

13. "Outbreak! Tamiflu 'Useless' Against Avian Flu," World Net Daily, 4 December 2005, www.worldnetdaily.com/news/article.asp?ARTICLE_ID=47725.

14. R. R. Regoes and S. Bonhoeffer, "Emergence of Drug-Resistant Influenza virus: Population Dynamical Considerations," *Science*, Vol. 312, No. 5772, 21 April 2006, pp. 389–91.

15. "Health Canada Looking at Tamiflu Data after Reports of Deaths in Japan," Canadian Press, 17 November 2005, www.canada.com/health/story.html?id=d155eac6-df71-4639-a222-aee4d88f426c.
16. "FDA Probes Japan Deaths Possibly Linked to Tamiflu," *USA Today*, 17 November 2005.
17. "Paranoia, Bird Flu and the World Health Org," *Maclean's*, 22 May 2006.
18. Michael Gormley, "Toxins Killing Birds," *Associated Press*, 3 June 2001.
19. Peter Doshi, "Are U.S. flu death figures more PR than science?" *British Medical Journal*, 10 December 2005, 331:1412.
20. R. E. Shope, 1936, *Journal of Experimental Medicine*, Vol. 63, pp. 669–684; P. A. Lewis, R. E. Shope, 1931, *Journal of Experimental Medicine*, Vol. 54, pp. 361–371; R. E. Shope, 1931, *Journal of Experimental Medicine*, Vol. 54, pp. 373–385.
21. Ibid.
22. W. E. P. Beyer, et al., "Influenza-epidemie in een verpleeghuis door een virus dat niet in het vaccin was opgenomen," *Nederlands Tijdschrift Voor Geneeskunde*, 1993; 137/39, pp. 1,973–7.
23. L. Altman, "Vaccine is Said to Fail to Protect against Flu Strain," *New York Times*, 15 January 2004.
24. P. Szilagyi, et al., "Influenza Vaccine Effectiveness Among Children 6 to 59 Months of Age During 2 Influenza Seasons," Archives of Pediatric & Adolescent Medicine, October 2008, 162(10), pp. 943–951.
25. T. Jefferson, "Influenza Vaccination: Policy Versus Evidence," *British Medical Journal*, 28 October 2006, 333(7574), pp. 912–5.
26. L. Simonsen, Ph.D., et al., "Mortality benefits of influenza vaccination in elderly people: an ongoing controversy," *The Lancet Infectious Diseases*, October 2007, 7(10), pp. 658–666.
27. http://en.wikipedia.org/wiki/Swine_influenza.
28. Janine Roberts, *Fear of the Invisible*, Impact Investigative Media Productions, 2008, p. 93–4.
29. http://www.wanttoknow.info/health/1976_swine_flu_vaccine_60_minutes_transcript; or http://www.examiner.com/x-6495-US-Intelligence-Examiner~y2009m7d10-CBS-60-Minutes-300-death-claims-from-1976-swine-flu-vaccine-only-one-death-from-flu.
30. Joseph Mercola, D.O., *The Great Bird Flu Hoax*, Nelson Books, Copyright 2006, p. 19.
31. Ibid.
32. http://www.wanttoknow.info/health/1976_swine_flu_vaccine_60_minutes_transcript.
33. H. Coulter, B. L. Fisher, *A Shot In The Dark*, Avery Press, 1991, p. 167.
34. http://www.wanttoknow.info/health/1976_swine_flu_vaccine_60_minutes_transcript.
35. A. H. Ropper, M. Victor, "Influenza Vaccination and the Guillain-Barré syndrome," *New England Journal of Medicine*, 17 December 1998, 339(25), pp. 1,845–6.
36. http://www.cdc.gov/h1n1flu/vaccination/providers_qa.htm; also http://wonder.cdc.gov/wonder/prevguid/m0052500/m0052500.asp.
37. A. S. Goldman, et al., "What was the cause of Franklin Delano Roosevelt's paralytic illness?" *Journal of Medical Biography*, November 2003; 11 (4), pp. 232–40.
38. Hugh Fundenberg, M.D., Founder and Director of Research, NeuroImmuno Therapeutic Research Foundation. Information is from Dr. Fundenberg's speech at the NVIC International Vaccine Conference, Arlington, VA, September 1997.
39. *Physicians' Desk Reference*, 63rd Edition, 2009, Fluarix: pp. 1,446–7; Flulaval: pp. 1,448–9.
40. http://www.fda.gov/downloads/BiologicsBloodVaccines/Vaccines/ApprovedProducts/UCM123704.pdf, p. 11.
41. http://www.cispimmunize.org/ill/Flu/Influenza%20Recommendations.pdf.
42. *Physicians' Desk Reference*, 63rd Edition, 2009, p. 1,945.
43. http://www.worldchiropracticalliance.org/news/immunityreferences.htm.
44. P. Brennan, Ph.D., et al., "Enhanced Phagocytic Cell Respiratory Burst Induced by Spinal Manipulation: Potential Role of Substance P," *Journal of Manipulative and Physiological Therapeutics*, Vol. 14, No. 7, September 1991, pp. 399–408.
45. P. Brennan, Ph.D., et al., "Enhanced Neutrophil Respiratory Burst as a Biological Marker for Manipulation Forces: Duration of the Effect and Association with Substance P and Tumor Necrosis Factor," *Journal of Manipulative and Physiological Therapeutics*, Vol. 15, No. 2, pp. 83–89.

46. P. Brennan, Ph.D., et al., "Lymphocyte Profiles in Patients with Chronic Low Back Pain Enrolled in a Clinical Trial," *Journal of Manipulative and Physiological Therapeutics*, Vol. 17, No. 4, May 1994, pp. 219–227.
47. D. D. Palmer, "The Flu and You," Published by the Palmer College of Chiropractic, 1919.
48. *Men's Health*, June 2005.

Chapter 14: Viruses: Message in a Bottle, Or Attack of the Living Dead?

1. Janine Roberts, *Fear of the Invisible*, Impact Investigative Media Productions, 2008, p. 219.
2. Y. Fang, N. Wu, X. Gan, W. Yan, J. C. Morrell, S. J. Gould, "Higher-order oligomerization targets plasma membrane proteins and HIV gag to exosomes," *PLoS Biology*, June 2007, 5(6):e 158.
3. K. Denzer, M. J. Kleijmeer, H. F. Heijnen, W. Stoorvogel, H. J. Geuze, "Exosome: from internal vesicle of the multivesicular body to intercellular signaling device," *Journal of Cell Science*, October 2000;113 Pt 19, pp. 3,365–74.
4. Janine Roberts, *Fear of the Invisible*, Impact Investigative Media Productions, 2008, p. 226.
5. Frank P. Ryan, "Human endogenous retroviruses in health and disease: a symbiotic perspective," *Journal of the Royal Society of Medicine*, December 2004; 97(12), pp. 560–565.
6. S. J. Gould, J. E. Hildreth, "The Trojan Exosome Hypothesis," *Proceedings of the National Academy of Sciences USA*, 16 September 2003, 100(19), pp. 10,592–7.
7. A. Pelcher-Mathews, G. Raposo, M. Marsh, "Endosomes, exosomes and Trojan Viruses," *Trends in Microbiology*, 12 July 2004, (7), pp. 310–6.
8. W. Wells, "When is a virus an exosome?" *The Journal of Cell Biology*, Vol. 162, No. 6, pp. 960–960.
9. Y. Fang, N. Wu, X. Gan, W. Yan, J. C. Morrell, S. J. Gould, "Higher-order oligomerization targets plasma membrane proteins and HIV gag to exosomes," *PLoS Biology*, June 2007; 5(6):e 158.
10. Arielle R. Rosenberg, Lélia Delamarre, Claudine Pique, Isabelle Le Blanc, Graziella Griffith, and Marie-Christine Dokhélar, "Early Assembly Step of a Retroviral Envelope Glycoprotein: Analysis Using a Dominant Negative Assay," *The Journal of Cell Biology*, 5 April 1999, 145(1) pp. 57–68.
11. Luis P. Villarreal, http://newsarchive.asm.org/oct01/feature1.asp; Based on a presentation at the annual meeting of the American Society for the Advancement of Science, January 2001; See also: http://en.wikipedia.org/wiki/Endogenous_retrovirus.
12. G. Tyrsted, B. Munch-Petersen, "Early effects of phytohemagglutinin on induction of DNA polymerase, thymidine kinase, deoxyribonucleoside triphosphate pools and DNA synthesis in human lymphocytes," *Nucleic Acids Research*, August 1977; 4(8), pp. 2,713–23.
13. A. E. Boycott, "The transition from life to death; the nature of filterable viruses," *Proceedings of the Royal Society of Medicine*, 1928, 22, pp. 55–69.
14. Sloan-Kettering Institute for Cancer Research, "Progress Report XV, Viruses and Cancer," January 1963.
15. "Measles' Risks Found Reduced by Vitamin A" *New York Times*, 22 July 1990, Section 1, p. 23.
16. D. Stephens, P. L. Jackson, Y. Gutierrez, "Subclinical vitamin A deficiency: a potentially unrecognized problem in the United States," *Pediatric Nursing*, Sept–Oct 1996. 22(5). pp. 377–89, p. 456.

Appendix A: How Big Business Took Over Medicine

1. Kenny Ausubel, *When Healing Becomes a Crime*, Healing Arts Press, Rochester, Vermont, 2000, p. 290.
2. Ibid, p. 287. Citing Harris Coulter and the *Journal of the American Medical Association*, Vol. XLI, 1903, p. 263 and Vol. XXXIX, 1902, p. 1,061.
3. F. H. Todd, "Organization," *Journal of the American Medical Association*, 25 October 1902; XXXIX (17), p. 1,061.
4. Kenny Ausubel, *When Healing Becomes a Crime*, Healing Arts Press, Rochester, Vermont, 2000, p. 287.

5. Ibid, p. 288.

6. G. Edward Griffin, *World without Cancer*, American Media, 1996, p. 267.

Appendix B: A Comparison of Medical & Chiropractic Education

1. Terry Rondberg, D.C., *Chiropractic First*, Published by *The Chiropractic Journal*, 1996.

2. Chester A. Wilk, *Medicine, Monopolies, and Malice*, Avery Publishing Group, Garden City Park, New York, 1996, p. 121.

Index

prevention of disease, natural
   methods for, 139–41
"preventive healthcare," as defined
   by Western medicine, 274
Prevnar, 253–54, 267–69
Price, Weston A., 102, 443
Prilosec, 83–84, 90
Primum non nocere, 55
Principiis obsta: sero medicina curator, 55
prions, 159, 161, 165. *See also* microzymas
prisoners, polio vaccine testing on, 232
The Private Science of Louis Pasteur
   (Geison), 146, 171
probiotic supplement, 178–79,
   196, 197, 441
processed foods, 437, 440
profit motive of Big Pharma cartel, 64–65,
   77–78, 117–20, 189, 272–73,
   280–81, 417–18, 422–24
propaganda to suppress natural
   therapies, 19, 21
proteolytic enzymes, for parasite
   infestation, 201
protits, 158. *See also* microzymas
protozoa parasites, 201
Prozac, 84–85
psychic abilities, and DNA
   communication, 451
psychological depression, as
   cause of disease, 163
Public Health Service, and thimerosal
   cover-up, 298–99
Public Readiness and Emergency
   Preparedness Act (PREP), 314–15
pubmed.gov, 187
puerperal sepsis, 35
Pure Food and Drug Act, 101
"pustular eczema," and smallpox
   vaccine cover-up, 216
PutChildrenFirst.org, survey on
   mercury, 316–17

Q
Qi, 44
"quackery," as suppressive label, 19,
   27–29, 51, 65, 463–64
Quadrigen, 253

R
rabbit tissue experiment of Naessens, 162
rabies vaccine, 146
radiation, 112, 133–34, 138

rapid heart rate, as adverse reaction
   to Hib vaccine, 262
rash, as DPT adverse reaction, 254–55
Rasio, Debora, 135
The Rat Theory of Garbage, 167–68
Reagan, Ronald, 382, 423
recombinant DNA in vaccines, 274
Recombivax HB, 272, 275
Reconnective Healing, 442
recreational drugs, as risk factor for
   AIDS, 354–57, 389–90
regulation of drug prices, 97–99
Reich, Wilhelm, 158
Reiter's syndrome, as adverse reaction
   to hepatitis B vaccine, 277
religion
   similarity to organized medicine,
      32–33, 40, 110
   suppressive influence of,
      24–28, 33–37
religious exemption to school
   immunization programs, 337–38
*Remarkable Aloe: Aloe Through the
   Ages* (Danhoff), 112
reproductive toxicity, caused
   by thimerosal, 312
research and development of drugs, as
   excuse for high drug prices, 94–96
research facilities, control by Big Pharma,
   22, 92, 117, 362–63, 466–68
respiratory flora, adverse effect
   of antibiotics on, 182
respiratory tract infections, as DPT
   adverse reaction, 254–55
responsibility for one's own health,
   138–41, 177–79, 334–35
rethinkingaids.com, 385–86, 415
retrotransposons, 453–54
retroviruses, 369, 373–77, 377–85, 452–55
reverse transcriptase, 373–75, 405
Reye's syndrome, and live virus
   vaccines, 239
Rezulin, 119, 138
RFID chips, 427–28
rheumatic heart disease, and antibiotic
   use in dentistry, 184–86
Rh-negative women, RhoGAM shots for,
   295, 307, 310
RhoGAM injections, mercury
   in, 295, 307, 310
Rife, Royal, 61, 154–58, 164, 170–71
The River: A Journey to the Source

silver fillings in teeth, mercury
  in, 310, 323–24
"Simian Retroviruses, Polio Vaccine,
  and the Origin of AIDS," 238
Simian Virus #40 (SV40), as cancer-
  causing virus, 232–39
Simmons, George Henry, 51, 463–64
Sinclair, Upton, 101
sinfulness, as cause of disease, 24–26
Singh, Vijendra, 327
single-celled protozoa, 201
sinusitis, antibiotics ineffective treatment
  for, 179–80, 189, 193
skin brushing, as health strategy, 441
sleep disorders, mercury as cause, 300
Slikker, William, Jr., 300
"slim disease," 410
smallpox vaccine, 79–80, 212–18
Smithburn, K.C., 291
Smith, Dorothy, 135
Smith, Lendon, 198
Smith, Ralph Lee, 67
SMON, 387
"snake oil salesman," as suppressive
  label, 27–28
social anxiety disorder, as disease
  invention, 83–84
socially responsible investments, 124–25
sodium chloride, in vaccines, 211
somatids, 161–66, 190–92. *See
  also* microzymas
Somotoscope of Naessens, 160, 166
Sonnabend, Joseph, 359–60
sorbitol, in vaccines, 211
"Sore Throat," informant on AMA, 69
sore throats, antibiotics ineffective
  treatment for, 179
soy products, as unfit food
  for humans, 344
Spanish Black Radish, 196, 197
Spanish flu pandemic of 1918, 430, 438
speech and language disorders,
  mercury as cause, 300
spinal manipulation, 43–44, 181,
  197, 268, 438–39, 441
spirit-nurturing strategies for health, 443
spirochetes, as parasites, 201
spit test for *Candida* overgrowth,
  193–94, 197
spongiform encephalopathy diseases, 159
spontaneous generation theory, 149
spore stage of pleomorphism, 162

"spurious" smallpox, and smallpox
  vaccine cover-up, 216
Stabenow, Debbie, 307
staff of Hermes, 26
Standard Process natural supplements,
  196, 197, 345, 443–44
statins (cholesterol medications),
  80–83, 87
statistics manipulation, 429–30, 438
Statton, Kathleen, 304
stealth amendments, to protect
  Big Pharma from lawsuits,
  307–8, 314–15
steroids, and *Candida* overgrowth, 195
Still, Andrew, 53, 58, 59
stomach-stapling surgery, as
  unnecessary, 132
"straights" and "mixers," 62
streptomycin, in polio vaccines, 246
stress, as cause of disease, 163
stress reduction, options for, 179
strokes, 104–8, 281–82
Sudafed, 109–10
Sudden Infant Death Syndrome
  (SIDS), as adverse reaction
  to vaccine, 254–55, 267
sugar, 194, 344, 438
suicide rate among medical
  doctors, 9, 39–40, 463
sunshine, as health protocol, 442
superbugs
  and antibiotic use, 175–79, 182, 188
  from vaccine use, 211, 268, 423–24
Surgeon General, and polio
  vaccine cover-up, 236
surgery
  history of, 29–31
  iatrogenic deaths from, 132–34, 138
  as legal cancer treatment, 112, 138
SV40 (Simian Virus #40), as cancer-
  causing virus, 232–39
swine flu debacle of 1976,
  79–80, 432–33, 458
symbiosis and evolution,
  pleomorphism and, 171
symptoms, as body's attempt
  to heal, 47–49
symptom suppression, as basis
  of Western medicine, 45,
  47–48, 80–82, 87, 140
synchronicity, and DNA
  communication, 451

HELP SPREAD THE WORD!

Share your newfound knowledge by sending a copy of *Thugs, Drugs and the War on Bugs* to a friend.

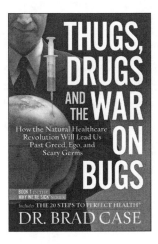

Call: 1-800-BOOKLOG (1-800-266-5564)
Or order online at: www.HealthIsNatural.com

To send copies to your Congressional representatives for just $15.00 each Call: 831-915-6783

We will mail any number of books directly to your representative(s) along with a letter letting them know that you would like them to read the book and vote according to the principals outlined within. We will also mail you a receipt when your book has been sent. This may qualify as a tax deduction. Please check your state laws.

More By Dr. Case

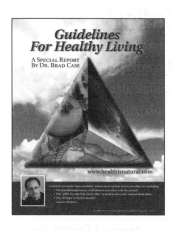

Guidelines For Healthy Living

Want more information on how to live a healthy life including The pHIL Up and Slim Down Diet™, the natural foods diet Dr. Case recommends?

To get your <u>free</u> copy of Dr. Case's E-Book *Guidelines For Healthy Living* Go to www.HealthIsNatural.com

101 Great Ways To Improve Your Health

With chapters by Dr. Case, Joseph Mercola, Julian Whitaker, Stephen Sinatra, Susan Lark, Gary Craig, and many more of today's leading experts on health.

Available at www.HealthIsNatural.com
For just $14.95

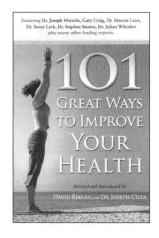